Current management of polycystic ovary syndrome

RCOG PRESS

Since 1973 the Royal College of Obstetricians and Gynaecologists has regularly convened Study Groups to address important growth areas within obstetrics and gynaecology. An international group of eminent clinicians and scientists from various disciplines is invited to present the results of recent research and to take part in in-depth discussions. The resulting volume, containing enhanced versions of the papers presented, is published within a few months of the meeting and provides a summary of the subject that is both authoritative and up to date.

SOME PREVIOUS STUDY GROUP PUBLICATIONS AVAILABLE

Menopause and Hormone Replacement
Edited by Hilary Critchley, Ailsa Gebbie and Valerie Beral

Disorders of the Menstrual Cycle
Edited by PMS O'Brien, IT Cameron and AB MacLean

Infection and Pregnancy
Edited by AB MacLean, L Regan and D Carrington

Pain in Obstetrics and Gynaecology
Edited by A MacLean, R Stones and S Thornton

Incontinence in Women
Edited by AB MacLean and L Cardozo

Maternal Morbidity and Mortality
Edited by AB MacLean and J Neilson

Lower Genital Tract Neoplasia
Edited by Allan B MacLean, Albert Singer and Hilary Critchley

Pre-eclampsia
Edited by Hilary Critchley, Allan MacLean, Lucilla Poston and James Walker

Preterm Birth
Edited by Hilary Critchley, Phillip Bennett and Steven Thornton

Implantation and Early Development
Edited by Hilary Critchley, Iain Cameron and Stephen Smith

Contraception and Contraceptive Use
Edited by Anna Glasier, Kaye Wellings and Hilary Critchley

Multiple Pregnancy
Edited by Mark Kilby, Phil Baker, Hilary Critchley and David Field

Heart Disease and Pregnancy
Edited by Philip J Steer, Michael A Gatzoulis and Philip Baker

Teenage Pregnancy and Reproductive Health
Edited by Philip Baker, Kate Guthrie, Cindy Hutchinson, Roslyn Kane and Kaye Wellings

Obesity and Reproductive Health
Edited by Philip Baker, Adam Balen, Lucilla Poston and Naveed Sattar

Renal Disease in Pregnancy
Edited by John M Davison, Catherine Nelson-Piercy, Sean Kehoe and Philip Baker

Cancer and Reproductive Health
Edited by Sean Kehoe, Eric Jauniaux, Pierre Martin-Hirsch and Philip Savage

Reproductive Ageing
Edited by Susan Bewley, William Ledger and Dimitrios Nikolaou

Reproductive Genetics
Edited by Sean Kehoe, Lyn Chitty and Tessa Homfray

Maternal and Infant Deaths: Chasing Millennium Development Goals 4 and 5
Edited by Sean Kehoe, James P Neilson and Jane E Norman

Current management of polycystic ovary syndrome

Edited by

Adam Balen, Stephen Franks, Roy Homburg
and Sean Kehoe

RCOG
PRESS

Adam Balen MD FRCOG
Professor of Reproductive Medicine and Surgery, Leeds Centre for Reproductive Medicine, Seacroft Hospital, York Road, Leeds LS14 6UH

Stephen Franks MD FmedSci
Professor of Reproductive Endocrinology, Institute of Reproductive and Developmental Biology, Imperial College London, Hammersmith Hospital, London W12 0NN

Roy Homburg MB BS FRCOG
Professor of Reproductive Medicine, Barzilai Medical Centre, Ashkelon, Israel, and Head of Research, Homerton Fertility Centre, Homerton University Hospital, London

Sean Kehoe MD FRCOG
Convenor of Study Groups, Lead Consultant in Gynaecological Oncology, Oxford Gynaecological Cancer Centre, John Radcliffe Hospital, Headington, Oxford OX3 9DU

Published by the **RCOG Press** at the Royal College of Obstetricians and Gynaecologists, 27 Sussex Place, Regent's Park, London NW1 4RG

www.rcog.org.uk

Registered charity no. 213280

First published 2010

ISBN 978-1-906985-41-7

A machine-readable catalogue record for this publication can be obtained from the British Library [www.bl.uk/catalogue/listings.html]

Cover image: Magnetic resonance imaging of polycystic ovaries © GustoImages/Science Photo Library

RCOG Editor: Andrew Welsh
Original design by Karl Harrington, FiSH Books, London
Typesetting by Andrew Welsh
Index by Jan Ross (Merrall-Ross International Ltd)

Contents

Participants

Adam Balen
Professor of Reproductive Medicine and Surgery, Leeds Centre for Reproductive Medicine, Seacroft Hospital, York Road, Leeds LS14 6UH, UK.

Julian H Barth
Consultant in Chemical Pathology and Metabolic Medicine, Clinical Biochemistry, Leeds General Infirmary, Great George Street, Leeds LS1 3EX, UK.

Tim Child
Consultant Gynaecologist and Sub-specialist in Reproductive Medicine and Surgery, Oxford Fertility Unit and the University of Oxford, Institute of Reproductive Sciences, Oxford Business Park North, Oxford OX4 2HW, UK.

Gerard Conway
Consultant Endocrinologist, Department of Endocrinology, University College London Hospital, London NW1 2PQ, UK.

Didier Dewailly
Head of Pole de Gynécologie, Lille University Hospital, Hôpital Jeanne de Flandre, Avenue Eugène Avinée, Lille 59037, France.

David Dunger
Professor of Paediatrics, Department of Paediatrics, Box 116 Level 8, University of Cambridge, Addenbrooke's Hospital, Hills Road, Cambridge CB2 0QQ, UK.

Bart JCM Fauser
Chair of Division of Woman & Baby, University Medical Centre Utrecht (UMC Utrecht), Heidelberglaan 100, 3584 CX Utrecht, The Netherlands.

Stephen Franks
Professor of Reproductive Endocrinology, Institute of Reproductive and Developmental Biology, Imperial College London, Hammersmith Hospital, London W12 0NN, UK.

Roy Homburg
Professor of Reproductive Medicine, Barzilai Medical Centre, Ashkelon, Israel, and Head of Research, Homerton Fertility Centre, Homerton University Hospital, London, UK.

Georgina Jones
Senior Lecturer (Non-clinical), Health Services Research Section, School of Health and Related Research, University of Sheffield, Regent Court, 30 Regent Street, Sheffield S1 4DA, UK.

Sean Kehoe
Convenor of Study Groups, Lead Consultant in Gynaecological Oncology, Oxford Gynaecological Cancer Centre, John Radcliffe Hospital, Headington, Oxford OX3 9DU, UK.

Alison M Layton
Consultant Dermatologist, Department of Dermatology, Harrogate and District Foundation Trust, Lancaster Park Road, Harrogate HG2 7SX, UK.

Carel W le Roux
Reader in Metabolic Medicine, Imperial Weight Centre, 9th Floor, Imperial College London, Charing Cross Hospital, Fulham Palace Road, London W6 8RF, UK.

Richard S Legro
Professor of Obstetrics and Gynecology, Milton S. Hershey Medical Center, Penn State College of Medicine, 500 University Drive, H103, Hershey, PA 17033, USA.

Renato Pasquali
Head of Division of Endocrinology, Policlinico S. Orsola-Malpighi, Via Massarenti 9, Bologna 40138, Italy.

Elisabet Stener-Victorin
Associate Professor, Institute of Neuroscience and Physiology, Department of Physiology/Endocrinology, Box 434, Göteborg SE–405 30, Sweden.

Chandrika N Wijeyaratne
Professor in Reproductive Medicine, Department of Obstetrics and Gynaecology, Faculty of Medicine, University of Colombo, PO Box 271, Kynsey Road, Colombo, Sri Lanka.

Additional contributors

Charles N Antonypillai
Senior Registrar in Endocrinology, National Hospital of Sri Lanka, Colombo 10, Sri Lanka.

Helen P Field
Clinical Scientist, Clinical Biochemistry, Leeds General Infirmary, Great George Street, Leeds LS1 3EX, UK.

Alessandra Gambineri
Clinical Lecturer, Division of Endocrinology, Policlinico S. Orsola-Malpighi, Via Massarenti 9, Bologna 40138, Italy.

GJ Chaminda Garusinghe
Senior Registrar in Endocrinology, Diabetes and Endocrine Unit, National Hospital of Sri Lanka, Colombo 10, Sri Lanka.

Vindya Kumarapeli
Consultant Community Physician, Non-Communicable Diseases Unit, Ministry of Healthcare and Nutrition, No 385, Baddegama Wimalawansa Mawatha, Colombo, Sri Lanka.

Alexander D Miras
Specialist Registrar in Endocrinology and Diabetes, St Helier Hospital, Wrythe Lane, Carshalton SM5 1AA, UK.

Ruwanthi de A Seneviratne
House Officer, Castle Street Hospital for Women, Colombo 8, Sri Lanka.

S Rohini de A Seneviratne
Professor in Community Medicine, Department of Community Medicine, Faculty of Medicine, University of Colombo, PO Box 271, Kynsey Road, Colombo, Sri Lanka.

Rachel Williams
Clinical Lecturer in Paediatric Endocrinology and Diabetes, Department of Paediatrics, Box 116, University of Cambridge, Addenbrooke's Hospital, Hills Road, Cambridge CB2 0QQ, UK.

S Chandrika Yapa
Visiting Obstetrician and Gynaecologist, Base Hospital, Dehiattakandiya, Sri Lanka.

Ephia Yasmin
Specialist Registrar, Obstetrics and Gynaecology, Bradford Royal Infirmary, Bradford LS6 3DD, UK.

DECLARATIONS OF PERSONAL INTEREST

All contributors to the Study Group were invited to make a specific Declaration of Interest in relation to the subject of the Study Group. This was undertaken and all contributors complied with this request. Adam Balen has received sponsorship from Ferring Pharmaceuticals and Organon/Schering Plough. His department has received financial support from Ferring, Organon/Schering Plough and Merck Serono. He is a consultant to or member of Infertility Network UK (INUK), PCOS UK and Verity. He has received feed for editorial work on *BJOG*. Tim Child has received sponsorship to attend meetings plus honoraria from Merck-Serono, Organon and Ferring. His department has unrestricted educational grants from Merck-Serono and Ferring. Gerard Conway is a consultant to the Daisy Network (ovarian failure), the Turner Syndrome Support Society and the Androgen Insensitivity Syndrome Support Group. Didier Dewailly's department has received research grants from Merck Serono, Schering-Plough, Ferring and Genevrier. He is the Chief Editor of *Medecine de la Reproduction, Gynécologie, Endocrinologie* at John Libbey, Paris. Bart Fauser's department has received research grants from commercial organisations related to obstetrics and gynaecology. He has received fees and grant support from the following companies: Andromed, Ardana, Ferring, Genovum, Merck Serono, Organon, Pantharel Bioscience, PregLem, Schering, Schering Plough, Serono and Wyeth. Stephen Franks is a medical adviser to Verity (a PCOS patient support group), to its health professionals arm PSOC UK, and to Infertility Network UK (all honorary). Georgina Jones is a member of the Executive Board of PCOS UK. Alison Layton is a member of the executive council of PCOS UK; this is an unpaid position. She has received some travel expenses for attendance at meetings via the organisation. Richard Legro is an Associate Editor on the journals *Fertility and Sterility* and *Human Reproduction*. He is on the Program Committee for the Annual Meeting of the American Society for Reproductive Medicine. Chandrika Wijeyaratne is a member of the Women's Health Committee, Sri Lanka Medical Association.

Preface

Polycystic ovary syndrome (PCOS) is a heterogeneous collection of signs and symptoms that, gathered together, form a spectrum of a disorder with a mild presentation in some, whereas in others there may be a severe disturbance of reproductive, endocrine and metabolic function. The definition of the syndrome has been much debated, with key features including menstrual cycle disturbance, hyperandrogenism and obesity. The pathophysiology of PCOS appears to be multifactorial and polygenic and is still being actively researched. PCOS is the most common endocrine disturbance and affects 10–15% of women in the UK. The clinical findings of hirsutism, acne, alopecia and obesity do not always correlate with the serum biochemistry, which itself may be difficult to assess. There is no doubt that PCOS has a significant effect on quality of life and psychological morbidity and, as many specialists may be involved in its management, a multidisciplinary approach is required.

The 59th RCOG Study Group brought together a wide range of experts who treat women with PCOS and the clinical conditions related to the syndrome. The actual definition, the accuracy of diagnostic investigations, the particular challenges in adolescent diagnosis and management, the relationship with ethnicity and issues relating to the clinical care of women with PCOS are all covered in this comprehensive book.

Importantly, there is a critical evaluation of current approaches to therapy, a discussion on the potential individualisation of therapy (regarding the identification of those who will – or will not – respond to fertility interventions) and a chapter on the role of alternative therapies, which are employed in managing some aspects of this syndrome.

For those caring for women with PCOS, be it in primary or secondary care, this book should prove both interesting and a valuable tool in increasing the knowledge base and facilitating the decision-making process.

Adam Balen
Stephen Franks
Roy Homburg
Sean Kehoe *(Convenor of RCOG Study Groups)*

Chapter 1

Overview and definitions of polycystic ovary syndrome and the polycystic ovary

Adam Balen

Introduction

Polycystic ovary syndrome (PCOS) is a heterogeneous collection of signs and symptoms that, gathered together, form a spectrum of a disorder with a mild presentation in some but a severe disturbance of reproductive, endocrine and metabolic function in others. The pathophysiology of PCOS appears to be multifactorial and polygenic. The definition of the syndrome has been much debated, with key features including menstrual cycle disturbance, hyperandrogenism and obesity (see Box 1.1). There are many extra-ovarian aspects to the pathophysiology of PCOS but ovarian dysfunction is central.

The joint European Society of Human Reproduction and Embryology (ESHRE)/ American Society for Reproductive Medicine (ASRM) consensus meeting in 2003 agreed a refined definition of PCOS, namely the presence of two of the following three criteria:[1] (1) oligo-ovulation and/or anovulation, (2) hyperandrogenism (clinical and/or biochemical), (3) polycystic ovaries; with the exclusion of other causes of menstrual cycle disturbance or androgen excess (see Table 1.1).

The morphology of the polycystic ovary has been defined as an ovary with 12 or more follicles measuring 2–9 mm in diameter and/or an increased ovarian volume (more than 10 cm^3).[2]

There is considerable heterogeneity of symptoms and signs among women with PCOS and, for an individual, these may change over time.[3] PCOS appears to be familial and various aspects of the syndrome may be differentially inherited.[4] Polycystic ovaries can even exist without clinical signs of the syndrome, which may then become expressed over time. There are a number of interlinking factors that may affect expression of PCOS. For example, a gain in weight is associated with a worsening of symptoms, while weight loss may ameliorate the endocrine and metabolic profile and symptomatology.[5]

Various factors influence ovarian function, and fertility is adversely affected by an individual being overweight or having elevated serum concentrations of luteinising hormone (LH). Strategies to induce ovulation include weight loss, oral anti-estrogens (principally clomifene citrate), parenteral gonadotrophin therapy and laparoscopic ovarian surgery.

The features of obesity, hyperinsulinaemia and hyperandrogenaemia that are commonly seen in PCOS are also known to be factors that confer an increased risk

Box 1.1 Signs and symptoms of polycystic ovary syndrome
Symptoms: • hyperandrogenism (acne, hirsutism, alopecia – *not* virilisation) • menstrual disturbance • infertility • obesity • sometimes: asymptomatic, with polycystic ovaries on ultrasound scan
Serum endocrinology: • increasing fasting insulin (not routinely measured; insulin resistance or impaired glucose tolerance assessed by oral glucose tolerance test) • increasing androgens (testosterone and androstenedione) • increasing luteinising hormone, usually normal follicle-stimulating hormone • decreasing sex hormone-binding globulin, results in elevated 'free androgen index' • increasing estradiol and estrone (neither measured routinely as there is a very wide range of values) • increasing prolactin
Possible late sequelae: • diabetes • dyslipidaemia • hypertension • cardiovascular disease • endometrial carcinoma • breast cancer (although data are conflicting)

of cardiovascular disease and type 2 diabetes (see Table 1.2).[6] There are studies which indicate that women with PCOS have an increased risk for these diseases that pose long-term risks for health, and this evidence has prompted debate as to the need for screening women for polycystic ovaries.

Elevated serum concentrations of insulin are more common in both lean and obese women with PCOS than in weight-matched women without the syndrome. Indeed, it is hyperinsulinaemia that seems to be key to the pathogenesis for many women with PCOS as insulin stimulates androgen secretion by the ovarian stroma and appears to affect the normal development of ovarian follicles, both by the adverse effects of androgens on follicular growth and possibly also by suppressing apoptosis and permitting the survival of follicles otherwise destined to disappear. The realisation of an association between hyperinsulinaemia and PCOS has resulted in the use of insulin-sensitising agents such as metformin, although they have not provided the benefit that was originally hoped.[7]

What is polycystic ovary syndrome?

Polycystic ovaries are commonly detected by ultrasound or other forms of pelvic imaging, with estimates of the prevalence in the general population being of the order of 20–33%.[8,9] However, not all women with polycystic ovaries demonstrate the clinical and biochemical features that define the syndrome. While it is now clear that ultrasound provides an excellent technique for the detection of polycystic ovarian morphology, identification of polycystic ovaries by ultrasound does not automatically confer a diagnosis of PCOS.

Table 1.1 Investigations for polycystic ovary syndrome

Test	Normal range (may vary with local laboratory assays)	Additional points
Pelvic ultrasound		To assess ovarian morphology and endometrial thickness; a transabdominal scan is usually adequate in women who are not sexually active (depends on body habitus)
Testosterone (T)	0.5–3.5 nmol/litre	A total T measurement is adequate for general screening; it is unnecessary to measure other androgens unless the total testosterone is more than 5 nmol/litre, in which case referral is indicated
Sex hormone-binding globulin (SHBG)	16–119 nmol/litre	Insulin suppresses SHBG, resulting in a high FAI in the presence of a normal total T; the measurement of SHBG is not required in routine practice and will not affect management
Free androgen index (FAI): T × 100/SHBG	<5	
Estradiol		Measurement is generally unhelpful to make diagnosis; estrogenisation may be confirmed by endometrial assessment
Luteinising hormone (LH)	2–10 IU/litre	FSH and LH are best measured during days 1–3 of a menstrual bleed; if oligomenorrhoeic or amenorrhoeic, then random samples are taken
Follicle-stimulating hormone (FSH)	2–8 IU/litre	
Antimüllerian hormone (AMH)	Assays differ and still being evaluated	AMH is a good representative of the number of antral follicles[47]
Prolactin	<500 mU/litre	Measures if the woman is oligomenorrhoeic or amenorrhoeic
Thyroid-stimulating hormone (TSH) for thyroid function	0.5–5 IU/litre	
Fasting insulin	<30 mU/litre	Not routinely measured; insulin resistance can be assessed by an oral glucose tolerance test

Table 1.2 Definitions of glucose tolerance

	Test	
	Fasting glucose (mmol/litre)	2-hour glucose (mmol/litre)
Diabetes	≥7.0	≥11.1
Impaired glucose tolerance (IGT)	<7.0	≥7.8 and <11.1
Impaired fasting glycaemia	≥6.1 and <7.0	<7.8

A 75 g oral glucose tolerance test should be performed in women with PCOS and body mass index (BMI) > 30 kg/m²; it has been suggested that South Asian women should have an assessment of glucose tolerance if their BMI is greater than 25 kg/m² because of the greater risk of insulin resistance at a lower BMI than seen in the white population

Despite the ESHRE/ASRM consensus meeting and definitions, controversy still exists in some quarters over a precise definition of the syndrome and whether or not the diagnosis should require confirmation of polycystic ovarian morphology. The original case series of Stein and Leventhal[10] in 1935 described seven women who had enlarged polycystic ovaries and amenorrhoea. Over the years, it was appreciated that the cardinal symptoms are chronic anovulation (oligomenorrhoea or amenorrhoea) and hyperandrogenism (usually hirsutism and acne, and sometimes alopecia). The 1990 National Institutes of Health (NIH) conference on PCOS recommended that the diagnostic criteria should include evidence of hyperandrogenism and ovulatory dysfunction, in the absence of non-classic adrenal hyperplasia, and that evidence of polycystic ovarian morphology was not essential (in a paper that is in book form only and no longer readily available).[11] In Europe and Australasia, ovarian imaging by ultrasound became an important component in the diagnosis, largely because ovarian morphology was part of the original disease description. Despite a degree of concordance between the NIH definition and the addition of ovarian imaging, it became necessary to try to gain transatlantic harmony with a new consensus held under the auspices of the ESHRE and the ASRM, which resulted in the 'Rotterdam criteria'.[1]

The generally accepted view in Europe and much of the world is that a spectrum exists that ranges from women with polycystic ovarian morphology and no overt abnormality at one end to those with polycystic ovaries associated with severe clinical and biochemical disorders at the other end.

A new group, the Androgen Excess and PCOS Society (AEPS), has more recently proposed that PCOS should be further redefined.[12] The latest suggestion is that two criteria are required: hyperandrogenism (clinical hirsutism and/or biochemical hyperandrogenaemia) and ovarian dysfunction (oligo-ovulation or anovulation and/or polycystic ovaries) after exclusion of other causes of androgen excess or related disorders.

The arguments for a 'tighter definition' include the potential for better prospects for providing genetic and proteomic causes of PCOS and concerns about avoiding overdiagnosis because of 'potential lifelong and insurability implications', yet the latest consensus 'recognises that there may be a number of women who have features suggestive of PCOS but who do not fulfil the criteria'.[12] Furthermore, there appears not to have been complete consensus, as some members of the AEPS group 'disagreed with the strong emphasis placed on hyperandrogenism', particularly as there is a high degree of inaccuracy in both the clinical and biochemical assessment of androgen excess.[12,13]

The latest proposed definition also raises concerns about allowing the presence of polycystic ovaries as a separate defining feature. We recognise that polycystic ovaries are detected in 19–33% of women in the general population, of whom approximately 80% have symptoms of PCOS, albeit often mild.[9] The biochemical features of the syndrome, namely elevated serum concentrations of testosterone, androstenedione, LH and insulin, may vary between individuals and change with time. The ovary is the source of excess androgens, which result from dysregulation of steroidogenesis combined with an excess of external promoters, principally LH and insulin.

Many consider that insulin resistance and hyperinsulinaemia are at the heart of the pathophysiology of PCOS but these features are clearly not essential in the development of the syndrome, particularly in lean women. Nevertheless, even if insulin resistance/hyperinsulinaemia is not the initiating cause, it is certainly an amplifier of hyperandrogenism in those who gain weight. The common association of PCOS and obesity has a synergistic deleterious impact on glucose homeostasis and can worsen both hyperandrogenism and anovulation. Hyperinsulinaemia also decreases the synthesis of sex hormone-binding globulin (SHBG) by the liver, leading to an increase in circulating free testosterone.

There are likely to be many routes to the development of PCOS, including genetic predisposition, environmental factors and disturbances of a number of endocrine pathways. There also appear to be significant racial differences in the expression of

PCOS, for example women from South Asia have worse symptoms, hormonal and metabolic disturbance and a greater likelihood of developing type 2 diabetes.[14]

PCOS is a well-recognised and common condition that causes considerable morbidity. A pragmatic approach is required in making the diagnosis and excluding other causes of menstrual cycle disturbance and hyperandrogenism.[15] Too exclusive a definition would leave many women at the milder end of the PCOS spectrum without a diagnosis even though they have an equal right to medical care and management of their symptoms. Indeed, there is significant psychological morbidity and negative impact on quality of life related to PCOS, even in adolescence,[16] whether related to the dermatological manifestations, disturbed menstrual cycle and subsequent infertility or associated obesity and metabolic problems. The diagnosis of mild PCOS or even the presence of polycystic ovaries alone may alert the individual and allow the physician to offer advice, for example about lifestyle, that may potentially help prevent a worsening of the syndrome and increased long-term morbidity.[17] In conclusion, the Rotterdam consensus definition of PCOS satisfies these criteria and allows a pragmatic approach for both diagnosis and management.

Defining the polycystic ovary: historical and histopathological considerations

Historically, the detection of a polycystic ovary required visualisation of the ovaries at laparotomy and histological confirmation following biopsy.[10] As further studies identified the association of certain endocrine abnormalities in women with histological evidence of polycystic ovaries, biochemical criteria became the mainstay for diagnosis. Raised serum levels of LH, testosterone and androstenedione, in association with low or normal levels of follicle-stimulating hormone (FSH) and abnormalities of estrogen secretion, described an endocrine profile that many believed to be diagnostic of PCOS. Well-recognised clinical presentations included menstrual cycle disturbances (oligomenorrhoea/amenorrhoea), obesity, and hyperandrogenism manifesting as hirsutism, acne or androgen-dependent alopecia. These definitions proved inconsistent, however, as clinical features were noted to vary considerably between women, and indeed some women with histological evidence of polycystic ovaries consistently failed to display any of the common symptoms. Likewise, the biochemical features associated with PCOS were not consistent in all women. Thus consensus on a single biochemical or clinical definition for PCOS was thwarted by the heterogeneity of presentation of the disorder.

Numerous descriptions have been made of the morphology of the polycystic ovary and these have been refined over time, alongside advances in imaging technology. The histology of the polycystic ovary was an ovary with prominent theca, fibrotic thickening of the tunica albuginea and multiple cystic follicles.[10] The number of antral follicles (2–6 mm in diameter) was described as 'excessive' by Goldzieher and Green in 1962 but not quantified.[18] Good correlation has been shown between ultrasound diagnoses of polycystic morphology and the histopathological criteria for polycystic ovaries by studies examining ovarian tissue obtained at hysterectomy or after wedge resection.[19] The histological data of Hughesdon[20] indicated a two- to three-fold increase in the follicle number in polycystic ovaries, from the stage of primary follicles up to tertiary follicles, and identified the cystic structures as follicles as opposed to pathological cysts. A more recent study of ovarian cortical biopsies described a lower proportion of healthy primordial follicles in polycystic ovaries compared with normal ovaries and a greater proportion of primary follicles that had started growing, indicating abnormalities in folliculogenesis.[21]

Ultrasound descriptions of the polycystic ovary

The advent of high-resolution ultrasound scanning has provided a non-invasive technique for the assessment of ovarian size and morphology. Although the ultrasound criteria for the diagnosis of polycystic ovaries have not been universally agreed, the characteristic features are accepted as being an increase in the number of follicles and the amount of stroma as compared with normal ovaries. Ultrasound was initially used to describe the ovarian appearance in women classified as having PCOS (by symptoms and serum endocrinology) rather than to make the diagnosis. There was often no record of timing of the scan in relation to the menstrual cycle in either women with suspected PCOS or those in a control group.

The transabdominal ultrasound criteria of Adams *et al.*[22] defined a polycystic ovary as one that contains, in one plane, at least ten follicles (usually between 2 and 8 mm in diameter) arranged peripherally around a dense core of ovarian stroma or scattered throughout an increased amount of stroma. Polycystic ovaries were found to have a higher volume ($14.6 \pm 1.1\ cm^3$) than either multicystic ($8.0 \pm 0.8\ cm^3$) or normal ovaries ($6.4 \pm 0.4\ cm^3$).[23] Uterine cross-sectional area was also greater in women with PCOS than those with multicystic or normal ovaries ($26.0 \pm 1.4\ cm^2$ versus $13.1 \pm 0.9\ cm^2$ versus $22.4 \pm 1.0\ cm^2$), which is a reflection of the degree of estrogenisation.

Multicystic and polycystic ovaries

The multicystic ovary is one in which there are multiple (at least six) cysts, usually 4–10 mm in diameter, with normal stromal echogenicity.[23] This is the characteristic appearance during puberty and in women recovering from hypothalamic amenorrhoea – both situations being associated with follicular growth without consistent recruitment of a dominant follicle. There may be confusion among inexperienced ultrasonographers, radiologists and gynaecologists, hence the need for careful consideration of the clinical picture and endocrinology. Polycystic ovaries may be evident in adolescent girls as a distinct entity from multicystic ovaries.[24] Indeed, it appears that PCOS manifests for the first time during the adolescent years, which are critical for future ovarian and metabolic function.

Transvaginal ultrasound

Transabdominal ultrasound has been largely superseded by transvaginal scanning because of greater resolution and, in many cases, patient preference, as the need for a full bladder is avoided, which saves time and may be more comfortable.

A study that set out to assess variability in the detection of polycystic and normal ovaries demonstrated intra-observer agreement of 69.4% and inter-observer agreement of 51%.[25] This suggests either that the diagnostic criteria are too subjective or that their measurement is too insensitive. Amer *et al.*[25] concluded that the use of three-dimensional ultrasound might provide a more reliable and reproducible diagnostic tool, although they did not perform a similar evaluation of observer variability.

The Rotterdam consensus definition[2] was based largely on the paper by Jonard *et al*,[26] who studied 214 women with PCOS and 112 with normal ovaries to determine the importance of follicle number per ovary (FNPO). Three different categories of follicle size were analysed separately (2–5, 6–9 and 2–9 mm). The mean FNPO was similar between normal and polycystic ovaries in the 6–9 mm range but significantly higher in the polycystic ovaries in both the 2–5 and 2–9 mm ranges.[26] Within the 2–5 mm range, there were significant positive correlations with serum testosterone, androstenedione and LH concentrations. There was an inverse correlation within the 6–9 mm range between FNPO and testosterone, body mass index and fasting insulin concentrations, and a positive correlation with inhibin B concentrations. The mean FNPO in the 2–5 mm range was significantly greater in the polycystic ovaries than in those of women in the control group, while it was similar in the 6–9 mm range. The authors suggest that intra-ovarian hyperandrogenism promotes excessive early follicular growth up to 2–5 mm, with more follicles able to enter the growing cohort which then become arrested at the 6–9 mm size. An FNPO of 12 or more follicles of 2–9 mm gave the best threshold for the diagnosis of PCOS (sensitivity 75%; specificity 99%).[26]

The Rotterdam consensus definition of the polycystic ovary proposed the presence of 12 or more follicles of 2–9 mm diameter (as a mean of both ovaries) and/or increased ovarian volume (more than 10 cm^3).[2] Further work by Jonard *et al.*[27] has suggested reducing the threshold volume to 7 cm^3. The same group reported a series of 457 women with polycystic ovaries and found that the number of 2–5 mm follicles gave the strongest correlation with the severity of follicular arrest, followed by age and then fasting insulin concentration.[28]

Stromal echogenicity

The increased echodensity of the polycystic ovary is a key histological feature[20] but is a subjective assessment that may vary depending on the settings of the ultrasound machine and the patient's body habitus. Stromal echogenicity has been described in a semi-quantative manner with a score of 1 for normal, 2 for moderately increased and 3 for frankly increased.[29] In this study, the total follicle number of both ovaries combined correlated significantly with stromal echogenicity. Follicle number also correlated significantly with free androgen index. A further study comparing women with PCOS with women in a control group found that the sensitivity and specificity of ovarian stromal echogenicity in the diagnosis of polycystic ovaries were 94% and 90%, respectively.[30]

Echogenicity has been quantified as the sum of the product of each intensity level (ranging from 0 to 63 on the scanner) and the number of pixels for that intensity level divided by the total number of pixels in the measured area:

$$\text{mean} = \left(\sum x_i f_i\right)/n$$

where n = total number of pixels in the measured area, x = intensity level (from 0 to 63) and f = number of pixels corresponding with the level.[31] The stromal index was calculated by dividing the mean stromal echogenicity by the mean echogenicity of the entire ovary to correct for cases in which the gain was adjusted to optimise image definition.[31]

Another approach used a 7.5 MHz transvaginal probe with histogram measurement of echogenicity.[32] The mean echogenicity was defined as the sum of the product of each intensity level (from 0 to 63) using the same formula as Al-Took *et al.*[31] Women with PCOS had greater total ovarian volume, stromal volume and peak stromal blood flow compared with normal ovaries, yet mean stromal echogenicity was similar. The stromal index was higher in PCOS owing to the finding of a reduced mean echogenicity of the entire ovary.[32] The inference was that the subjective impression of increased stromal echogenicity was due both to increased stromal volume and reduced echogenicity of the multiple cysts. Morever, the increased stromal blood flow was suggested as a more relevant predictor of ovarian function.[32]

A large study compared 80 women with oligomenorrhoea/amenorrhoea and PCOS with a control group of 30 women using a 6.5 MHz transvaginal probe.[33] Based on mean ± 2 SD data from the control group, the cut-off values were calculated for ovarian volume (13.21 cm^3), ovarian total area (7.00 cm^2), ovarian stromal area (1.95 cm^2) and stromal : ovarian area ratio (0.34). The sensitivities of these parameters for the diagnosis of PCOS were 21%, 4%, 62% and 100%, respectively, suggesting that a stromal : ovarian area ratio above 0.34 is diagnostic of PCOS.[33] Further studies of a series of 418 women described stromal : ovarian area ratio as the most significant predictor of biochemical androgen excess, with above 0.32 as the best cut-off.[34,35]

Three-dimensional ultrasound, Doppler and MRI

Three-dimensional ultrasound requires longer time for storage and data analysis, increased training and more expensive equipment, yet good correlations have been found between stromal volume and serum androstenedione concentrations.[36] Three-dimensional ultrasound has been shown to be a good tool for the accurate measurement of ovarian volume and more precise than two-dimensional ultrasound. Stromal volume also positively correlated with serum androstenedione concentrations in PCOS.[36] The higher sensitivity of three-dimensional ultrasound has also suggested that an FNPO of more than 20 is a more accurate cut-off for the diagnosis of polycystic ovaries.[37]

Stromal hypertrophy itself appears to be secondary to increased blood flow.[38] A number of studies of colour Doppler measurement of uterine and ovarian vessel blood flow have demonstrated a low resistance index in the stroma of polycystic ovaries (that is, increased flow) and correlations with endocrine changes. Battaglia *et al.*[39] reported a good correlation between both the serum androstenedione concentration and the LH : FSH ratio and the number of small follicles, and the LH : FSH ratio also correlated well with the stromal artery pulsatility index. Ovarian blood flow has also been shown to correlate not only with sex steroid concentrations but also with the degree of insulin resistance.[40] The combination of three-dimensional ultrasound and assessment of stromal vascularisation are therefore important tools in the assessment of functional and endocrine disturbances in PCOS.[41,42]

The use of magnetic resonance imaging (MRI) for the visualisation of the structure of pelvic organs has been claimed to have even greater sensitivity than ultrasound for the detection of polycystic ovaries.[43] MRI may also be useful in adolescent girls, particularly in those who are obese with ovaries that may be difficult to visualise by transabdominal ultrasound.[44] However, the substantial cost and practical problems involved with this imaging technique may limit its use as an easily accessible diagnostic tool for use in general clinical practice.

Exclusion of related disorders

To establish the diagnosis of PCOS it is important to exclude other disorders with a similar clinical presentation, such as congenital adrenal hyperplasia, Cushing syndrome and androgen-secreting tumours.[1] The measurement of total testosterone is usually sufficient in most populations. In some populations, however, 21-hydroxylase-deficient non-classic adrenal hyperplasia is more prevalent than in others and this can be excluded by measuring a basal morning 17-hydroxyprogesterone level.[45]

The routine exclusion of thyroid dysfunction in women deemed to be hyper-androgenic is of limited value, as the incidence of this disorder among women with hyperandrogenism is no higher than that in normal women of reproductive age (approximately 5% of the female population). The measurement of thyroid-stimulating hormone may, therefore, be a useful screening test but is certainly not obligatory in the diagnosis of PCOS.

If the woman presents with oligo-ovulation/anovulation, it is necessary to measure serum FSH, LH and estradiol (E_2) levels to exclude hypogonadotrophic hypogonadism (low FSH, LH and E_2) or premature ovarian failure (high FSH and LH and low E_2). PCOS is part of the spectrum of normogonadotrophic normo-estrogenic anovulation (WHO group II).[46] A measurement of prolactin should also be performed to exclude hyperprolactinaemia, although women with PCOS as a sole diagnosis may sometimes have moderately elevated serum prolactin concentrations.[3]

There may be clinical suspicions of syndromes of severe insulin resistance (for example, for the diagnosis of the hyperandrogenic insulin-resistant acanthosis nigricans [HAIR-AN] syndrome), Cushing syndrome, androgen-secreting neoplasms or the use of high-dose exogenous androgens and, if so, these should be excluded.

Conclusion

PCOS is a syndrome with varied manifestations both within different populations and between different populations. With recent increases in the understanding of the pathophysiology of PCOS and the recognition of the importance of ultrasound in defining the morphology of the polycystic ovary, the syndrome has now been defined as the presence of two of the following three criteria: (1) oligo-ovulation and/or anovulation, (2) hyperandrogenism (clinical and/or biochemical), (3) polycystic ovaries; with the exclusion of other aetiologies of menstrual disturbance and androgen excess.

Key points

- There is considerable heterogeneity of symptoms and signs and these may change over time.
- The morphology of the polycystic ovary has been defined as an ovary with 12 or more follicles measuring 2–9 mm in diameter and/or increased ovarian volume (> 10 cm^3). A stromal : ovarian area ratio of more than 0.32 correlates with the degree of hyperandrogenism. The use of three-dimensional ultrasound technology may increase the cut-off to 20 follicles.
- Polycystic ovaries are commonly detected by ultrasound, with a prevalence in the general population of 20–33%, of whom approximately three-quarters will exhibit clinical features of the syndrome.
- Elevated serum concentrations of insulin are more common in both lean and obese women with PCOS than weight-matched women without PCOS and hyperinsulinaemia is a component of the pathogenesis of PCOS.
- Clinical hyperandrogenism is difficult to quantify and there are racial variations. Biochemical hyperandrogenism is assessed by a variety of assays, the methodology for which is fraught with problems.
- To establish the diagnosis of PCOS, it is important to exclude other disorders with a similar clinical presentation, such as congenital adrenal hyperplasia, Cushing syndrome and androgen-secreting tumours.

References

1. Fauser B, Tarlatzis B, Chang J, Azziz R, Legro R, Dewailly D, *et al*; The Rotterdam ESHRE/ASRM-sponsored PCOS consensus workshop group. Revised 2003 consensus on diagnostic criteria and long-term health risks related to polycystic ovary syndrome (PCOS). *Hum Reprod* 2004;19:41–7.
2. Balen AH, Laven JS, Tan SL, Dewailly D. Ultrasound assessment of the polycystic ovary: international consensus definitions. *Hum Reprod Update* 2003;9:505–14.
3. Balen AH, Conway GS, Kaltsas G, Techatrasak K, Manning PJ, West C, *et al*. Polycystic ovary syndrome: the spectrum of the disorder in 1741 patients. *Hum Reprod* 1995;10:2107–11.
4. Franks S, Gharani N, McCarthy M. Candidate genes in polycystic ovary syndrome. *Hum Reprod Update* 2001;7:405–10.
5. Clark AM, Ledger W, Galletly C, Tomlinson L, Blaney F, Wang X, *et al*. Weight loss results in significant improvement in pregnancy and ovulation rates in anovulatory obese women. *Hum Reprod* 1995;10:2705–12.
6. Rajkowha M, Glass MR, Rutherford AJ, Michelmore K, Balen AH. Polycystic ovary syndrome: a risk factor for cardiovascular disease? *Br J Obstet Gynaecol* 2000;107:11–18.
7. Tang T, Lord JM, Norman RJ, Yasmin E, Balen AH. Insulin-sensitising drugs (metformin, rosiglitazone, pioglitazone, D-chiro-inositol) for women with polycystic ovary syndrome, oligo amenorrhoea and subfertility. *Cochrane Database Syst Rev* 2010;(1):CD003053.
8. Polson DW, Adams J, Wadsworth J, Franks S. Polycystic ovaries – a common finding in normal women. *Lancet* 1988;1:870–2.
9. Michelmore KF, Balen AH, Dunger DB, Vessey MP. Polycystic ovaries and associated clinical and biochemical features in young women. *Clin Endocrinol (Oxf)* 1999;51:779–86.
10. Stein I, Leventhal M. Amenorrhea associated with bilateral polycystic ovaries. *Am J Obstet Gynecol* 1935;29:181–5.
11. Zawadzki JK, Dunaif A. Diagnostic criteria for polycystic ovary syndrome: towards a rational approach. In: Dunaif A, Givens JR, Haseltine F, editors. *Polycystic Ovary Syndrome*. Boston: Blackwell Scientific; 1992. p. 377–84.
12. Azziz R, Carmina E, Dewailly D, Diamanti-Kandarakis E, Escobar-Morreale HF, Futterweit W, *et al*. The Androgen Excess and PCOS Society criteria for the polycystic ovary syndrome: the complete task force report. *Fertil Steril* 2009;91:456–88.
13. Barth J, Yasmin E, Balen AH. The diagnosis of polycystic ovary syndrome: the criteria are insufficiently robust for clinical research. *Clin Endocrinol (Oxf)* 2007;67:811–15.
14. Wijeyaratne CN, Balen AH, Barth J, Belchetz PE. Clinical manifestations and insulin resistance (IR) in polycystic ovary syndrome (PCOS) among South Asians and Caucasians: is there a difference? *Clin Endocrinol (Oxf)* 2002;57:343–50.
15. Franks S. Diagnosis of polycystic ovarian syndrome: in defense of the Rotterdam Criteria. *J Clin Endocrinol Metab* 2006;91:786–9.
16. Jones GL, Hall JM, Balen AH, Ledger W. Health-related quality of life measurement in women with polycystic ovary syndrome: a systematic review. *Hum Reprod Update* 2008;14:15–25.
17. Balen AH, Homburg R, Franks S. Defining polycystic ovary syndrome. *BMJ* 2009;338:426.
18. Goldzieher MW, Green JA. The polycystic ovary. I. Clinical and histologic features. *J Clin Endocrinol Metab* 1962;22:325–38.
19. Takahashi K, Eda Y, Abu Musa A, Okada S, Yoshino K, Kitao M. Transvaginal ultrasound imaging, histopathology and endocrinopathy in patients with polycystic ovarian syndrome. *Hum Reprod* 1994;9:1231–6.
20. Hughesdon PE. Morphology and morphogenesis of the Stein-Leventhal Ovary and of so-called "hyperthecosis". *Obstet Gynecol Survey* 1982;37:59–77.
21. Webber LJ, Stubbs S, Stark J, Trew GH, Margara R, Hardy K, *et al*. Formation and early development of follicles in the polycystic ovary. *Lancet* 2003;362:1017–21.
22. Adams J, Polson DW, Franks S. Prevalence of polycystic ovaries in women with anovulation and idiopathic hirsutism. *Br Med J* 1986;293:355–9.

23. Adams J, Polson DW, Abdulwahid N, Morris DV, Franks S, Mason HD, *et al.* Multifollicular ovaries: clinical and endocrine features and response to pulsatile gonadotropin releasing hormone. *Lancet* 1985;2:1375–9.
24. Herter LD, Magalhaes JA, Spritzer PM. Relevance of the determination of ovarian volume in adolescent girls with menstrual disorders. *J Clin Ultrasound* 1996;24:243–8.
25. Amer SA, Li TC, Bygrave C, Sprigg A, Saravelos H, Cooke ID. An evaluation of the inter-observer and intra-observer variability of the ultrasound diagnosis of polycystic ovaries. *Hum Reprod* 2002;17:1616–22.
26. Jonard S, Robert Y, Cortet-Rudelli C, Decanter C, Dewailly D. Ultrasound examination of polycystic ovaries: is it worth counting the follicles? *Hum Reprod* 2003;18:598–603.
27. Jonard S, Robert Y, Dewailly D. Revisiting the ovarian volume as a diagnostic criterion for polycystic ovaries. *Hum Reprod* 2005;20:2893–8.
28. Dewailly D, Catteau-Jonard S, Reyss AC, Maunoury-Lefebvre C, Poncelet E, Pigny P. The excess in 2–5mm follicles seen at ovarian ultrasonography is tightly associated to the follicular arrest of the polycystic ovary syndrome. *Hum Reprod* 2007;22:1562–6.
29. Pache TD, Hop WC, Wladimiroff JW, Schipper J, Fauser BC. Transvaginal sonography and abnormal ovarian appearance in menstrual cycle disturbances. *Ultrasound Med Biol* 1991;17:589–93.
30. Pache TD, Wladimiroff JW, Hop WC, Fauser BC. How to discriminate between normal and polycystic ovaries: transvaginal ultrasound study. *Radiology* 1992;183:421–3.
31. Al-Took S, Watkin K, Tulandi T, Tan SL. Ovarian stromal echogenicity in women with clomiphene citrate-sensitive and clomiphene citrate-resistant polycystic ovary syndrome. *Fertil Steril* 1999;71:952–4.
32. Buckett WM, Bouzayen R, Watkin KL, Tulandi T, Tan SL. Ovarian stromal echogenicity in women with normal and polycystic ovaries. *Hum Reprod* 1999;14:618–21.
33. Fulghesu AM, Ciampelli M, Belosi C, Apa R, Pavone V, Lanzone A. A new ultrasound criterion for the diagnosis of polycystic ovary syndrome: the ovarian stroma:total area ratio. *Fertil Steril* 2001;76:326–31.
34. Belosi C, Selvaggi L, Apa R, Guido M, Romualdi D, Fulghesu AM, *et al.* Is the PCOS diagnosis solved by ESHRE/ASRM 2003 consensus or could it include ultrasound examiniation of the ovarian stroma? *Hum Reprod* 2006;21:3108–15.
35. Fulghesu AM, Angioni S, Frau E, Belosi C, Apa R, Mioni R, *et al.* Ultrasound in polycystic ovary syndrome – the measuring of ovarian stroma and relationship with circulating androgens: results of a multicentric study. *Hum Reprod* 2007;22:2501–8.
36. Kyei-Mensah A, Tan SL, Zaidi J, Jacobs HS. Relationship of ovarian stromal volume to serum androgen concentrations in patients with polycystic ovary syndrome. *Hum Reprod* 1998;13:1437–41.
37. Allemand MC, Tummon IS, Phy JL, Foong SC, Dumesic DA, Session DR. Diagnosis of polycystic ovaries by three-dimensional transvaginal ultrasound. *Fertil Steril* 2006;85:214–19.
38. Zaidi J, Campbell S, Pittrof R, Kyei-Mensah A, Jacobs HS, Tan SL. Ovarian stromal blood flow in women with polycystic ovaries – a possible new marker for diagnosis? *Hum Reprod* 1995;10:1992–6.
39. Battaglia C, Genazzani AD, Salvatori M, Giulini S, Artini PG, Genazzani AR, *et al.* Doppler, ultrasonographic and endocrinological environment with regard to the number of small subcapsular foillicles in polycystic ovary syndrome. *Gynecol Endocrinol* 1999;13:123–9.
40. Carmina E, Orio F, Palomba S, Longo RA, Lombardi G, Lobo RA. Ovarian size and blood flow in women with polycystic ovary syndrome and their correlations with endocrine parameters. *Fertil Steril* 2005;84:413–19.
41. Lam PM, Johnson IR, Raine-Fenning NJ. Three-dimensional ultrasound features of the polycystic ovary and the effect of different phenotypic expressions on these parameters. *Hum Reprod* 2006;21:2209–15.
42. Lam PM, Johnson IR, Raine-Fenning NJ. The role of 3-D ultrasonography in polycystic ovary syndrome. *Hum Reprod* 2007;22:3116–23.
43. Faure N, Prat X, Bastide A, Lemay A. Assessment of ovaries by magnetic resonance imaging in patients presenting with polycystic ovarian syndrome. *Hum Reprod* 1989;4:468–72.

44. Yoo RY, Sirlin CB, Gottschalk M, Chang RJ. Ovarian imaging by magnetic resonance in obese adolescent girls with polycystic ovary syndrome: a pilot study. *Fertil Steril* 2005;84:985–95.
45. Azziz R, Hincapie LA, Knochenhauer ES, Dewailly D, Fox L, Boots LR. Screening for 21-hydroxylase deficient non-classic adrenal hyperplasia among hyperandrogenic women: a prospective study. *Fertil Steril* 1999;72:915–25.
46. Laven JS, Imani B, Eijkemans MJ, Fauser BC. New approaches to PCOS and other forms of anovulation. *Obstet Gynecol Surv* 2002;57:755–67.
47. Pigny P, Merlen E, Robert Y, Cortet-Rudelli C, Decanter C, Jonard S, *et al.* Elevated serum level of anti-mullerian hormone in patients with polycystic ovary syndrome: relationship to the ovarian follicle excess and to the follicular arrest. *J Clin Endocrinol Metab* 2003;88:5957–62.

2

Chapter 2

Genetics and pathogenesis of polycystic ovary syndrome

Stephen Franks

Introduction

Despite the fact that polycystic ovary syndrome (PCOS) is by far the most common endocrine disorder in women, affecting an estimated 5–10% of women of reproductive age, its aetiology and pathogenesis remain uncertain. PCOS usually presents during adolescence and is a heterogeneous syndrome that is classically characterised by features of anovulation (amenorrhoea, oligomenorrhoea, irregular cycles) together with symptoms of androgen excess (hirsutism, acne, alopecia).[1] The most consistent biochemical abnormality is elevation of serum androgen concentrations. Luteinising hormone (LH) concentrations are often also raised, whereas levels of follicle-stimulating hormone (FSH) are normal. It is now well established that PCOS is also characterised by metabolic abnormalities, particularly insulin resistance and hyperinsulinaemia, which are associated with an increased risk of developing type 2 diabetes in later life.[2,3] It is important to emphasise, however, that the syndrome is by nature heterogeneous and that the spectrum of presentation of PCOS includes women with anovulation who have no symptoms of androgen excess (although most have raised serum androgen concentrations) as well as those with hyperandrogenism but regular menses.[2,4] The recognition of this heterogeneity underpins the revision of the diagnostic criteria for PCOS that resulted from the joint consensus meeting of the European Society for Human Reproduction and Embryology (ESHRE) and the American Society for Reproductive Medicine (ASRM). Thus the so-called 'Rotterdam' diagnostic criteria[5] are defined by the presence of two of the three following features:

- polycystic ovaries
- anovulation
- androgen excess (clinical and/or biochemical).

The Rotterdam criteria are still controversial[6,7] but they have been widely adopted in clinical practice, particularly in Europe. The principal concern that has been expressed is the inclusion of women with polycystic ovaries and anovulation but with neither clinical nor biochemical evidence of androgen excess. The argument about diagnostic criteria is likely to continue, at least until the underlying pathogenesis is clearly understood, but it is important to point out that, whether using the narrower National Institutes of Health (NIH) or the broader Rotterdam definition, we are still dealing with a heterogeneous presentation, both clinically and biochemically. For example, although women with both hyperandrogenism and anovulation are more likely to have insulin resistance than those with only one of those abnormalities, this is by no means invariable. This is significant with regard to pathogenesis since it makes it unlikely that hyperinsulinaemia per se is *the* underlying cause of PCOS. In addition, from a clinical management viewpoint, it is useful to be able to interpret the clinical presentation in terms of risk of metabolic abnormalities and thence the consequences for long-term health of PCOS.[8–10]

Obesity is probably more common in women with PCOS than in the general population but we lack large population studies to verify this. The prevalence of overweight and obesity reported in the literature varies widely (35–80%) and this is probably related to the type of clinic to which the woman is first referred.[2,3,11] There is no doubt that overweight/obesity increases the clinical severity of PCOS and the attendant risk of metabolic dysfunction. Women with PCOS become disproportionately more insulin resistant with increasing body mass index (BMI) than those without PCOS (and have a greater risk of impaired glucose tolerance). Alarmingly, the prevalence of impaired glucose tolerance in obese young women with PCOS has been estimated to be as high as 30–40%, with an additional 5–10% having frank diabetes.[12,13] The current level of obesity in the population therefore has very serious implications for the long-term health of women with PCOS.

Developmental origin of PCOS

Perhaps the most plausible hypothesis for the origin of PCOS is that it represents an abnormality of developmental programming resulting from exposure to excess androgen in prenatal life or, possibly, during postnatal maturation of the hypothalamic–pituitary–ovarian axis. The presentation of PCOS in adolescence suggests that there is an underlying predisposition to the typical ovarian (and perhaps metabolic) abnormalities that has its origins well before the onset of puberty. There is clear evidence that there is a major genetic component of PCOS (see below) and one hypothesis is that PCOS is a genetically determined ovarian disorder characterised by excessive androgen production in which the heterogeneity of PCOS can be explained by the interaction of this disorder with environmental factors, notably dietary.[14,15] This hypothesis is based primarily on the observations of Abbott and colleagues, who have reported the effects of prenatal exposure of excess androgen in female rhesus monkeys. If these animals are exposed to high concentrations of testosterone *in utero*, they develop, as adults, many of the typical features of PCOS such as hypersecretion of LH, ovarian hyperandrogenism, anovulation in relation to increased body weight and insulin resistance.[16–18] It therefore seems likely that the clinical and biochemical features of PCOS are the result of effects of androgen excess and that the hypothalamic–pituitary–ovarian axis is 'programmed' by androgen in prenatal life. The rhesus monkeys were, however, given very large doses of testosterone, high enough to saturate circulating concentrations of sex hormone-binding globulin (SHBG) and to swamp placental aromatase activity (which efficiently converts maternal androgen to estrogens). Because of these barriers, it is unlikely that maternal androgens, even in women with PCOS, are able to cross the placenta in significant amounts in human pregnancy to expose the fetus to inappropriate levels of androgen.[19] It is therefore important to consider the possible source of excess androgen in PCOS. The most likely origin of excess androgen is the fetal ovary, although the adrenal gland may also play a role since clinical and biochemical manifestations of PCOS (including excess *ovarian* androgen production) have been noted in young adults with non-classical congenital adrenal hyperplasia due to 21-hydroxylase deficiency.[20]

Although it was previously thought that the fetal ovary is steroidogenically inactive, there is now evidence suggesting that the ovary has the capacity to synthesise androgen in prenatal life.[21] However, even if the fetal ovary does not produce significant amounts of androgen, the ovary may hypersecrete androgen in infancy when the hypothalamic–pituitary axis is activated physiologically or at puberty (or both). The consequences of this increased exposure to androgen include abnormalities of LH secretion[22] and insulin secretion and action[14,15] that manifest themselves during adolescence (Figure 2.1). The idea that the genesis of PCOS is prepubertal is supported by the observations that polycystic ovarian morphology[23] and even clinical manifestations of androgen excess[24] have been reported in prepubertal girls. Premature adrenarche and premature pubarche have been linked to the aetiology of PCOS; both are associated with increased risk of PCOS during adolescence.[24,25]

Full expression of PCOS depends on the maturation of the hypothalamic–pituitary–ovarian axis that occurs during puberty. The increase in circulating levels of LH that are characteristic of normal puberty are exaggerated in girls with a predisposition to PCOS and this further amplifies ovarian androgen production.[24] The presentation of PCOS during adolescence may also be affected by metabolic changes that are closely related

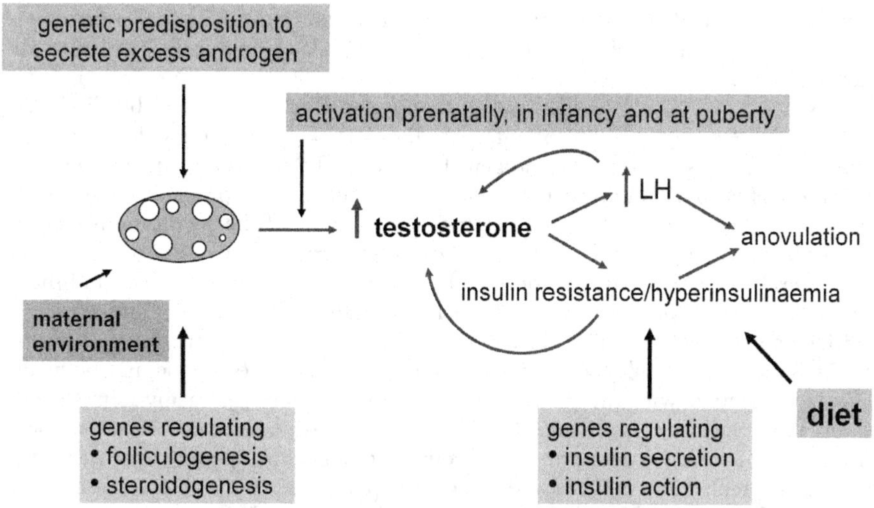

Figure 2.1 Proposed developmental aetiology of polycystic ovary syndrome; it is proposed that the ovary is genetically predisposed to hypersecrete androgens, perhaps as early as intrauterine life but certainly during the activation of the hypothalamic–pituitary–ovarian axis that occurs transiently in infancy and in a sustained manner at puberty; higher than normal circulating levels of testosterone 'programme' the hypothalamic–pituitary unit to produce high tonic levels of luteinising hormone (LH) and also amplify the physiological insulin resistance of puberty; higher than normal concentrations of LH and insulin further enhance ovarian androgen production and may contribute to the mechanism of anovulation; adapted and revised with permission from Abbott *et al*,[14] Franks *et al.*[15] and Franks[82]

to changes in body fat distribution. Normal puberty and adolescence are characterised by a physiological increase in insulin resistance together with an increase in serum concentrations of fasting insulin.[26] There is a reciprocal fall in SHBG driven by the increasing insulin levels and this serves to amplify the effects of sex steroids. Insulin also has a direct gonadotrophic action on ovarian steroidogenesis. These events are part of the normal cadence of puberty and provide a mechanism by which nutritional status can influence reproductive development. In girls with polycystic ovaries, the physiological hyperinsulinaemia of puberty may affect the genesis of both ovarian hyperandrogenism and anovulation. Insulin has been shown to amplify the steroidogenic response of both theca cells[27,28] and granulosa cells[29,30] to LH in the human ovary. Higher than normal insulin levels, whether due to a genetic predisposition or excessive weight gain (or both), would be expected to exaggerate these potentially adverse effects.[31] It may seem paradoxical that insulin appears to contribute to abnormal ovarian follicular function in PCOS – a state of peripheral insulin resistance – but data suggest that insulin resistance in the ovary is signalling pathway specific.[32–34]

Genes and PCOS

There is now compelling evidence that genetic factors play a major part in the aetiology of PCOS.[35–38] There is familial clustering of cases[35,36] and, critically, a greater concordance of symptoms of PCOS in identical twins compared with non-identical twins.[38] There is also evidence for heritability of endocrine and metabolic features of PCOS.[36,39] The mode of inheritance remains unclear;[35,37,40] an autosomal dominant disorder has been proposed, suggesting a single-gene effect,[41,42] but the more likely proposition is that PCOS is a complex endocrine disorder involving more than one, and probably several, genes.[35,43,44] The search for candidate genes in PCOS has so far proved elusive.

It is not too difficult to identify biochemical pathways that may be disrupted in PCOS. There is evidence for intrinsic disorders of ovarian folliculogenesis,[45–47] constitutive hypersecretion of androgens by theca cells[48,49] and disordered secretion and action of insulin[50] (Figure 2.1). There are, however, obvious problems in searching for candidate genes in PCOS: the heterogeneous nature of the syndrome has given rise to disagreement about definition and diagnostic criteria; in addition, expression of features of PCOS occurs predominantly in women of reproductive age and there is no clear male phenotype – both of which make family-based studies difficult.[35,37]

Many genes have been investigated as possible susceptibility loci (Box 2.1) but, if PCOS is indeed a complex genetic disorder, the effect of any one gene may be small. This fact, together with the problem of ethnic heterogeneity of many populations, means that conclusive case–control (or family-based) studies require large numbers of cases and controls (at least 300 per group), homogeneous populations and, very importantly, replication in other, independent populations.[37,44,51–54] To date, nearly 100 genes have been studied but few of the published studies (including some of our own initial studies) have satisfied the rigorous criteria of appropriate population selection and size, correction for comparison of multiple markers within any one population, and replication in independent populations. For a comprehensive catalogue and evaluation of candidate genes investigated to date, see the reviews by Urbanek[54] and by Simoni *et al.*[55]

Work from our own laboratory illustrates the problems related to interpretation of earlier (and which we now know to be underpowered) studies. Based on the evidence for a primary abnormality in theca cell steroidogenesis,[48,49] we investigated

Box 2.1 Candidate pathways and examples of candidate genes involved in the aetiology of polycystic ovary syndrome

Steroid hormone production and metabolism:
- *CYP11a* (P450scc)
- *CYP17* (P450c17)
- *CYP19* ($P450_{arom}$)

Metabolic (insulin secretion and action; obesity):
- β-cell function – *TCF7L2, KCNJ11*
- insulin resistance – *IR, PPARg*
- obesity – *FTO*

Androgen action:
- androgen receptor

Ovarian follicle development:
- follistatin; *FBN3*

a polymorphism (a pentanucleotide repeat sequence) in the promoter of *CYP11A* (coding for P450 cholesterol side-chain cleavage, the rate-limiting enzyme at the origin of the steroidogenic pathway) in a relatively small case–control series and a family-based study. We found evidence for linkage and association with PCOS and testosterone levels at the *CYP11A* locus.[56] The preliminary findings of a subsequent study by Urbanek *et al.*[57] were consistent with our results. When, however, we repeated the analysis in two large case–control populations, we could no longer find evidence of association of the polymorphism with PCOS or serum testosterone.[58]

Two promising candidate genes have, however, so far emerged from an enormous list of potential genes. The first is a locus on chromosome 19p13.2 (D19S884), which is close to, but not in linkage disequilibrium with, the insulin receptor gene.[59,60] The candidate locus maps to an intron of the fibrillin 3 gene (*FBN3*),[44] the function of which remains uncertain. However, fibrillins are transforming growth factor-beta (TGFβ) binding proteins and, since growth factors of the TGFβ family have been implicated in early follicle development and theca formation in the ovary,[61] this presents an intriguing link to the proposed primary ovarian abnormality. The second is the *FTO* (fat mass and obesity-associated) gene that is associated with obesity in the general population.[62] In a 2008 publication, Barber *et al.*[63] reported a significant association of polymorphisms in the *FTO* gene with PCOS in a study of 463 women with PCOS and 1336 women without in a UK population of British/Irish origin. This association was largely related to women with PCOS being more obese than those in the control group but, interestingly, it remained significant even after adjustment for BMI, suggesting an effect of *FTO* on the phenotype of PCOS that is independent of its influence on obesity. However, it is important that these studies, implicating the chromosome 19 locus and *FTO*, be confirmed in other large populations from independent groups. The candidate gene approach remains valid but the return has so far proved very low. Genome-wide association studies, of the kind that has yielded positive results in another complex endocrine trait, type 2 diabetes,[64] may well be the most informative approach, given the now-available catalogue of genetic variation and the feasibility of high-volume phenotyping.[44] That approach will, however, require thousands of cases and controls in homogeneous populations and, ideally, the pooling of resources in an international initiative.

Role of the intrauterine environment

It seems unlikely that exposure to excess maternal androgens during fetal life can directly influence the development of PCOS in the child, as discussed above. It remains possible, however, that maternal metabolic abnormalities during pregnancy have an effect, although there are no direct data to support this hypothesis.[65] Notably, however, intrauterine growth restriction and low birth weight have been linked to an increased risk of PCOS in adolescents and adults.[25,66] On the other hand, a survey of a large population in the north of Finland concluded that there was no association between birth weight and symptoms of PCOS in adolescents and adults.[67] For the time being, then, it is important to keep an open mind about the possible non-genetic, intrauterine factors that could affect development of PCOS.

Role of the external environment: diet, obesity and PCOS

There is little doubt that dietary factors interact with the putative genetic influences to affect the phenotype of PCOS. Insulin resistance is a common but by no means invariable feature of PCOS and, although it is arguable that in most cases of PCOS there is an underlying primary ovarian abnormality, there is clearly an important interaction of insulin resitance/hyperinsulinaemia with the ovarian disorder.[14] The clinical and biochemical abnormalities are amplified by overweight and obesity.[2,3] In a series of nearly 300 women with PCOS presenting to a single reproductive endocrine clinic, we found that the prevalence of hirsutism and of ovulatory dysfunction was significantly greater in overweight and obese women than in lean women.[68] We have recently repeated this analysis, with similar results, in a larger population ($n = 650$) of women with PCOS. Increasing body weight is, not surprisingly, related to worsening metabolic indices. Insulin sensitivity is negatively correlated with BMI and fasting and glucose-stimulated plasma insulin concentrations positively associated with BMI.[50,69] Hyperandrogenism is also exaggerated in overweight women with PCOS. Hyperinsulinaemia suppresses production of SHBG by the liver,[70] leading to higher concentrations of free testosterone, but total testosterone is also positively correlated with BMI,[71,72] probably reflecting the effect of insulin on theca cell androgen production. Hyperinsulinaemia has also been implicated in the mechanism of anovulation.[73,74] As mentioned above, insulin is able to amplify the effect of LH not only on androgen production by theca cells but also on granulosa cell steroidogenesis. This phenomenon is associated with premature terminal differentiation of granulosa cells[75] and arrest of antral follicles. Calorie restriction (and lifestyle modification) in obese women with PCOS results in improvement in metabolic indices and in fertility with as little as a 5% reduction in body weight.[76–80]

The increasing prevalence of overweight and obesity in children has given rise to numerous concerns about short-term and longer term effects. It is even more problematic for girls with a predisposition to PCOS.[24] Although there are, at the time of writing, no formal studies to chart the increasing prevalence of PCOS in adolescents, more and more clinics are dealing with obese teenagers with troublesome symptoms of PCOS. Hirsutism, persistent acne and menstrual disturbances are very distressing symptoms for adults and have even more impact in adolescent girls. Overweight and obese girls with PCOS have at least a three-fold increase in risk of developing type 2 diabetes in later life and, alarmingly, impaired glucose tolerance and even overt diabetes have been reported in teenagers with PCOS.[81] Another alarming but not altogether unexpected finding from the northern Finland cohort study was that girls who were obese at the age of 14 were very likely to be obese at age 31, and had a greater chance of developing symptoms of PCOS by age 31. The highest free androgen index was found in adults who were obese at the age of 14.[67]

Summary

There is strong evidence that genetic factors play an important part in the aetiology of PCOS. Studies in animal models of PCOS, notably in the rhesus monkey, have given rise to the hypothesis that PCOS has its origin in fetal life and that, in human females, exposure to excess androgen at any stage from fetal development of the ovary to the onset of puberty leads to many of the characteristic features of PCOS, including abnormalities of LH secretion and insulin resistance. In postnatal life, the natural history of PCOS can be further modified by factors affecting insulin secretion and/or action, most importantly nutrition. In the search for genes involved in the aetiology of PCOS, the focus has been on genes implicated in folliculogenesis (but about which little is known), those involved in the androgen biosynthetic pathway and those affecting insulin secretion or action. However, the candidate gene approach has, to date, proved disappointing. Even those studies that have been sufficiently well powered to either identify or exclude candidate susceptibility loci (and these have been very few) have produced few positive findings. The exceptions are the recent reports of a candidate locus on chromosome 19p13.2 (the *FBN3* gene) and the *FTO* locus on chromosome 16. While the search for candidate genes is bound to continue, it seems increasingly likely that genome-wide association studies (of the kind that has paid dividends in the search for genes in type 2 diabetes) are the approach that is most likely to uncover the genes contributing to PCOS, even though this will require considerable resources and very large case–control populations.

References

1. Zawadzki J, Dunaif A. Diagnostic criteria for polycystic ovary syndrome: towards a rational approach. In: Dunaif A, Givens JR, Haseltine FP, Merriam GR, editors. *Polycystic Ovary Syndrome.* Oxford: Blackwell Scientific Publications; 1992. p. 377–84.
2. Franks S. Polycystic ovary syndrome. *N Engl J Med* 1995;333:853–61.
3. Ehrmann DA. Polycystic ovary syndrome. *N Engl J Med* 2005;352:1223–36.
4. Adams J, Polson DW, Franks S. Prevalence of polycystic ovaries in women with anovulation and idiopathic hirsutism. *Br Med J (Clin Res Ed)* 1986;293:355–9.
5. Rotterdam ESHRE/ASRM-Sponsored PCOS consensus workshop group. Revised 2003 consensus on diagnostic criteria and long-term health risks related to polycystic ovary syndrome (PCOS). *Hum Reprod* 2004;19:41–7.
6. Azziz R. Controversy in clinical endocrinology: diagnosis of polycystic ovarian syndrome: the Rotterdam criteria are premature. *J Clin Endocrinol Metab* 2006;91:781–5.
7. Franks S. Controversy in clinical endocrinology: diagnosis of polycystic ovarian syndrome: in defense of the Rotterdam criteria. *J Clin Endocrinol Metab* 2006;91:786–9.
8. Dewailly D, Catteau-Jonard S, Reyss AC, Leroy M, Pigny P. Oligoanovulation with polycystic ovaries but not overt hyperandrogenism. *J Clin Endocrinol Metab* 2006;91:3922–7.
9. Welt CK, Gudmundsson JA, Arason G, Adams J, Palsdottir H, Gudlaugsdottir G, *et al.* Characterizing discrete subsets of polycystic ovary syndrome as defined by the Rotterdam criteria: the impact of weight on phenotype and metabolic features. *J Clin Endocrinol Metab* 2006;91:4842–8.
10. Barber TM, Wass JA, McCarthy MI, Franks S. Metabolic characteristics of women with polycystic ovaries and oligo-amenorrhoea but normal androgen levels: implications for the management of polycystic ovary syndrome. *Clin Endocrinol* 2007;66:513–17.

11. Franks S. Polycystic ovary syndrome: a changing perspective. *Clin Endocrinol (Oxf)* 1989;31:87–120.
12. Ehrmann DA, Barnes RB, Rosenfield RL, Cavaghan MK, Imperial J. Prevalence of impaired glucose tolerance and diabetes in women with polycystic ovary syndrome. *Diabetes Care* 1999;22:141–6.
13. Legro RS, Kunselman AR, Dodson WC, Dunaif A. Prevalence and predictors of risk for type 2 diabetes mellitus and impaired glucose tolerance in polycystic ovary syndrome: a prospective, controlled study in 254 affected women. *J Clin Endocrinol Metab* 1999;84:165–9.
14. Abbott DH, Dumesic DA, Franks S. Developmental origin of polycystic ovary syndrome – a hypothesis. *J Endocrinol* 2002;174:1–5.
15. Franks S, McCarthy MI, Hardy K. Development of polycystic ovary syndrome: involvement of genetic and environmental factors. *Int J Androl* 2006;29:278–85; discussion 286–90.
16. Dumesic DA, Abbott DH, Eisner JR, Herrmann RR, Reed JE, Welch TJ, *et al.* Pituitary desensitization to gonadotropin-releasing hormone increases abdominal adiposity in hyperandrogenic anovulatory women. *Fertil Steril* 1998;70:94–101.
17. Eisner JR, Dumesic DA, Kemnitz JW, Abbott DH. Timing of prenatal androgen excess determines differential impairment in insulin secretion and action in adult female rhesus monkeys. *J Clin Endocrinol Metab* 2000;85:1206–10.
18. Eisner JR, Barnett MA, Dumesic DA, Abbott DH. Ovarian hyperandrogenism in adult female rhesus monkeys exposed to prenatal androgen excess. *Fertil Steril* 2002;77:167–72.
19. McClamrock HD, Adashi EY. Gestational hyperandrogenism. *Fertil Steril* 1992;57:257–74.
20. Barnes RB, Rosenfield RL, Ehrmann DA, Cara JF, Cuttler L, Levitsky LL, *et al.* Ovarian hyperandrogynism as a result of congenital adrenal virilizing disorders: evidence for perinatal masculinization of neuroendocrine function in women. *J Clin Endocrinol Metab* 1994;79:1328–33.
21. Cole B, Hensinger K, Maciel GA, Chang RJ, Erickson GF. Human fetal ovary development involves the spatiotemporal expression of p450c17 protein. *J Clin Endocrinol Metab* 2006;91:3654–61.
22. Eagleson CA, Gingrich MB, Pastor CL, Arora TK, Burt CM, Evans WS, *et al.* Polycystic ovarian syndrome: evidence that flutamide restores sensitivity of the gonadotropin-releasing hormone pulse generator to inhibition by estradiol and progesterone. *J Clin Endocrinol Metab* 2000;85:4047–52.
23. Bridges NA, Cooke A, Healy MJ, Hindmarsh PC, Brook CG. Standards for ovarian volume in childhood and puberty. *Fertil Steril* 1993;60:456–60.
24. Rosenfield RL. Clinical review: identifying children at risk for polycystic ovary syndrome. *J Clin Endocrinol Metab* 2007;92:787–96.
25. Ibañez L, Potau N, Francois I, de Zegher F. Precocious pubarche, hyperinsulinism, and ovarian hyperandrogenism in girls: relation to reduced fetal growth. *J Clin Endocrinol Metab* 1998;83:3558–62.
26. Hannon TS, Janosky J, Arslanian SA. Longitudinal study of physiologic insulin resistance and metabolic changes of puberty. *Pediatr Res* 2006;60:759–63.
27. Bergh C, Carlsson B, Olsson JH, Billig H, Hillensjo T. Effects of insulin-like growth factor I and growth hormone in cultured human granulosa cells. *Ann N Y Acad Sci* 1991;626:169–76.
28. Nahum R, Thong KJ, Hillier SG. Metabolic regulation of androgen production by human thecal cells in vitro. *Hum Reprod* 1995;10:75–81.
29. Willis D, Franks S. Insulin action in human granulosa cells from normal and polycystic ovaries is mediated by the insulin receptor and not the type-I insulin-like growth factor receptor. *J Clin Endocrinol Metab* 1995;80:3788–90.
30. Willis D, Mason H, Gilling-Smith C, Franks S. Modulation by insulin of follicle-stimulating hormone and luteinizing hormone actions in human granulosa cells of normal and polycystic ovaries. *J Clin Endocrinol Metab* 1996;81:302–9.
31. Franks S. Adult polycystic ovary syndrome begins in childhood. *Best Pract Res Clin Endocrinol Metab* 2002;16:263–72.
32. Lin Y, Fridstrom M, Hillensjo T. Insulin stimulation of lactate accumulation in isolated human granulosa-luteal cells: a comparison between normal and polycystic ovaries. *Hum Reprod* 1997;12:2469–72.

33. Fedorcsak P, Storeng R, Dale PO, Tanbo T, Abyholm T. Impaired insulin action on granulosa-lutein cells in women with polycystic ovary syndrome and insulin resistance. *Gynecol Endocrinol* 2000;14:327–36.
34. Rice S, Christoforidis N, Gadd C, Nikolaou D, Seyani L, Donaldson A, *et al.* Impaired insulin-dependent glucose metabolism in granulosa-lutein cells from anovulatory women with polycystic ovaries. *Hum Reprod* 2005;20:373–81.
35. Franks S, Gharani N, Waterworth D, Batty S, White D, Williamson R, *et al.* The genetic basis of polycystic ovary syndrome. *Hum Reprod* 1997;12:2641–8.
36. Legro RS, Driscoll D, Strauss JF 3rd, Fox J, Dunaif A. Evidence for a genetic basis for hyperandrogenemia in polycystic ovary syndrome. *Proc Natl Acad Sci U S A* 1998;95:14956–14960.
37. Franks S, McCarthy M. Genetics of ovarian disorders: polycystic ovary syndrome. *Rev Endocr Metab Disord* 2004;5:69–76.
38. Vink JM, Sadrzadeh S, Lambalk CB, Boomsma DI. Heritability of polycystic ovary syndrome (PCOS) in a Dutch twin-family study. *J Clin Endocrinol Metab* 2006;91:2100–4.
39. Legro RS, Bentley-Lewis R, Driscoll D, Wang SC, Dunaif A. Insulin resistance in the sisters of women with polycystic ovary syndrome: association with hyperandrogenemia rather than menstrual irregularity. *J Clin Endocrinol Metab* 2002;87:2128–33.
40. Hague WM, Adams J, Reeders ST, Peto TE, Jacobs HS. Familial polycystic ovaries: a genetic disease? *Clin Endocrinol (Oxf)* 1988;29:593–605.
41. Ferriman D, Purdie AW. The inheritance of polycystic ovarian disease and a possible relationship to premature balding. *Clin Endocrinol (Oxf)* 1979;11:291–300.
42. Carey AH, Chan KL, Short F, White D, Williamson R, Franks S. Evidence for a single gene effect causing polycystic ovaries and male pattern baldness. *Clin Endocrinol (Oxf)* 1993;38:653–8.
43. Simpson JL. Elucidating the genetics of polycystic ovary syndrome. In: Dunaif A, Givens JR, Haseltine FP, Merriam GR, editors. *Polycystic Ovary Syndrome* . Oxford: Blackwell Scientific Publications; 1992. p. 59–77.
44. Stewart DR, Dombroski BA, Urbanek M, Ankener W, Ewens KG, Wood JR, *et al.* Fine mapping of genetic susceptibility to polycystic ovary syndrome on chromosome 19p13.2 and tests for regulatory activity. *J Clin Endocrinol Metab* 2006;91:4112–17.
45. Webber LJ, Stubbs S, Stark J, Trew GH, Margara R, Hardy K, *et al.* Formation and early development of follicles in the polycystic ovary. *Lancet* 2003;362:1017–21.
46. Maciel GA, Baracat EC, Benda JA, Markham SM, Hensinger K, Chang RJ, *et al.* Stockpiling of transitional and classic primary follicles in ovaries of women with polycystic ovary syndrome. *J Clin Endocrinol Metab* 2004;89:5321–7.
47. Webber LJ, Stubbs SA, Stark J, Margara RA, Trew GH, Lavery SA, *et al.* Prolonged survival in culture of preantral follicles from polycystic ovaries. *J Clin Endocrinol Metab* 2007;92:1975–8.
48. Gilling-Smith C, Willis DS, Beard RW, Franks S. Hypersecretion of androstenedione by isolated thecal cells from polycystic ovaries. *J Clin Endocrinol Metab* 1994;79:1158–65.
49. Nelson VL, Qin KN, Rosenfield RL, Wood JR, Penning TM, Legro RS, *et al.* The biochemical basis for increased testosterone production in theca cells propagated from patients with polycystic ovary syndrome. *J Clin Endocrinol Metab* 2001;86:5925–33.
50. Dunaif A. Insulin resistance and the polycystic ovary syndrome: mechanism and implications for pathogenesis. *Endocr Rev* 1997;18:774–800.
51. Editorial. Freely associating. *Nat Genet* 1999;22:1–2.
52. Cardon LR, Bell JI. Association study designs for complex diseases. *Nat Rev Genet* 2001;2:91–9.
53. Nam Menke M, Strauss JF 3rd. Genetics of polycystic ovarian syndrome. *Clin Obstet Gynecol* 2007;50:188–204.
54. Urbanek M. The genetics of the polycystic ovary syndrome. *Nat Clin Pract Endocrinol Metab* 2007;3:103–11.
55. Simoni M, Tempfer CB, Destenaves B, Fauser BC. Functional genetic polymorphisms and female reproductive disorders: Part I: polycystic ovary syndrome and ovarian response. *Hum Reprod Update* 2008;14:459–84.
57. Urbanek M, Legro RS, Driscoll DA, Azziz R, Ehrmann DA, Norman RJ, *et al.* Thirty-seven candidate genes for polycystic ovary syndrome: strongest evidence for linkage is with follistatin. *Proc Natl Acad Sci U S A* 1999;96:8573–8.

58. Gaasenbeek M, Powell BL, Sovio U, Haddad L, Gharani N, Bennett A, *et al.* Large-scale analysis of the relationship between CYP11A promoter variation, polycystic ovarian syndrome, and serum testosterone. *J Clin Endocrinol Metab* 2004;89:2408–13.
59. Tucci S, Futterweit W, Concepcion ES, Greenberg DA, Villanueva R, Davies TF, *et al.* Evidence for association of polycystic ovary syndrome in caucasian women with a marker at the insulin receptor gene locus. *J Clin Endocrinol Metab* 2001;86:446–9.
60. Urbanek M, Woodroffe A, Ewens KG, Diamanti-Kandarakis E, Legro RS, Strauss JF 3rd, *et al.* Candidate gene region for polycystic ovary syndrome on chromosome 19p13.2. *J Clin Endocrinol Metab* 2005;90:6623–9.
61. Matzuk MM. Revelations of ovarian follicle biology from gene knockout mice. *Mol Cell Endocrinol* 2000;163:61–6.
62. Frayling TM, Timpson NJ, Weedon MN, Zeggini E, Freathy RM, Lindgren CM, *et al.* A common variant in the *FTO* gene is associated with body mass index and predisposes to childhood and adult obesity. *Science* 2007;316:889–94.
63. Barber TM, Bennett AJ, Groves CJ, Sovio U, Ruokonen A, Martikainen H, *et al.* Association of variants in the fat mass and obesity associated (*FTO*) gene with polycystic ovary syndrome. *Diabetologia* 2008;51:1153–8.
64. Zeggini E, Weedon MN, Lindgren CM, Frayling TM, Elliott KS, Lango H, *et al.* Replication of genome-wide association signals in UK samples reveals risk loci for type 2 diabetes. *Science* 2007;316:1336–41.
65. Franks S. Genetic and environmental origins of obesity relevant to reproduction. *Reprod Biomed Online* 2006;12:526–31.
66. Cresswell JL, Barker DJ, Osmond C, Egger P, Phillips DI, Fraser RB. Fetal growth, length of gestation, and polycystic ovaries in adult life. *Lancet* 1997;350:1131–5.
66. Gharani N, Waterworth DM, Batty S, White D, Gilling-Smith C, Conway GS, *et al.* Association of the steroid synthesis gene *CYP11a* with polycystic ovary syndrome and hyperandrogenism. *Hum Mol Genet* 1997;6:397–402.
67. Laitinen J, Taponen S, Martikainen H, Pouta A, Millwood I, Hartikainen AL, Ruokonen A, *et al.* Body size from birth to adulthood as a predictor of self-reported polycystic ovary syndrome symptoms. *Int J Obes Relat Metab Disord* 2003;27:710–15.
68. Kiddy DS, Sharp PS, White DM, Scanlon MF, Mason HD, Bray CS, *et al.* Differences in clinical and endocrine features between obese and non-obese subjects with polycystic ovary syndrome: an analysis of 263 consecutive cases. *Clin Endocrinol (Oxf)* 1990;32:213–20.
69. Holte J, Bergh T, Berne C, Lithell H. Serum lipoprotein lipid profile in women with the polycystic ovary syndrome: relation to anthropometric, endocrine and metabolic variables. *Clin Endocrinol (Oxf)* 1994;41:463–71.
70. Singh A, Hamilton-Fairley D, Koistinen R, Seppala M, James VH, Franks S, *et al.* Effect of insulin-like growth factor-type I (IGF-I) and insulin on the secretion of sex hormone binding globulin and IGF-I binding protein (IBP-I) by human hepatoma cells. *J Endocrinol* 1990;124: R1–3.
71. Conway GS, Honour JW, Jacobs HS. Heterogeneity of the polycystic ovary syndrome: clinical, endocrine and ultrasound features in 556 patients. *Clin Endocrinol (Oxf)* 1989;30:459–70.
72. Conway GS, Jacobs HS. Clinical implications of hyperinsulinaemia in women. *Clin Endocrinol (Oxf)* 1993;39:623–32.
73. Franks S, Mason H, Willis D. Follicular dynamics in the polycystic ovary syndrome. *Mol Cell Endocrinol* 2000;163:49–52.
74. Franks S, Stark J, Hardy K. Follicle dynamics and anovulation in polycystic ovary syndrome. *Hum Reprod Update* 2008;14:367–78.
75. Willis DS, Watson H, Mason HD, Galea R, Brincat M, Franks S. Premature response to luteinizing hormone of granulosa cells from anovulatory women with polycystic ovary syndrome: relevance to mechanism of anovulation. *J Clin Endocrinol Metab* 1998;83:3984–91.
76. Kiddy DS, Hamilton-Fairley D, Bush A, Short F, Anyaoku V, Reed MJ, *et al.* Improvement in endocrine and ovarian function during dietary treatment of obese women with polycystic ovary syndrome. *Clin Endocrinol (Oxf)* 1992;36:105–11.

77. Clark AM, Ledger W, Galletly C, Tomlinson L, Blaney F, Wang X, *et al.* Weight loss results in significant improvement in pregnancy and ovulation rates in anovulatory obese women. *Hum Reprod* 1995;10:2705–12.
78. Clark AM, Thornley B, Tomlinson L, Galletley C, Norman RJ. Weight loss in obese infertile women results in improvement in reproductive outcome for all forms of fertility treatment. *Hum Reprod* 1998;13:1502–5.
79. Huber-Buchholz MM, Carey DG, Norman RJ. Restoration of reproductive potential by lifestyle modification in obese polycystic ovary syndrome: role of insulin sensitivity and luteinizing hormone. *J Clin Endocrinol Metab* 1999;84:1470–4.
80. Moran L, Norman RJ. Understanding and managing disturbances in insulin metabolism and body weight in women with polycystic ovary syndrome. *Best Pract Res Clin Obstet Gynaecol* 2004;18:719–36.
81. Palmert MR, Gordon CM, Kartashov AI, Legro RS, Emans SJ, Dunaif A. Screening for abnormal glucose tolerance in adolescents with polycystic ovary syndrome. *J Clin Endocrinol Metab* 2002;87:1017–23.
82. Franks S. Polycystic ovary syndrome in adolescents. *Int J Obes (Lond)* 2008;32:1035–41.

Chapter 3

Ethnic variations in the expression of polycystic ovary syndrome

Chandrika N Wijeyaratne, Vindya Kumarapeli, Ruwanthi de A Seneviratne, Charles N Antonypillai, S Rohini de A Seneviratne, GJ Chaminda Garusinghe, S Chandrika Yapa and Adam Balen

Introduction

Polycystic ovary syndrome (PCOS) is the most common endocrine problem affecting women of reproductive age and is reported from many regions of the world.[1–4] Some reports indicate ethnic differences in its manifestation. This chapter examines the evidence for ethnic variation in the PCOS phenotype and explores the possible basis of this phenomenon.

Despite having a relatively recent ancestry, the species of modern *Homo sapiens sapiens* is a non-homogeneous group, as is evident from their differing physical, behavioural and social characteristics. Such variation has the potential to affect the prevalence and presentation of common diseases. Every human being has a unique inherited (genetic) make-up that can be affected by many environmental (non-genetic) influences during life that can modify external features and manifestations. Spielman *et al.*[5] demonstrated that the expression of some genes differs significantly among different ethnic groups. Phenotypic variations in human populations may be caused by natural selection and adaptation to environmental conditions. Recent genome-wide studies have identified a few loci that contribute to differentiation of disease-related phenotypic diversity.[6]

Researchers studying PCOS in depth need to decipher any ethnic variations of its genotype and phenotype. This requires sound epidemiological evidence that can characterise risks, both at an individual and a population level, to enable effective planning of prevention and treatment strategies. Such an analysis must also consider variations in normal traits, risk factors for comorbidities, response to treatment and effects of pharmacological agents.[7]

Defining race and ethnicity

The word 'race' is attributed to an 18th century European outlook of a group of individuals with a common characteristic. 'Ethnicity' denotes a wider concept that is based on one's history, language, religion and ancestral heritage and that is closely linked to geography, geo-politics and culture. Ethnicity encompasses culture, diet, religion, dress, customs, kinship systems and historical and territorial identity.[7,8] The accepted classification of ethnic groups in the USA for biomedical research includes black or African-American, white (Hispanic and non-Hispanic), Asian, Native Hawaiian or other Pacific Islander, American Indian and Alaskan Native, which are all mainly based on the geographic location of their ancestry.

Genetic differentiation depends on the degree and duration of geographic segregation of one's ancestors. Geographic isolation and inbreeding (endogamy) due to social and/or cultural forces over extended time periods create and enhance genetic differentiation, whereas migration and inter-mating reduce it. Numerous human population genetics studies have concluded that genetic differentiation is greatest when defined on a continental basis: African, Caucasian (Europe and Middle East), Asian, Pacific Islander (Australian, New Guinean and Melanesian) and Native American.[8,9] This does not take into account the diversity and vast differences that exist within specific groups or across the largest continent, Asia. For instance, a drawback of this classification is that South East Asians from countries east of India and south of China and South Asians predominantly from the Indian subcontinent are not distinctively identified. Another criticism is the distinction based on skin colour, which is superficial and makes no allowance for genetic interchange. Furthermore, genetics research that involves making broad comparisons between populations can inaccurately stereotype racial and ethnic groups by extrapolating findings of a section of the group to the entire group of individuals. This can have major implications on some sectors of the community by an overemphasis on health differences, which can shift attention away from established contributors to health disparities.[9]

An ethnic difference in the frequency of an aspect of the phenotype of a disease may be the first clue to its aetiology. Without suitable classification, the underlying factors may not be adequately investigated. To disentangle genetic from environmental causes, studies on the effects of migration are required. Assuming that the ethnic group being studied is homogeneous, migrant studies need to compare the frequency of a trait between people with the same ethnic origin who live in different environments.[8] A review of PCOS research published in the past three decades reveals that the main focus of its epidemiological, biomedical, genetic and social aspects are based on studies of predominantly Western women of white European origin, although more recent large studies carried out in predominantly mixed populations in the USA have attempted to identify the ethnic origin of subgroups. The link between insulin resistance and PCOS is strong and is a main determinant of the phenotypic presentation and response to management protocols. Recent epidemiological analysis of type 2 diabetes reveals its frequent detection in children and adolescents among American Indian and African-American people, and among Hispanic/Latino American people earlier than in non-Hispanic white people.[10] This disparity exists even after controlling for population age differences. However, the propensity for type 2 diabetes among young South Asian people is not reflected in these US-based studies, possibly owing to South Asian migrants forming a relatively insignificant proportion of the population. The effects of social determinants of health are also contingent upon ethnicity.[7] Given the known health consequences of obesity and recent trends towards increasing body mass in young women from some ethnic groups, the impact of ethnicity on disparities in phenotypic expression of PCOS requires in-depth study.

Evidence for ethnic variations in the expression of PCOS

Evaluating ethnic variations in the expression of PCOS requires systematic review of the strength of the evidence, preferably from population-based data or from large samples in the clinic setting. This includes studying the possible links with:

- racial determinants of manifestation
- cultural determinants of presentation and diagnosis
- body configuration and propensity to obesity, insulin resistance and metabolic risk.

This chapter evaluates reports of differing expression of hyperandrogenism, obesity, insulin resistance and metabolic manifestations. The reports discussed mainly comprise comparative and case–control studies providing level III evidence. Relevant research papers were identified from a literature search using MEDLINE, PubMed and BioMed Central using the keywords 'PCOS', 'phenotype', 'ethnicity', 'insulin resistance' and 'metabolic syndrome'.

PCOS is a polygenic disorder. Critical appraisal of epidemiological data therefore requires careful and uniform phenotyping, with the study of sufficiently large representative cohorts from differing backgrounds and populations. In view of the heterogeneity of the PCOS phenotype, such an appraisal must also evaluate possible links between the androgenic, reproductive and metabolic phenotypes of PCOS, together with the ovarian characteristics. To determine ethnic variation, phenotypic evidence of hyperandrogenism, oligomenorrhoea/amenorrhoea, infertility, age of manifestation, anthropometry, insulin resistance and the metabolic syndrome, family history, community prevalence and impact of migration must be determined.

The available data show variations in the PCOS phenotype among Caribbean Hispanic, Mexican American, Japanese, indigenous Chinese/Taiwanese, migrant versus indigenous South Asian, Thai, Malay, southern European, indigenous Canadian and migrant Arab women. Unpublished data of indigenous South Asian women that address some aspects of the phenotype, metabolic correlates, diagnostic criteria of polycystic ovaries, quality of life, health-seeking behaviour and new dimensions of metabolic problems will also be detailed. Finally, the effects of migration and urbanisation on type 2 diabetes and probable links to PCOS will be discussed.

Historical background

In 1992, Carmina and co-workers[11] studied women with hyperandrogenic anovulation from three distinct ethnic backgrounds, namely 25 Japanese women, 25 Italian women and 25 Hispanic American women, and compared them with normal women from each ethnic group (Table 3.1). The participants were characterised based on clinical features, endocrine status that included insulin sensitivity, and ovarian ultrasound scans. The Japanese women had less hirsutism but comparable hyperandrogenaemia, and lower body mass index (BMI) but a similar degree of insulin resistance when compared with white European women. Dunaif *et al.*[12] compared insulin sensitivity (determined by the euglycaemic clamp method) in Caribbean Hispanic and non-Hispanic white women with a control group of women matched for age, BMI and ethnicity.[12] They reported in 1993 that PCOS and ethnicity had an independent but additive effect, with the Caribbean Hispanic women with PCOS being the most insulin resistant. In 1995, Norman *et al.*[13] reported their comparison of glucose-induced insulin response in white and South Asian (Indian) women with and without PCOS in South Africa. A significantly greater insulin response was observed in the

Table 3.1 Ethnic variations of polycystic ovary syndrome reported among various ethnic groups in both migrant and indigenous settings

Source	Ethnic group(s) studied	Sample size, study design and study setting	Characteristics of comparison groups	Summary of findings
Multi-ethnic groups within and outside the USA				
Carmina *et al.* (1992)[11]	Japanese	$n = 75$ (25 in each arm)	Italian and US-based white women	Japanese women were less hirsute but had similar androgen levels, and were less obese but had similar insulin resistance to white women
Dunaif *et al.* (1993)[12]	Caribbean Hispanic	PCOS: 13 vs 10; controls: 5 versus 8	Non-Hispanic white women; PCOS vs control groups	Normal Caribbean Hispanic women had greater insulin resistance than non-Hispanic white women and PCOS had an additive effect
Norman *et al.*(1995)[13]	South Africa: South Asian (Indian)	11 in each of 4 groups	White women; PCOS vs control groups	South Asian Indian women (PCOS and controls) had greater insulin response to glucose provocation than matched white women
Rodin *et al.* (1998)[14]	UK: South Asian	212 screened	Four groups with and without polycystic ovaries and/or type 2 diabetes, 12–15 women per group	Prevalence of polycystic ovaries in South Asian women was 52% (versus 20–33% in white women); insulin resistance of South Asian women with polycystic ovaries alone was the same as that of South Asian women with type 2 diabetes alone
Williamson *et al.* (2001)[15]	New Zealand: South Asian (Indian), Maori, Pacific Islander	$n = 162$ (total)	Compared with 1996 census data	Infertility was more common among indigenous groups and they had higher BMI, insulin resistance and SBP but lower SHBG; they had less perception of obesity
Kauffman *et al.* (2002)[16]	Mexican American	PCOS $n = 83$; controls $n = 19$	37 Mexican Americans versus 65 white Europeans	Mexican American women had higher insulin resistance and BMI; insulin resistance occurred in 73% of Mexican American women with PCOS versus 44% of white women with PCOS
Goodarzi *et al.* (2005)[17]	Mexican American	156 women screened	Selected group with family history of coronary artery disease	A high prevalence (13%) of PCOS in Mexican American women; higher insulin resistance in women with PCOS

Source	Ethnic group(s) studied	Sample size, study design and study setting	Characteristics of comparison groups	Summary of findings
Kauffman *et al.* (2006)[18]	Mexican American	PCOS $n=50$	White women with PCOS $n=111$	Mexican American women had higher insulin resistance than white women but lower DHEAS; similar testosterone levels between groups
Wijeyaratne *et al.* 2002)[19]	UK: South Asian (Pakistani)	PCOS $n=47$; controls $n=11$	White women: PCOS $n=40$, controls $n=22$	South Asian women with PCOS presented at a younger age, had earlier symptoms, more infertility and acanthosis nigricans, greater insulin resistance and lower SHBG
Wijeyaratne *et al.* (2004)[20]	Sri Lanka: indigenous South Asian	PCOS $n=80$, mean age 26 years, mean BMI 26 kg/m^2	British South Asian (Pakistani) women with PCOS $n=47$, mean age 26 years, mean BMI 30 kg/m^2; hyperandrogenism in 66%	Lower BMI, more central obesity and acanthosis nigricans, higher insulin resistance, lower FG score, similar testosterone and lower SHBG; high homocysteine correlating with insulin resistance
Aruna *et al.* (2004)[21]	South Asian (Indian)	PCOS $n=50$		Lower BMI, more central obesity than white European women
Weerakiet *et al.* (2007)[22]	Indigenous Thai	PCOS $n=170$	Mean age 28.8 years, mean BMI 27 kg/m^2	Metabolic syndrome in 35%
Charnvises *et al.* (2005)[23]	Indigenous Thai	PCOS $n=121$	Mean age 29 years, mean BMI 27 kg/m^2	AGT in 42%, acanthosis nigricans was an important predictor
Saundararaman *et al.* (2003)[24]	South Asian (south Indian)	Case–control	PCOS BMI 26 kg/m^2 versus controls BMI 23 kg/m^2	Greater insulin resistance and intima–media thickness in women with PCOS; insulin resistance correlated with waist circumference
Kalra *et al.* (2009)[25]	South Asian (Indian)	Body fat mass by MRI	Mean age 21 years, mean BMI 26 kg/m^2	Total and subcutaneous fat volumes, not global obesity, measured by BMI; linked to family history of type 2 diabetes

Table 3.1 (*cont.*) Ethnic variations of polycystic ovary syndrome reported among various ethnic groups in both migrant and indigenous settings

Source	Ethnic group(s) studied	Sample size, study design and study setting	Characteristics of comparison groups	Summary of findings
US-based multi-ethnic groups				
Apridonidze *et al.* (2005)[32]	White $n=98$, African-American $n=8$	Retrospective cohort, $n=106$	Clinic-based, NCEP ATP III criteria	Metabolic syndrome in 43% (NIH criteria) of women with PCOS; acanthosis nigricans more frequent in women with the metabolic syndrome
Lo *et al.* (2006)[26]	White 34.2%, black 5%, Asian/Pacific 10%, Hispanic 12%, Other 3%, unknown 34.7%	PCOS $n=11\,035$, PCOS prevalence 2.6%, five age-matched controls selected for every case	Community-based, multi-ethnic, Kaiser Permanente	Women with PCOS, compared with white women: black and Hispanic women were more likely to be obese and Asian women less likely, Asian and Hispanic women were more likely to have diabetes, black women were more likely to have hypertension
Ehrmann *et al.* (2006)[27]	Clinic-based multi-ethnic groups	PCOS $n=394$, multicentre data	Metabolic syndrome in women with PCOS: white 34%, African-American 26%, Hispanic 31%, Asian 50%, mixed ancestry 43%	No statistically significant ethnic difference; African-American women had greater waist circumference and insulin resistance, and low prevalence of elevated triglycerides
Legro *et al.* (2006)[28]	Clinic-based multi-ethnic groups	Anovulatory PCOS $n=626$	Mean age 28 years, mean BMI 35.2 kg/m², polycystic ovaries in 90%	As an women had a milder phenotype, and white and African-American women were similar
Welt *et al.* (2006)[29]	Clinic-based multi-ethnic groups	PCOS: Boston $n=262$, Iceland $n=105$	White women in both countries and, in Boston, African-American $n=44$, Hispanic $n=25$, Asian $n=21$	White women were taller; African-American women had greater BMI and type 2 diabetes; FG score and LH were lower in Icelandic women
Far East Asian groups				
Iwasa *et al.* (2007)[58]	Japanese	PCOS $n=46$, controls $n=50$; High LH diagnostic criterion (JSOG 1993)	Normal cycling, ovulatory, euthyroid women with normal prolactin and ovaries	Clinical and biochemical hyperandrogenism less prevalent at 10.2%; testosterone was not diagnostic
Lin *et al.* (2005)[59]	Taiwanese (Hoklo and Hakka)	PCOS $n=47$, controls $n=40$	Mean age 26 years, mean BMI 28 kg/m², acanthosis nigricans in 31%	AGT in 46.8%; both insulin resistance and AGT in more than 82%
Li *et al.* (2007)[60]	South China	PCOS $n=273$, retrospective clinic based	Mean age 24.8 years, mean BMI 22.2 kg/m², polycystic ovaries in 97%	Hyperandrogenism, obesity and insulin resistance were lower than in women from other races also with PCOS

Source	Ethnic group(s) studied	Sample size, study design and study setting	Characteristics of comparison groups	Summary of findings
Chen *et al.* (2008)[61]	South China	n=915, Guangzhou community	Mean age 30 years, FG score was 1–3, 7.5% were overweight, 1.3% were obese	Women with PCOS: prevalence was 2.2%; low rates of hirsutism; hyperandrogenism was age and BMI dependent
Yu Ng and Ho (2008)[62]	Asian (review)	Fertile Chinese women versus clinic-based infertile women	Polycystic ovaries in 5.6% versus 12.2%; women with PCOS had lower antral follicle counts	Women with polycystic ovaries: IGT in 20.5%; type 2 diabetes in 1.9%; 30% were overweight; insulin resistance in 12.8%
Other groups – Arab, Mediterranean and Eastern European				
Al-Fozan *et al.* (2005)[47]	Canada-based immigrant Arab women	PCOS n=92: white Europeans n=41, Arab (Middle Eastern) women n=18, others n=33	BMI-matched ethnic groups; insulin response to oral glucose tolerance test	Those of Middle Eastern origin had greatest response
Al-Ruhaily *et al.* (2008)[48]	Saudi Arab women	n=101 women with hirsutism: PCOS n=83, idiopathic hirsutism n=11; clinic based		79% of the women with PCOS were overweight or obese, 51% had BMI > 30 kg/m²; no difference in metabolic phenotype (both groups high)
Schmid *et al.* (2004)[49]	Vienna-based Muslim immigrant women	PCOS n=49	Quality of life in terms of symptoms, compared with white women	Greater impact of infertility on health-related quality of life in Muslim immigrant women
Vural *et al.* (2005)[53]	Turkey	PCOS n=43, controls n=43	Mean age 21 years, mean BMI 23 kg/m²	Women with PCOS: hyperandrogenism in 88%, median FG score 13; insulin resistance greater; carotid intima–media thickness greater
Vrbikova *et al.* (2003)[54]	Czech Republic-based	PCOS n=69, controls n=73	Age-matched controls, randomly selected	Women with PCOS: cardiovascular disease risk worse than women in the control group and not explained by obesity alone; IGT in 12%

AGT = abnormal glucose tolerance; BMI = body mass index; DHEAS = dehydroepiandrosterone sulfate; FG = Ferriman–Gallwey measure of hirsutism; IGT = impaired glucose tolerance; JCOG = Japan Society of Obstetrics and Gynecology; LH = luteinising hormone; MRI = magnetic resonance imaging; NCEP ATP = National Cholesterol Education Program Adult Treatment Panel; NIH = National Institutes of Health; PCOS = polycystic ovary syndrome; SBP = systolic blood pressure; SHBG = sex hormone-binding globulin

Indian women, both in the PCOS and the reference groups, compared with the white women. This highlighted the ethnic differences, particularly with regard to metabolic status, evident even among normal Indian women.

These reports prompted researchers in other regions of the world to study specific aspects of PCOS in different ethnic groups. They addressed variations in phenotypic manifestation, age of presentation, community prevalence and impact on quality of life linked to cultural and social issues.

Ethnic variations of obesity, insulin resistance and the metabolic syndrome in PCOS

Insulin resistance is central to the pathogenesis of PCOS and any ethnic variation is likely to be reflected in its manifestation among ethnic groups. Those studied so far include UK-based, New Zealand-based and indigenous South Asian women, and Maori, Pacific Islander, Mexican American and South East Asian women (Table 3.1).[14–25] A link between ethnicity and variation in the metabolic phenotype of PCOS (obesity, acanthosis nigricans and insulin resistance) has been identified and, to a lesser extent, between ethnicity and the androgenic phenotype.

The Asian perspective

A comparative study reported that more severe manifestations of PCOS occur in younger and more insulin-resistant UK-based South Asian women of Pakistani origin compared with white European women.[19] Others have suggested greater prevalences of polycystic ovaries among migrant South Asian women in the UK[14] and of PCOS among Mexican American women[17] that are probably linked to their ethnic propensity to insulin resistance.

No doubt such reports of ethnic variation could be confounded by heterogeneity of clinical presentation, controversies in diagnostic definitions that existed until 2004, inadequately powered samples, selection bias in recruitment from varying clinical settings, effects of migration, etc. Furthermore, accuracy of self-reported ancestry, ethnic variation in body configuration, propensity to obesity and insulin resistance, lack of standardised definitions of insulin resistance, equivocal family history and differing cultural perceptions of clinical manifestations are potential confounders. Some drawbacks were addressed in large multicentre national trials in the USA that identified geographically and ethnically diverse groups (Table 3.1).[26–29] However, migrant Asian women comprised fewer than 10% of each cohort, without details of their exact geographic origins within Asia. Constant features of Asian women with PCOS are that they are shorter, have lower BMI and have a 'milder' phenotype in terms of hyperandrogenism, but that they have the highest prevalence of the metabolic syndrome, affecting as much as 50% of one subgroup.[27] Another supporting feature of an ethnic basis is a family history of type 2 diabetes within groups that correlates with glucose intolerance of PCOS.

Consistent data indicate an earlier age of manifestation of PCOS among migrant and indigenous South Asian women (Table 3.1), which mirrors their ethnic propensity to insulin resistance and type 2 diabetes. South Asia is now identified as having an exponential increase of type 2 diabetes, with more young adults having the condition.[30] It is noteworthy that young South Asian women with PCOS consistently demonstrate a lower mean BMI of around 26 kg/m^2 but have greater insulin resistance and a higher prevalence of the metabolic syndrome than older and more obese white women.[20,24,25]

In fact, for South Asian women it is central obesity rather than BMI that correlates with insulin resistance and metabolic problems. This highlights the importance of measuring waist circumference of women from high-risk ethnic groups to help identify their risk of abnormal glucose tolerance (AGT), which should be specifically addressed at diagnosis and during follow-up. Furthermore, measuring total plasma testosterone alone is unlikely to identify an impact of ethnicity on hyperandrogenism, as sex hormone-binding globulin (SHBG), a surrogate marker of insulin resistance, is significantly lower in South Asian women than white women.[15,19,20] This supports the recommendation to measure plasma SHBG at initial evaluation of high-risk ethnic groups such as South Asian women and the need to emphasise lifestyle modification and weight reduction from diagnosis even though the women might have a 'lower' BMI. Greater awareness and application of ethnicity-specific BMI cut-off points is also recommended.[31]

It is noteworthy that indigenous Thai women with PCOS attending tertiary clinics with a mean age of 29 years had a higher mean BMI (27 kg/m^2) than South Asian women but had comparable prevalence of the metabolic syndrome.[22,23] A common clinical indicator of greater metabolic risk in South Asian and Thai women is acanthosis nigricans, although this is not included as a clinical marker in diagnosing PCOS. This supports the recommendation to adopt a policy of training primary health caregivers, particularly in resource-limited countries in South East Asia, on the need to evaluate young women complaining of irregular menses and hyperandrogenism, with or without infertility, for PCOS. This should be combined with risk assessment for metabolic disease by measuring waist circumference and blood pressure and identifying acanthosis nigricans to enable preventive care. It is interesting that US-based 'Asians' (not identified by geographic origin) with PCOS have a relatively large waist circumference despite smaller body configuration with similar risk for the metabolic syndrome that correlates with acanthosis nigricans[32] and family history of type 2 diabetes.[27]

Thus it is essential that a detailed family history of type 2 diabetes and assessment of cardiovascular risks is included in the baseline evaluation of young South Asian women with PCOS, and this should be linked to planning their long-term metabolic management. Their greater risk of gestational diabetes and premature type 2 diabetes should also be evaluated by incorporating baseline 75 g oral glucose tolerance testing, especially before ovulation induction.[33–35] Maintaining databases of high-risk ethnic groups for longitudinal follow-up of long-term cardiovascular and metabolic endpoints should be encouraged.

With regard to East Asian women, Chen *et al.*[36] reported AGT occurring in 22.4% of Chinese women with PCOS as opposed to the US figure of 38.5%.[28] However, in another study of 197 Chinese women diagnosed with PCOS by the Rotterdam criteria, with 125 having anovular hyperandrogenism (National Institutes of Health [NIH] criteria), and with a mean age of 26 years and median BMI of 26 kg/m^2, 60% had central obesity and 48% had insulin resistance, of whom more than two-thirds had AGT.[37] A larger study of 883 Chinese women with PCOS reported that hyperandrogenaemia, not hirsutism, was independently associated with the risk of type 2 diabetes (OR 5.7; P=0.028).[38] Another study of 804 Chinese women with PCOS demonstrated hyperandrogenism-related metabolic syndrome, with its highest prevalence of 28.5% being in the well-characterised phenotype of PCOS.[39] However, an unpublised study of indigenous Sri Lankan women seeking treatment from an endocrine service (n=469) found that the distribution of the four PCOS phenotypes by the Rotterdam criteria were:

- classical with hyperandrogenism, oligomenorrhoea and polycystic ovaries (H+O+P): 54.6%
- anovulatory and hyperandrogenism (O+H): 17.5%
- hyperandrogenism with polycystic ovaries (H+P) but with regular cycles: 7.7%
- anovulatory with polycystic ovaries but without hyperandrogenism (O+P): 20.3%.

The median BMI was 25 kg/m^2 but the group of women with normal cycles had a significantly lower median BMI of 21 kg/m^2 (P<0.001). However, the prevalence of the metabolic syndrome (National Cholesterol Education Program [NCEP] criteria) within each phenotype showed no significant difference ($\chi^2 = 0.394$):

- H+O+P: 34.7%
- O+H: 31.7%
- H+P: 20.0%
- O+P: 23.5%.

This observation in South Asian women is different to the relationship between hyperandrogenism and the metabolic syndrome evident in white European[40–42] and Chinese women.[43] This suggests a South Asian propensity to the metabolic syndrome that is independent of the hyperandrogenism of PCOS. Another insight into metabolic manifestations of PCOS in this South Asian cohort was that non-alcoholic hepatic steatosis affected about 52% of a consecutive series of 110 women, of mean age 25 years, attending the clinic (unpublished data).

Non-Asians

In contrast, a US-based study[40] of 258 women with PCOS whose ethnic origins, although not detailed, had a family history of type 2 diabetes of more than 47% reported a higher prevalence of metabolic syndrome, about 40%, in hyperandrogenic women versus 20% in normoandrogenic women, and AGT in one-fifth of hyperandrogenic women. Their mean age was 29 years, and BMI above 30 kg/m^2 was associated with the metabolic syndrome. African-American women with PCOS generally have higher BMI and blood pressure than US-based Asian women,[26–29] although their degree of insulin resistance does not mirror this difference. Compared with other racial groups, African-American women bear a disproportionate burden of cardiovascular disease risk factors of hypertension, obesity and the metabolic syndrome, which is reflected in their greater age-adjusted death rates than white women.[40,44] Consistent data demonstrate that African-American women with and without PCOS are more obese than other racial groups, with a higher likelihood of hypertension. However, their clinical manifestation of PCOS is reported to be similar to that of white women[45] in age, hyperandrogenism and infertility, despite greater body weight, central obesity and insulin resistance. Interestingly, African-American and white women with PCOS appeared to have a worse metabolic phenotype than US-based Asian women with PCOS.[28] Ehrmann *et al.*[27] reported no significant racial/ethnic differences but larger waist circumference among the African-American women, which was linked to their greater insulin resistance. Nevertheless, their low prevalence of elevated fasting triglycerides remains unexplained.[27,46] This brings into focus possible genetic- or ethnic-based variations in manifesting PCOS among African-American women that might be due to genetic modification over generations. Unfortunately, there are no published reports from their indigenous counterparts residing in their countries of origin.

There are sparse reports of PCOS in Arab women, although the few available suggest a similarity to South Asian women. There are reports of an even greater prevalence of metabolic problems among clinic-based Arab women with PCOS, although not different from those with idiopathic hirsutism.[47–49] White European women with PCOS manifest symptoms and seek medical help at an older age than South Asian women and have less acanthosis nigricans and less insulin resistance based on fasting plasma glucose and insulin measurements, despite a higher mean BMI (30 kg/m^2).[19] The prevalence of the metabolic syndrome among white women with PCOS shows wide variation: 43–47% in the USA,[32,50,51] 28% in Brazilian women,[41] 2–8% among Turkish, Czech and southern Italian women[53–55] and 16% in Dutch women,[41] with a 12% rate of impaired glucose tolerance among Czech women.[54] Furthermore, white women with PCOS living in Iceland differ from their Boston-based counterparts by having lower high-density lipoprotein (HDL) cholesterol and less severe hirsutism and acne.[29] Migration, different environments, cultures and lifestyles, and diet-induced genetic modifications might explain such wide variation within this group with a supposedly common ancestry. Further study is thus recommended to determine any variation of the metabolic syndrome among white Europeans living in different geographic locations.

Ethnic variation of hyperandrogenism in PCOS

Hirsutism, the main hyperandrogenism feature of PCOS, is a function of the individual's genetically determined response to circulating androgens. Testosterone acts on the pilosebaceous unit through androgen receptors responsive to the active metabolite dihydrotestosterone formed by 5α-reductase-driven conversion of testosterone in hair follicles. Reports on the degree of hyperandrogenism in PCOS in women from different regions of the world are varied, as they are based on various diagnostic criteria, clinical settings, age and ethnic origins.

East Asians

East Asian people are typically less hairy than European people despite having no major differences in androgen concentration.[56,57] Chinese and Japanese women have a lower prevalence of hirsutism despite fulfilling the diagnostic criteria of PCOS (Table 3.2).[58–62] This may be explained by low 5α-reductase activity in their skin. Such an ethnic difference will also have an effect on the diagnosing of PCOS, particularly when NIH diagnostic criteria are applied. Lam *et al.*[63] found that the Rotterdam criteria for diagnosing PCOS are more applicable to Hong Kong Chinese women than the NIH criteria, since fewer than half those with PCOS had clinical or biochemical hyperandrogenism. Chen *et al.*[61] reported the mean modified Ferriman–Gallwey hirsutism score in southern Chinese women with PCOS as 3–4 and only 63% of Chinese women with PCOS diagnosed by the Rotterdam criteria fulfilled the NIH criteria. Moreover, Hsu *et al.*[43] reported that Taiwanese Chinese women with hyperandrogenism had more severe metabolic problems of PCOS, with dyslipidaemia affecting more than 50%. The hyperandrogenism manifesting in Chinese women with PCOS appears to be age and BMI dependent.

The exact pathophysiology of the interrelationship between obesity/insulin resistance and androgenic problems of PCOS remains unresolved. Obesity, which is reported in 40% of Taiwanese women with PCOS, correlates with testosterone concentration. Hence, using obesity as the Asian 'cut-off' rather than hyperandrogenism to identify the more severe form of PCOS should be encouraged. However, the BMI of Taiwanese

Table 3.2 Ethnic variations of hyperandrogenism and metabolic problems in polycystic ovary syndrome

Source	Ethnicity	Number of women with PCOS	Findings
Hyperandrogenic manifestations in Far East Asian women with PCOS			
Lam *et al.* (2005)[63]	Hong Kong Chinese	90	Clinical or biochemical hyperandrogenism in 48.9%
Li *et al.* (2007)[60]	Southern Han Chinese	273	Hirsutism in 34%, acne in 45%
Iwasa *et al.* (2007)[58]	Japanese	46	Hirsutism only in 10%; need to rely on luteinising hormone and testosterone concentrations
Chen *et al.* (2008)[61]	South Chinese	2.2% of 915	Mild hirsutism; FG score low (≤ 3)
Welt *et al.* (2006)[29]	Boston-based Asian	21 Asian women of 262	Hirsutism in 66%, far less than in white and African-American women
Legro *et al.* (2006)[28]	US-based Asian	2.7% Asian of 626	Milder phenotype and testosterone lower than in white European women
Obesity, insulin resistance and abnormal glucose tolerance in women with PCOS			
Carmina *et al.* (1992)[55]	Japanese	25	Less obese but similar insulin resistance compared with Italian and US white women
Lam *et al.* (2005)[63]	Hong Kong Chinese	90	Insulin resistance in 40%
Welt *et al.* (2006)[29]	Boston-based Asian	21 Asian of 262	Shorter; mean BMI 26 kg/m² versus ≥ 30 kg/m² in others; waist circumference less; waist–hip ratio similar; insulin resistance/IGT less common than in white and Hispanic women
Lo *et al.* (2006)[26]	California-based Asian/ Pacific Islander	10% Asian/Pacific Islander of 11 035	Type 2 diabetes in 12%; BMI > 30 in 45% versus 67.5% in white, 80% in black and 74% in Hispanic women
Chen *et al.* (2006)[36]	Guangdong Chinese	102	IGT and type 2 diabetes in 22%; not BMI related
Li *et al.* (2007)[60]	Southern Han Chinese	273	Insulin resistance in 12.8–21.6%; BMI > 25 in 30%
Charnvises *et al.* (2005)[23]	Thai	121	Mean BMI 27 kg/m²; IGT and IFG in 33.9%; type 2 diabetes in 9.1%; acanthosis nigricans was an independent predictor
Weerakiet *et al.* (2007)[22]	Thai	170	Mean BMI 27 kg/m²; the metabolic syndrome (IDF definition) in 35%
Wijeyaratne *et al.* (unpublished)	South Asian (Sri Lankan)	460, clinic setting	Mean age 25 years; mean BMI 26 kg/m²; the metabolic syndrome (NCEP definition) in 38%
Kumarapeli *et al.* (unpublished)	South Asian (Sri Lankan)	170, community setting	Mean age 23 years; median BMI 24 kg/m²

AGT = abnormal glucose tolerance; BMI = body mass index; FG = Ferriman–Gallwey measure of hirsutism; IDF = International Diabetes Federation; IFG = impaired fasting glucose; IGT = impaired glucose tolerance; NCEP = National Cholesterol Education Program; PCOS = polycystic ovary syndrome women with simple obesity also correlates with the concentration of androgens[64] but shows negative correlation with luteinising hormone, which remains unexplained.

Other ethnic groups

A parallel difference – greater metabolic risk in those with hyperandrogenism – was observed among white women in the USA,[40] Bulgarian women[42] and Dutch women.[41] Women with PCOS attending US clinics, except for Asian women, had hirsutism in 60–70% of cases, without major differences between black and white women.[28] Interestingly, white women showed a difference in the degree of hirsutism based on residence in Iceland or in Boston: the Icelandic women were less androgenic with lower luteinising hormone concentrations and a taller body frame.[29] Further variations have been shown in that only 10.4% of selected Greek women[2] and 7.1% of unselected Spanish women had hyperandrogenism,[3] while 88% of clinic-based young Turkish women with PCOS were hyperandrogenic.[3] These differences do appear to mirror the variation in the metabolic syndrome.

In contrast, among the 6.3% of young Sri Lankan women with confirmed PCOS in a randomly selected community-based study[65] of 3030 women (of whom 2915 responded to the questionnaire), only 53% had hyperandrogenism, although this was significantly more than among the women without PCOS. These newly diagnosed women had a higher prevalence of the metabolic syndrome (32% versus 17%; $P=0.002$), hypertension (11% versus 4%; $P=0.02$) and central obesity (waist–hip ratio more than 0.85) (57% versus 41%; $P=0.01$) than age-matched women without PCOS from the same community. Their BMI and waist circumference correlated positively with insulin resistance, triglycerides and low-density lipoprotein (LDL) cholesterol ($P<0.001$), and negatively with SHBG and HDL cholesterol ($P<0.01$). The newly diagnosed women ($n=147$) were then compared with clinic attendees ($n=460$) from the same province (unpublished data). This revealed a graded increase in severity of manifestations from community to clinic, with hyperandrogenism-related symptoms rather than metabolic problems being the main determinant for seeking medical help. Seventy-three percent of this series of 460 women with PCOS, referred to earlier, had hyperandrogenism but there was a low prevalence of infertility as they were a predominantly (60%) unmarried group.

Ethnic interrelationships of metabolic problems and hyperandrogenism manifestations of PCOS

The correlation between metabolic problems of PCOS and hyperandrogenism and infertility is based on the concept that insulin resistance plays a central role in its pathogenesis and manifestations. Therefore any ethnic variation in insulin resistance is deemed to be the main determinant of the severity of manifestations, in particular hyperandrogenism. The question arises as to the role of obesity in hyperandrogenism, independently of PCOS.

It is interesting that 73% of Chinese women with PCOS in Taiwan (mean age 26.7 years) who met the Rotterdam criteria had oligo-ovulation/anovulation and 78% had hyperandrogenism, but only 28% had significant hirsutism, with 48% manifesting acne.[66] Liou *et al.*[66] reported that 93% of those women diagnosed by the Rotterdam criteria had polycystic ovaries and women with obesity had no significant difference in hirsutism when compared with lean women, despite having higher total testosterone. A discrepancy between body weight and hyperandrogenism in PCOS is further supported by affected Taiwanese women with obesity having significantly less acne than their non-obese counterparts (38% versus 54%; $P=0.009$).[64] Liou *et al.*[66] highlighted this, which parallels a report by Lin *et al.* in the Chinese language of nearly 200 Chinese women with PCOS who showed no significant difference in hirsutism between obese and non-obese subgroups. Such a discrepancy may be confined to East Asian women.

Interestingly, a study[67] of young Mediterranean women with PCOS revealed that AGT affected about 19%, which is lower than US and Asian figures, with hyperandrogenism being linked to insulin resistance and AGT, but with paradoxical skin manifestations like in Taiwanese women. Acne was more prevalent in normoglycaemic women with PCOS, at 25% in the obese subgroup and 58% in the non-obese subgroup.[67] This supports an ethnic difference in skin response to androgen stimulation that is independent of obesity and insulin resistance.[64] Liou *et al.*[66] suggested an explanation whereby an obesity-associated difference in androgen clearance might explain this relative 'ineffectiveness' of circulating androgens. An association between adipose tissue and the elevated testosterone of PCOS and a correlation between hyperandrogenism and metabolic complications have led to the hypothesis of androgen excess contributing to the development of insulin resistance, the metabolic syndrome and type 2 diabetes in PCOS.[68] However, ethnic diversity in manifesting hyperandrogenism and obesity, particularly in East Asian women, disallows direct comparison of data without making suitable adjustment for the ethnic origins of cohorts. Hence, it is recommended that any translation of these concepts to clinical practice should include awareness of an ethnic variation.

Additionally, differences in plasma homocysteine and other markers of premature atherosclerosis have been reported in South Asian women with PCOS,[20,24] as well as differing responses to ovarian stimulation that suggest a lower fertilisation capacity.[69] Such ethnic differences are mirrored by greater insulin resistance in South Asian children living in Britain,[70,71] which might be partly explained by their lower physical activity,[72] although greater insulin resistance with endothelial dysfunction and lipid abnormality in brothers of South Asian women with PCOS supports a genetic basis.[73] Such ethnic propensity to metabolic problems is also reflected in the rising prevalence of gestational diabetes in Asia,[74] with reports from the UK,[35] Thailand[34] and Sri Lanka[33] of gestational diabetes in Asian women being linked to PCOS. This favours a role for epigenetics in the development of PCOS.

Epidemiological variations of insulin resistance and the prevalence of PCOS – are they in parallel?

Epidemiological variations in obesity-related insulin resistance and metabolic disease are greater in non-white populations, who also appear to have more complications of diabetes. However, this might be due to confounding variables such as migration and socio-cultural disparities in health and disease management. Furthermore, Misra and Ganda[75] clearly demonstrated a step-wise increase in risks of the metabolic syndrome and type 2 diabetes in people from rural India (8.4%) to urban India (13.6%) to US-based Indian people (17.4%).[75] Heterogeneity of coronary artery disease risks within the South Asian group has also been noted, in that, despite being metabolically a disadvantaged group in comparison with white European people, Indian, Pakistani and Bangladeshi people differ in their individual coronary artery disease risk factors. The differences observed in manifestations of PCOS between Pakistani[19] and Sri Lankan[20] women support this. Therefore, pooling all South Asian data might prove misleading and should be discouraged.[76]

It would also be interesting to determine any ethnic variation in the prevalence of PCOS. Community prevalence in Sri Lanka using the Rotterdam criteria was found to be 6.3% (95% CI 5.9–6.8%) in women aged 15–39 years.[65] Other ethnic groups had similar results: 6.8% in white women in Greece,[2] 6.5% in white women in Spain[3] and 3–5% in white and black women in south-eastern USA (Table 3.3).[77] However, these prevalence rates are not directly comparable owing to different diagnostic criteria, methodologies and sampling. The Sri Lankan study conducted random sampling of a defined community of a younger age group. Other community-based assessments include a southern China report of 2% prevalence in a young population[61] and 5% in Thai women,[78] while a retrospective birth cohort of presumably diverse ethnicity from Australia suggests a higher prevalence of 11%.[79] Hence, the currently available data are inadequate to identify ethnic diversity in the prevalence of PCOS.

Ethnic differences in diagnostic thresholds for polycystic ovaries

In a review of the Rotterdam diagnostic criteria for polycystic ovaries, Jonard *et al.*[80] found that the best threshold for ovarian volume in white European women was 7 cm^3 rather than 10 cm^3, and they recommended follicle number greater than 12 to be the best diagnostic criterion to define polycystic ovaries. An endocrine clinic in Sri Lanka that performed early follicular ultrasound by a blinded single observer (one of the current authors, SCY) in consecutive women with classical PCOS ($n=337$) and women in a control group ($n=205$) found that the best cut-off value for ovarian volume was 6 cm^3 or more (sensitivity and specificity by receiver operating characteristic curves of 72% and 69%, respectively) and for follicles measuring 0.2–0.9 cm in diameter was 10 (sensitivity and specificity of 90% and 70%, respectively) (unpublished data). Chinese women with PCOS have also been reported to have significantly lower ovarian stromal volume and vascularity than white women with PCOS.[81] These variations suggest possible ethnic differences in ovarian volume and follicle number in polycystic ovaries that needs further study.

Ethnic differences in quality of life

PCOS causes significant psychological distress and leads to poor health-related quality of life as a result of physical changes in appearance, infertility, menstrual irregularity and obesity. Most published studies are on PCOS in Western women. An unpublished case–control study of newly diagnosed Sri Lankan women with PCOS revealed significant effects on their physical, psychological and social relationships-related quality of life when compared with women in an age-matched control group ($P=0.01$). Their psychological distress was based mainly on the severity of physical change, with one-third of the women being affected. It was their Ferriman–Gallwey hirsutism score and not obesity that emerged as the most significant predictor of their distress, which is different from the data in Western women with PCOS. Immigrant Arab women rated menstrual irregularities, infertility and hirsutism as bigger problems than being overweight,[49] suggesting that obesity might be considered unattractive only in Western cultures and when dressed in Western attire, while Eastern cultures might perceive obesity as a sign of prosperity. The Sri Lankan study also revealed that only 20% of women with PCOS who had psychological distress perceived that they had excess body weight, which supports this hypothesis. Hence, the impact of PCOS on psychological wellbeing appears to be determined by ethnicity and cultural backgrounds, and requires further study.

Table 3.3 Prevalence and specific features of polycystic ovary syndrome (PCOS) among various ethnic groups

Country and source	Method of selection	Ethnic group	Prevalence of PCOS	Findings
Greece; Diamanti-Kandarakis *et al.*(1999)[2]	Selected invitees	White	6.8%	Hyperandrogenism in 10.4%
Spain; Asuncion *et al.* (2000)[3]	Blood donors	White	6.5%	Hirsutism in 71%
USA; Knochenhauer *et al.* (1998)[77]	Pre-employment	White and black	3.4% and 4.7%, respectively	Black women were more obese
China; Chen *et al.* (2008)[61]	Community based	South Chinese	2%	Younger
USA; Goodarzi *et al.* (2005)[17]	Self-reporting	Mexican American	13%	Symptoms and insulin resistance greater
Sri Lanka; Kumarapeli *et al.* (2008)[65]	Community based, random selection	South Asian	6.3%	Younger; less insulin resistance than clinic-based women with PCOS only half sought help; oligomenorrhoea/amenorrhoea was the predominant feature

Summary and conclusion

Ethnic variation in PCOS does occur and appears to be linked to differing expression of hyperandrogenism and insulin resistance. Possible explanations include genetic and ethnic propensities to obesity and metabolic problems, possibly compounded by environmental and/or cultural factors. A variation within Asia is also evident. The variations have implications for screening and diagnosis, management priorities and response to intervention that indicate the need for ethnicity-specific guidelines where appropriate.

The variations of PCOS among different ethnic groups needs further assessment by larger studies of community prevalence among indigenous groups residing in their countries of origin, long-term follow up of ethnic cohorts and the study of the role of genetics, environmental factors and medication such as insulin sensitisers in such groups with a view to improving the health status of women from all regions and in all settings.

Acknowledgements

- Commonwealth Association of Universities
- special trustees of the Leeds General Infirmary
- Association of Physicians of Great Britain and Ireland
- National Science Foundation and National Research Council of Sri Lanka
- Dr Paul Belchetz and Dr Julian Barth
- consultants and staff of the assisted conception units of Leeds General Infirmary, Bradford Royal Infirmary and Halifax General Hospital
- Sri Lankan colleagues at the University of Colombo and the Ministry of Health, Sri Lanka
- patients and their families.

References

1. Franks S. Polycystic ovary syndrome: a changing perspective. *Clin Endocrinol* 1989;31:87–120.
2. Diamanti-Kandarakis E, Kouli CR, Bergiele AT, Filandra FA, Tsianateli TC, Spina GG, *et al.* A survey of the polycystic ovary syndrome in the Greek island of Lesbos: hormonal and metabolic profile. *J Clin Endocrinol Metab* 1999;84:4006–11.
3. Asuncion M, Calvo RM, San Millan JL, Sancho J, Avila S, Escobar-Morreale HF. A prospective study of the prevalence of the polycystic ovary syndrome in unselected Caucasian women from Spain. *J Clin Endocrinol Metab* 2000;85:2434–8.
4. Azziz R, Woods KS, Reyna R, Key TJ, Knochenhauer ES, Yildiz BO. The prevalence and features of the polycystic ovary syndrome in an unselected population. *J Clin Endocrinol Metab* 2004;89:2745–9.
5. Spielman RS, Bastone LA, Burdick JT, Morley M, Ewens WJ, Cheung VG. Common genetic variants account for differences in gene expression among ethnic groups. *Nat Genet* 2007;39:226–31.
6. Barreiro LB, Laval G, Quach H, Patin E, Quintana-Murci L. Natural selection has driven population differentiation in modern humans. *Nat Genet* 2008;40:340–5.
7. Race, Ethnicity, Genetics Working Group. The use of racial, ethnic, and ancestral categories in human genetics research. *Am J Hum Genet* 2005;77:519–32.
8. González Burchard E, Borrell LN, Choudhry S, Naqvi M, Tsai HJ, Rodriguez-Santana JR, *et al.* Latino populations: a unique opportunity for the study of race, genetics, and social environment in epidemiological research.*Am J Public Health* 2005;95:2161–8.

9. Risch N, Burchard E, Ziv E, Tang H. Categorization of humans in biomedical research: genes, race and disease. *Genome Biol* 2002;3:comment2007.
10. Zimmet PZ, McCarty DJ, de Courten MP. The global epidemiology of non-insulin-dependent diabetes mellitus and the metabolic syndrome. *J Diabetes Complications* 1997;11:60–8.
11. Carmina E, Koyama T, Chang L, Stanczyk FZ, Lobo RA. Does ethnicity influence the prevalence of adrenal hyperandrogenism and insulin resistance in polycystic ovary syndrome? *Am J Obstet Gynecol* 1992;167:1807–12.
12. Dunaif A, Sorbara L, Delson R, Green G. Ethnicity and polycystic ovary syndrome are associated with independent and additive decreases in insulin action in Caribbean-Hispanic women. *Diabetes* 1993;42:1462–8.
13. Norman RJ, Mahabeer S, Masters S. Ethnic differences in insulin and glucose response to glucose between white and Indian women with polycystic ovary syndrome. *Fertil Steril* 1995;63:58–62.
14. Rodin DA, Bano G, Bland JM, Taylor K, Nussey SS. Polycystic ovaries and associated metabolic abnormalities in Indian subcontinent Asian women. *Clin Endocrinol (Oxf)* 1998;49:91–9.
15. Williamson K, Gunn AJ, Johnson N, Milsom SR. The impact of ethnicity on the presentation of polycystic ovarian syndrome. *Aust N Z J Obstet Gynaecol* 2001;41:202–6.
16. Kauffman RP, Baker VM, Dimarino P, Gimpel T, Castracane VD. Polycystic ovarian syndrome and insulin resistance in white and Mexican American women: a comparison of two distinct populations. *Am J Obstet Gynecol* 2002;187:1362–9.
17. Goodarzi MO, Quiñones MJ, Azziz R, Rotter JI, Hsueh WA, Yang H. Polycystic ovary syndrome in Mexican-Americans: prevalence and association with the severity of insulin resistance. *Fertil Steril* 2005;84:766–9.
18. Kauffman RP, Baker VM, DiMarino P, Castracane VD. Hyperinsulinemia and circulating dehydroepiandrosterone sulfate in white and Mexican American women with polycystic ovary syndrome. *Fertil Steril* 2006;85:1010–16.
19. Wijeyaratne CN, Balen AH, Barth JH, Belchetz PE. Clinical manifestations and insulin resistance (IR) in polycystic ovary syndrome (PCOS) among South Asians and Caucasians: is there a difference? *Clin Endocrinol (Oxf)* 2002;57:343–50.
20. Wijeyaratne CN, Nirantharakumar K, Balen AH, Barth JH, Sheriff R, Belchetz PE. Plasma homocysteine in polycystic ovary syndrome: does it correlate with insulin resistance and ethnicity? *Clin Endocrinol (Oxf)* 2004;60:560–7.
21. Aruna J, Mittal S, Kumar S, Misra R, Dadhwal V, Vimala N. Metformin therapy in women with polycystic ovary syndrome. *Int J Gynaecol Obstet* 2004;87:237–41.
22. Weerakiet S, Bunnag P, Phakdeekitcharoen B, Wansumrith S, Chanprasertyothin S, Jultanmas R, *et al.* Prevalence of the metabolic syndrome in Asian women with polycystic ovary syndrome: using the International Diabetes Federation criteria. *Gynecol Endocrinol* 2007;23:153–60.
23. Charnvises K, Weerakiet S, Tingthanatikul Y, Wansumrith S, Chanprasertyothin S, Rojanasakul A. Acanthosis nigricans: clinical predictor of abnormal glucose tolerance in Asian women with polycystic ovary syndrome. *Gynecol Endocrinol* 2005;21:161–4.
24. Sundararaman PG, Manomani R, Sridhar GR, Sridhar V, Sundaravalli A, Umachander M. Risk of atherosclerosis in women with polycystic ovary syndrome: a study from South India. *Metab Syndr Relat Disord* 2003;1:271–5.
25. Kalra P, Bansal B, Nag P, Singh JK, Gupta RK, Kumar S, *et al.* Abdominal fat distribution and insulin resistance in Indian women with polycystic ovarian syndrome. *Fertil Steril* 2009;91:1437–40.
26. Lo JC, Feigenbaum SL, Yang J, Pressman AR, Selby JV, Go AS. Epidemiology and adverse cardiovascular risk profile of diagnosed polycystic ovary syndrome. *J Clin Endocrinol Metab* 2006;91:1357–63.
27. Ehrmann DA, Liljenquist DR, Kasza K, Azziz R, Legro RS, Ghazzi MN; for the PCOS/Troglitazone Study Group. Prevalence and predictors of the metabolic syndrome in women with PCOS. *J Clin Endocrinol Metab* 2006;91:48–53.
28. Legro RS, Myers ER, Barnhart HX; for the Reproductive Medicine Network. The Pregnancy in Polycystic Ovary Syndrome Study: baseline characteristics of the randomized cohort including racial effects. *Fertil Steril* 2006;86:914–33.
29. Welt CK, Arason G, Gudmundsson JA. Defining constant versus variable phenotypic features of women with polycystic ovary syndrome using different ethnic groups and populations. *J Clin Endocrinol Metab* 2006;91:4361–8.

30. Chan JC, Malik V, Jia W, Kadowaki T, Yajnik CS, Yoon KH, *et al.* Diabetes in Asia: epidemiology, risk factors, and pathophysiology. *JAMA* 2009;301:2129–40.
31. Misra A, Chowbey P, Makkar BM, Vikram NK, Wasir JS, Chadha D, *et al*; Consensus Group. Consensus statement for diagnosis of obesity, abdominal obesity and the metabolic syndrome for Asian Indians and recommendations for physical activity, medical and surgical management. *J Assoc Physicians India* 2009;57:163–70.
32. Apridonidze T, Essah PA, Iuorno MJ, Nestler JE. Prevalence and characteristics of the metabolic syndrome in women with polycystic ovary syndrome. *J Clin Endocrinol Metab* 2005;90:1929–35.
33. Wijeyaratne CN, Waduge R, Arandara D, Arasalingam A, Sivasuriam A, Dodampahala SH, *et al.* Metabolic and polycystic ovary syndromes in indigenous South Asian women with previous gestational diabetes mellitus. *BJOG* 2006;113:1182–7.
34. Weerakiet S, Srisombut C, Rojanasakul A, Panburana P, Thakkinstian A, Herabutya Y. Prevalence of gestational diabetes mellitus and pregnancy outcomes in Asian women with polycystic ovary syndrome. *Gynecol Endocrinol* 2004;19:134–40.
35. Kousta E, Cela E, Lawrence N, Penny A, Millauer B, White D, *et al.* The prevalence of polycystic ovaries in women with a history of gestational diabetes. *Clin Endocrinol (Oxf)* 2000;53:501–7.
36. Chen X, Yang D, Li L, Feng S,Wang L. Abnormal glucose tolerance in Chinese women with polycystic ovary syndrome. *Hum Reprod* 2006;21:2027–32.
37. Lam PM, Tam WH, Cheung LI. Higher metabolic risk in Chinese women fulfilling NIH diagnostic criteria for polycystic ovarian syndrome. *Fertil Steril* 2009;91:1493–5.
38. Zhao X, Zhong J, Mo Y, Chen X, Chen Y, Yang D. Association of biochemical hyperandrogenism with type 2 diabetes and obesity in Chinese women with polycystic ovary syndrome. *Int J Gynaecol Obstet* 2010;108:148–51.
39. Zhang HY, Zhu FF, Xiong J, Shi XB, Fu SX. Characteristics of different phenotypes of polycystic ovary syndrome based on the Rotterdam criteria in a large-scale Chinese population. *BJOG* 2009;116:1633–9.
40. Shroff R, Syrop CH, Davis W, Van Voorhis BJ, Dokras A. Risk of metabolic complications in the new PCOS phenotypes based on the Rotterdam criteria. *Fertil Steril* 2007;88:1389–95.
41. Goverde AJ, van Koert AJ, Eijkemans MJ, Knauff EA, Westerveld HE, Fauser BC, *et al.* Indicators for metabolic disturbances in anovulatory women with polycystic ovary syndrome diagnosed according to the Rotterdam consensus criteria. *Hum Reprod* 2009;24:710–17.
42. Pehlivanov B, Orbetzova M. Characteristics of different phenotypes of polycystic ovary syndrome in a Bulgarian population. *Gynecol Endocrinol* 2007;23:604–9.
43. Hsu MI, Liou TH, Chou SY, Chang CY, Hsu CS. Diagnostic criteria for polycystic ovary syndrome in Taiwanese Chinese women: comparison between Rotterdam 2003 and NIH 1990. *Fertil Steril* 2007; 88:727–9.
44. Mensah GA, Mokdad AH, Ford ES, Greenlund KJ, Croft JB. State of disparities in cardiovascular health in the United States. *Circulation* 2005;111:1233–41.
45. Finkelstein EA, Khavjou MA, Mobley LR, Haney DM, Will JC. Racial/ethic disparities in coronary heart disease risk factors among WISEWOMAN enrollees. *J Womens Health (Larchmt)* 2004;13:503–18.
46. Coney P, Ladson G, Sweet S, Legro RS. Does polycystic ovary syndrome increase the disparity in metabolic syndrome and cardiovascular-related health for African-American women? *Semin Reprod Med* 2008;26:35–8.
47. Al-Fozan H, Al-Futaisi A, Morris D, Tulandi T. Insulin responses to the oral glucose tolerance test in women of different ethnicity with polycystic ovary syndrome. *J Obstet Gynaecol Can* 2005;27:33–7.
48. Al-Ruhaily AD, Malabu UH, Sulimani RA. Hirsutism in Saudi females of reproductive age: a hospital-based study. *Ann Saudi Med* 2008;28:28–32.
49. Schmid J, Kirchengast S, Vytiska-Binstorfer E, Huber J. Psychosocial and sociocultural aspects of infertility – a comparison between Austrian women and immigrant women. *Anthropol Anz* 2004;62:301–9.
50. Glueck CJ, Papanna R, Wang P, Goldenberg N, Sieve-Smith L. Incidence and treatment of metabolic syndrome in newly referred women with confirmed polycystic ovarian syndrome. *Metabolism* 2003;52:908–15.

51. Dokras A, Bochner M, Hollinrake E, Markham S, Vanvoorhis B, Jagasia DH. Screening women with polycystic ovary syndrome for metabolic syndrome. *Obstet Gynecol* 2005;106:131–7.
52. Soares EM, Azevedo GD, Gadelha RG, Lemos TM, Maranhão TM. Prevalence of the metabolic syndrome and its components in Brazilian women with polycystic ovary syndrome. *Fertil Steril* 2008;89:649–55.
53. Vural B, Caliskan E, Turkoz E, Kilic T, Demirci A. Evaluation of metabolic syndrome frequency and premature carotid atherosclerosis in young women with polycystic ovary syndrome. *Hum Reprod* 2005;20:2409–13.
54. Vrbikova J, Vondra K, Cibula D, Dvorakova K, Stanicka S, Sramkova D, *et al.* Metabolic syndrome in young Czech women with polycystic ovary syndrome. *Hum Reprod* 2005;20:3328–32.
55. Carmina E, Napoli N, Longo RA, Rini GB, Lobo RA. Metabolic syndrome in polycystic ovary syndrome (PCOS): lower prevalence in southern Italy than in the USA and the influence of criteria for the diagnosis of PCOS. *Eur J Endocrinol* 2006;154:141–5.
56. Ewing JA, Rouse BA. Hirsutism, race and testosterone levels: comparison of East Asians and Euroamericans. *Hum Biol* 1978;50:209–15.
57. Lookingbill DP, Demers LM, Wang C, Leung A, Rittmaster RS, Santen RJ. Clinical and biochemical parameters of androgen action in normal healthy Caucasian versus Chinese subjects. *J Clin Endocrinol Metab* 1991;72:1242–8.
58. Iwasa T, Matsuzaki T, Minakuchi M, Tanaka N, Shimizu F, Hirata Y, *et al.* Diagnostic performance of serum total testosterone for Japanese patients with polycystic ovary syndrome. *Endocr J* 2007;54:233–8.
59. Lin TC, Yen JM, Gong KB, Kuo TC, Ku DC, Liang SF, *et al.* Abnormal glucose tolerance and insulin resistance in polycystic ovary syndrome amongst the Taiwanese population- not correlated with insulin receptor substrate-1 Gly972Arg/Ala513Pro polymorphism. *BMC Med Genet* 2006;7:36.
60. Li L, Yang D, Chen X, Chen Y, Feng S, Wang L. Clinical and metabolic features of polycystic ovary syndrome. *Int J Gynaecol Obstet* 2007;97:129–34.
61. Chen X, Yang D, Mo Y, Li L, Chen Y, Huang Y. Prevalence of polycystic ovary syndrome in unselected women from southern China. *Eur J Obstet Gynecol Reprod Biol* 2008;139:59–64.
62. Yu Ng EH, Ho PC. Polycystic ovary syndrome in asian women. *Semin Reprod Med* 2008;26:14–21.
63. Lam PM, Ma RC, Cheung LP, Chow CC, Chan JC, Haines CJ. Polycystic ovarian syndrome in Hong Kong Chinese women: patient characteristics and diagnostic criteria. *Hong Kong Med J* 2005;11:336–41.
64. Hsu MI, Liou TH, Liang SJ, Su HW, Wu CH, Hsu CS. Inappropriate gonadotropin secretion in polycystic ovary syndrome. *Fertil Steril* 2009;91:1168–74.
65. Kumarapeli V, Seneviratne Rde A, Wijeyaratne CN, Yapa RM, Dodampahala SH. A simple screening approach for assessing community prevalence and phenotype of polycystic ovary syndrome in a semi-urban population in Sri Lanka. *Am J Epidemiol* 2008;168:321–8.
66. Liou TH, Yang JH, Hsieh CH, Lee CY, Hsu CS, Hsu MI. Clinical and biochemical presentations of polycystic ovary syndrome among obese and nonobese women. *Fertil Steril* 2009;92:1960–5.
67. Gambineri A, Pelusi C, Manicardi E, Vicennati V, Cacciari M, Morselli-Labate AM, *et al.* Glucose intolerance in a large cohort of Mediterranean women with polycystic ovary syndrome: phenotype and associated factors. *Diabetes* 2004;53:2353–8.
68. Corbould A. Effects of androgens on insulin action in women: is androgen excess a component of female metabolic syndrome? *Diabetes Metab Res Rev* 2008;24:520–32.
69. Palep-Singh M, Picton HM, Vrotsou K, Maruthini D, Balen AH. South Asian women with polycystic ovary syndrome exhibit greater sensitivity to gonadotropin stimulation with reduced fertilization and ongoing pregnancy rates than their Caucasian counterparts. *Eur J Obstet Gynecol Reprod Biol* 2007;134:202–7.
70. Whincup PH, Gilg JA, Papacosta O, Seymour C, Miller GJ, Alberti KG, *et al.* Early evidence of ethnic differences in cardiovascular risk: cross sectional comparison of British South Asian and white children. *BMJ* 2002;324:635.
71. Whincup PH, Gilg JA, Owen CG, Odoki K, Alberti KG, Cook DG. British South Asians aged 13–16 years have higher fasting glucose and insulin levels than Europeans. *Diabet Med* 2005;22:1275–7.

72. Owen CG, Nightingale CM, Rudnicka AR, Cook DG, Ekelund U, Whincup PH. Ethnic and gender differences in physical activity levels among 9–10-year-old children of white European, South Asian and African-Caribbean origin: the Child Heart Health Study in England (CHASE Study). *Int J Epidemiol* 2009;38:1082–93.
73. Kaushal R, Parchure N, Bano G, Kaski JC, Nussey SS. Insulin resistance and endothelial dysfunction in the brothers of Indian subcontinent Asian women with polycystic ovaries. *Clin Endocrinol (Oxf)* 2004;60:322–8.
74. Ma RC, Chan JC. Pregnancy and diabetes scenario around the world: China. *Int J Gynaecol Obstet* 2009;104:S42–5.
75. Misra A, Ganda OP. Migration and its impact on adiposity and type 2 diabetes. *Nutrition* 2007;23:696–708.
76. Bhopal R, Unwin N, White M, Yallop J, Walker L, Alberti KG, *et al.* Heterogeneity of coronary heart disease risk factors in Indian, Pakistani, Bangladeshi, and European origin populations: cross sectional study. *BMJ* 1999;319:215–20.
77. Knochenhauer ES, Key TJ, Kahsar-Miller M, Waggoner W, Boots LR, Azziz R. Prevalence of the polycystic ovary syndrome in unselected black and white women of the southeastern United States: a prospective study. *J Clin Endocrinol Metab* 1998;83:3078–82.
78. Vutyavanich T, Khaniyao V, Wongtra-Ngan S, Sreshthaputra O, Sreshthaputra R, Piromlertamorn W. Clinical, endocrine and ultrasonographic features of polycystic ovary syndrome in Thai women. *J Obstet Gynaecol Res* 2007;33:677–80.
79. March WA, Moore VM, Willson KJ, Phillips DI, Norman RJ, Davies MJ. The prevalence of polycystic ovary syndrome in a community sample assessed under contrasting diagnostic criteria. *Hum Reprod* 2010;25:544–51.
80. Jonard S, Robert Y, Dewailly D. Revisiting the ovarian volume as a diagnostic criterion for polycystic ovaries. *Hum Reprod* 2005;20:2893–8.
81. Lam P, Raine-Fenning N, Cheung L, Haines C. Three-dimensional ultrasound features of the polycystic ovary in Chinese women. *Ultrasound Obstet Gynecol* 2009;34:196–200.

Chapter 4

Quality of life for women with polycystic ovary syndrome

Georgina Jones

Introduction

Polycystic ovary syndrome (PCOS) is the most common chronic endocrine disorder affecting women of reproductive age.[1] Depending on the definitions used for diagnosis, the prevalence of the condition is estimated to be between 4% and 25%.[2,3] The two main sets of symptoms typically associated with PCOS are disruption to fertility resulting from irregular menses (oligomenorrhoea) or absence of menstruation (anovulation) and clinical signs of hyperandrogenism (including hirsutism, acne and alopecia). There may be secondary metabolic problems related to obesity and insulin resistance.[4] This combination of outwardly visible and reproduction-inhibiting symptoms makes PCOS a particular distressing disorder suffered by a large number of women. For example, acne and hirsutism have been identified as major causes of social and emotional stress and psychological morbidity.[5–7] Irregular menses and infertility issues have been suggested to cause tensions within the family, altered self-perception, impaired sexual functioning and problems in the workplace.[8,9]

As there is currently no cure, the management of PCOS is directed towards improving the woman's health-related quality of life (HRQoL) by means of alleviation of symptoms and prevention of long-term complications. From patients' own perceptions, HRQoL provides the metric through which effectiveness of management of the disorder is assessed, rather than assessment of clinical efficacy. Given the nature of the condition, it is perhaps not surprising that in recent years there has been a growing interest in the impact of PCOS on the HRQoL of women with the condition. This literature has wider interest and provides both insight and a framework for considering how to assess which interventions have the most impact for people with other currently incurable disorders in what is currently an under-researched area.

This chapter provides a general overview of HRQoL measurement, describing in more detail what HRQoL actually is and how it is measured, a description of the instruments available for measuring HRQoL in PCOS, a review of the HRQoL literature in relation to PCOS and its associated symptoms, including mental health, fertility and obesity, and a summary of treatments for PCOS that have measured associated changes to HRQoL.

What is health-related quality of life?

HRQoL is a multidimensional concept that encompasses physical, emotional and social aspects associated with a specific disease or its treatment.[10] Through this range of measurements, HRQoL therefore provides a rounded set of important information on the benefits of medical therapies or interventions from the patient's perspective.[11] This is particularly important given that subjective clinical data often do not correlate with HRQoL.[12] HRQoL measurement also has an important role in measuring the impact of chronic disease[13] and in evaluative research as a measure of outcome, particularly in clinical trials where health status tools can assist in clinical decision making regarding treatment choice and policy decisions.

Measuring HRQoL

HRQoL can be measured using either a qualitative or a quantitative methodology. One way of collecting information on HRQoL using a qualitative methodology is to conduct in-depth interviews with patients with the condition of interest. The rationale behind this type of interviewing is that, compared with structured interviews in which all the questions are predetermined and most answers are fixed choices,[14] it allows people to describe their personal experiences in their own words. Such qualitative methodologies are increasingly being used in healthcare research and technological assessment.[15] The rationale for this approach is to understand people's subjective experiences and reasoning. For example, in understanding the impact of PCOS on HRQoL, two qualitative papers have been published by Kitzinger and Willmott[16] and by Snyder.[17] They have highlighted the negative impact infertility has on the lives of women with the condition: the actual or possible prospect of infertility has been described as 'crushing' and contributing to women's feelings of 'freakishness' and 'failure' owing to not conforming to the notions of femininity and womanhood.[16] However, despite the rich data that qualitative methods generate, their limitations mean that they are not suitable for large observational or randomised studies – those particularly favoured in medical research.

Consequently, quantitative methods have been more commonly adopted. In particular, there has been an increasing demand for the development of measurement tools in the form of questionnaires and interview schedules that can assess and systematically evaluate patients' experiences of health and illness or health status.[18] They are principally designed to provide information on patients' views of their own health. There are three types of questionnaire that can be chosen when assessing HRQoL:

- generic, which can be used to measure health status for any condition
- disease-specific, which can only be used for the disease for which they have been developed
- condition-specific, which have been developed to measure a particular condition such as obesity or pain.

One limitation of choosing generic questionnaires is that, because they are designed to measure health status across a wide range of illnesses, it is argued that they may not be sensitive enough to measure changes in specific illnesses.[19] Questionnaires designed specifically for patients with a given disease should be more responsive or sensitive to changes in health status because they contain items from relevant patient groups.[20] However, this depends on whether the patients have been directly involved in the process to derive or construct the items and whether the developers of the instrument have followed appropriate methodology and analyses.

Whichever type of questionnaire is chosen, the reliable assessment of HRQoL depends on the psychometric properties of the questionnaire (that is, the tests underlying the construction and evaluation of the questionnaire) and the statistical methods employed to analyse and interpret the data.[21] Although there are many tests that can be carried out to evaluate these properties, the general consensus is that they should be reliable, valid (measuring that which they are supposed to measure) and sensitive to change or responsive (able to detect changes in HRQoL over a period of time).[22] It is important, therefore, that any HRQoL questionnaire to be used is based on these psychometric properties.

Types of instrument available to measure quality of life in women with PCOS

There is currently only one disease-specific instrument available, the PCOSQ (Polycystic Ovary Syndrome Questionnaire).[23] To develop the questionnaire, the authors carried out semi-structured interviews with women with PCOS, a survey with health professionals who worked closely with women with PCOS and a literature review, from which 182 items potentially relevant to women with PCOS were identified. One hundred women with PCOS completed a questionnaire detailing which items were most relevant to them in their daily lives. Items for the final questionnaire were selected after considering both item impact (frequency and importance of the items) and the results of a factor analysis. The result of this study was the construction of a 26-item questionnaire measuring the following five areas of HRQoL:

1. emotions (eight items)
2. body hair (five items)
3. weight (five items)
4. infertility problems (four items)
5. menstrual problems (four items).

Each item is scored on a scale from 1 to 7, where 1 indicates maximum impairment in HRQoL (that is, worst health status) and 7 denotes no difficulties or problems on that item (that is, best health status). To present the domain scores on the PCOSQ, it is recommended that the mean score for each domain be calculated (that is, the sum of all items within each domain divided by the number of items within that domain).

Since its development, two studies have assessed and validated the psychometric properties of the PCOSQ[24,25] and it has now also been translated and validated in a Swedish sample of 69 women with PCOS.[26] In 2004, Jones *et al.*[24] evaluated the psychometric properties of the PCOSQ in a study of 82 women with PCOS recruited from an outpatient gynaecology clinic. The results of the study indicated that all five PCOSQ dimensions were internally reliable (that is, the questions within each domain were measuring the same underlying construct and exceeded the accepted Cronbach's α value of 0.70), test–re-test reliability was high, and concurrent validity was demonstrated by very high correlations for all comparisons of similar scales of the Short Form-36 (SF-36) and PCOSQ. In addition, the study highlighted the absence of questions related to acne in the questionnaire, which is an important symptom of PCOS that a better instrument should include. The study concluded that the

PCOSQ is a reliable and valid instrument with which to measure the HRQoL in women with PCOS, although it requires the incorporation of a dimension on acne to improve its validity.

In 2004, Guyatt *et al.*[25] analysed data from a randomised controlled trial (RCT) of troglitazone in 393 women with PCOS, 277 of whom completed the PCOSQ at baseline and again at 44 weeks. The body hair, weight, infertility and emotions domains demonstrated excellent internal reliability, with the menstrual problems domain performing poorly. Factor analysis proved largely consistent with the five-domain structure of the PCOSQ and the results of the study provided moderate support for the construct and longitudinal validity of the questionnaire.

The authors also carried out the only analysis to date to evaluate the responsiveness of the PCOSQ.[25] As mentioned earlier, outcome measures need to be evaluated in terms of their responsiveness or ability to detect change. In clinical settings especially, it is important to establish the ability of health status measures to detect and describe changes in patients' health status over time and whether these changes are clinically relevant.[27] Although the PCOSQ detected significant improvements in the emotions, infertility and menstruation domains (despite very limited evidence of a treatment effect on the physiological measures), the PCOSQ did not find a difference between treatment arms[25] and thus the responsiveness of the questionnaire was inconclusive.

Although not the primary focus of their study, Coffey *et al.*[28] derived similar results regarding the reliability of the PCOSQ as reported in the aforementioned studies. Both good concurrent validity (with the SF-36) and excellent discriminative validity were established.

Some limitations have been identified with the PCOSQ, such as the lack of an acne domain,[24] and its application in clinical research has been limited. A systematic review in 2008 revealed that it had been used in only seven studies.[29] From this review it was found that, as measured on the PCOSQ, weight appeared to be the area of most concern to women with the condition. Five cross-sectional studies that used the PCOSQ all found the weight domain to be the area most negatively affected. On a scale where 1 represents poorest functioning and 7 represents optimal functioning, mean PCOSQ weight scores were 2.1,[28] 2.6,[25] 2.33,[30] 2.86[31] and 2.94.[24] Since then a further paper has been published that also found the weight domain as measured on the PCOSQ to be the area of HRQoL most negatively affected.[32]

Generic questionnaires

As mentioned above, generic questionnaires can be used to measure the HRQoL of any disease. In specific relation to PCOS, the 2008 systematic review found that generic instruments were the most commonly used measure of HRQoL, with the SF-36 being the most frequently chosen.[29] The SF-36 is a reliable and widely validated generic instrument (including the reliability, validity and responsiveness of the questionnaire) that has been used in the assessment of HRQoL in a range of medical conditions, including PCOS. The SF-36 is composed of 36 items structured in the form of 11 questions. These 36 items form eight domains of HRQoL:[33]

1. general health perceptions (five items)
2. physical functioning (ten items)
3. role limitations due to physical factors (four items)
4. role limitations due to emotional factors (three items)
5. social functioning (two items)

6. bodily pain (two items)
7. energy and vitality (four items)
8. mental health (five items).

There is also a 'change in health' question (one item).[33] These domains can also be computed to produce two scales measuring physical and mental health: a Physical Component Summary scale (PCS) and a Mental Component Summary scale (MCS), respectively.

Besides the SF-36, the other most widely used generic questionnaire has been the Child Health Questionnaire Version CF-87 (CHQ-CF87). This has been specifically designed for measuring HRQoL in children and adolescents and has mainly been applied in studies of adolescents with PCOS.[34–36] However, other well-validated generic instruments have also been used in research into PCOS and include the WHOQOL-BREF,[37,38] Rosenberg Self-Esteem,[37,38] Sickness Impact Profile (SIP),[39] General Health Questionnaire (GHQ),[31] Health Utilities Index Mark III (HUI III)[39] and a German Fragebogen zur Lebenszufriedenheit (FLZ).[40] In contrast, only a small number of studies have used a condition-specific questionnaire. However, of these, the main condition-specific area that has been measured has been psychological wellbeing and the most commonly used one has been the validated Symptom Checklist 90 (SCL-90-R).[40–43]

No study has yet evaluated the responsiveness of the generic SF-36 questionnaire in a group of women with PCOS. However, the SF-36 has demonstrated responsiveness across a wide variety of non-gynaecological conditions such as osteoarthritis and rheumatoid arthritis[44] and gynaecological conditions such as endometriosis.[45,46] This would suggest that the SF-36 would be suitable for measuring the outcome of PCOS-associated treatments, although further studies in which the SF-36 is used as a supplement to the PCOSQ are needed to confirm this hypothesis.

Overall impact of PCOS on HRQoL

The body of research evidence overwhelmingly and consistently suggests that PCOS has a negative impact on HRQoL. When compared with healthy women (that is, without gynaecological disorders) or normative data, it appears that women with PCOS have a worse HRQoL. Ching *et al.*[31] found that SF-36 scores were significantly lower for their Australian sample of women with PCOS ($n=203$) compared with 173 age- and sex-matched Australian SF-36 normative data ($P<0.01$). Similarly, Hahn *et al.*[42] and Elsenbruch *et al.*[40] both compared 50 age-matched healthy women (recruited from a health screening programme for university employees) with 120 and with 50 women with PCOS, respectively. They both found a reduced HRQoL in the women with PCOS compared with the women in the control group, significantly in the areas of physical role function, bodily pain, vitality, social function, emotional role function and mental health as measured on the SF-36.

Coffey *et al.*[28] compared the SF-36 scores of people with asthma, epilepsy, diabetes, back pain, arthritis and coronary heart disease collected as part of the Oxford Health and Lifestyle Survey with the scores of 22 women with PCOS. Although the PCOS sample was small, the PCS for the PCOS group was comparable with those of the asthma, epilepsy, diabetes and back pain groups, and were higher (indicating better HRQoL) than those of the arthritis and coronary heart disease groups. However, the MCS indicated a much poorer psychological-related HRQoL in women with PCOS (more than 20% lower) than the women with any of the other conditions analysed.

Comparisons with controls (other gynaecological populations)

Studies that have compared the HRQoL of women with PCOS with that of other gynaecological populations have also reported worse HRQoL scores. For example, Coffey *et al.*[28] also compared their sample of 22 women with PCOS with a control group of 96 women attending a family planning clinic. They found significantly worse HRQoL scores on all domains of the PCOSQ and, with the exception of physical and social functioning, on all other six domains of the SF-36. Similarly, Trent *et al.*[34] carried out a cross-sectional study to examine HRQoL in 97 American adolescents with PCOS, compared with 186 healthy adolescents (presenting for routine or sports physicals, or treatment of minor medical problems in primary care; adolescents presenting for routine gynaecological care and contraceptive advice were also recruited). The results of the CHQ-CF87 indicated that HRQoL in the domains of general health perception, behaviour, physical function and family activities were significantly lower in those with PCOS than in the healthy adolescents ($P<0.05$). However, significantly higher scores in the domain of 'change in health' in the last year were found for adolescents with PCOS compared with their healthy counterparts. Later analyses focusing specifically on fertility concerns and sexual behaviour[35] and weight issues[36] also found significant differences between these groups and are discussed below.

PCOS and mental health

One area of HRQoL that is negatively affected in women with PCOS is emotional wellbeing. In particular, women with PCOS appear to suffer from anxiety and depression to a higher degree than their healthy counterparts. For example, Benson *et al.*[47] carried out an internet-based cross-sectional survey in 448 women with PCOS. Anxiety and depression were measured using the Hospital Anxiety and Depression Scale (HADS). Overall, they found that 34% of the women had clinically relevant HADS anxiety scores and 21% showed clinically relevant HADS depression scores. Interestingly, the risk for clinically relevant HADS anxiety scores was significantly enhanced in those women with acne and in those who had an unfulfilled wish to conceive.

When compared with a normative control group of women, levels of depression also appear to be higher in women with PCOS. For example, Mansson *et al.*[48] administered the MINI International Neuropsychiatric Interview to 49 women with PCOS and 49 age-matched women in a control group to assess whether the rate of clinical psychiatric disorders in PCOS differs from the normal population. Overall, they found a higher incidence of depressive episodes, social phobia and eating disorders in the women with PCOS. Suicide attempts were seven times more common in the PCOS group than in the control group. Lifetime usage, as well as current usage, of antidepressants and anxiolytic drugs was more common in the PCOS group.

Sundararaman *et al.*[49] carried out a study in a sample of 99 Indian women with PCOS who presented to an endocrinology clinic. Women presenting with PCOS had increased psychological distress (as measured using the Goldberg's GHQ 28 (General Health Questionnaire), which was related to smaller size of family and more severe physical manifestations of the condition.

Impact of PCOS-associated obesity on HRQoL

Overall, the symptoms typically associated with PCOS, including hirsutism and infertility, have been shown to lead to a significant reduction in quality of life. However, as mentioned above in many of the cross-sectional studies that have been carried out in this area, it is weight that appears to be the worst area of HRQoL affected by PCOS.[24,28]

The finding that weight issues have the most negative impact on HRQoL is perhaps not surprising. It is well known that overweight people find it very difficult to lose weight and, with the exception of surgery, interventions to lose weight are often unsuccessful and are associated with high rates of weight regain.[50] There is debate as to whether overweight women with PCOS have a different metabolic rate or control of satiety as compared with overweight women with normal ovaries.[51] Also, there is no clear evidence of benefit for different approaches to diet and weight loss for women with PCOS than for normal women. Thus it is perhaps not surprising that many women with PCOS report frustration in losing weight, low self-esteem and consequently a poor body image.[23] In relation to weight, a poor body image in women with PCOS may be compounded by cultural influences as it has been shown that android fat pattern, which is commonly associated with PCOS, is considered unattractive in many cultures.[52,53] However, other explanations found in the general population regarding women, such as societal expectations of thinness, may also be responsible.

This is particularly evident in relation to adolescent girls with PCOS. Dramusic *et al.*[54] found that, in a study of adolescents with PCOS in Singapore, 87.5% reported being 'unhappy about their body weight'. High 'drive for thinness' and 'body dissatisfaction' scores were also observed in adolescents with PCOS compared with their normative counterparts. However, two studies that have investigated the relationship between a clinical eating disorder (such as bulimia nervosa) and polycystic ovaries in a UK sample have reached different conclusions.[55,56] The psychological consequences of weight concerns for young women with PCOS is evident and suggests that more psychological support in this area is needed. There is currently no evidence on the existence of in-group discrimination between obese adolescents/women with PCOS but again this would be important to explore in future studies.

The role that BMI plays in the quality of life of women with PCOS is complex. Some studies have shown that reductions in HRQoL are associated with an elevated BMI. For example, one study found a significant correlation ($P<0.05$) between elevated BMI (25–30 kg/m^2) and worse SF-36 PCS scores compared with women with PCOS with a normal BMI (less than 25 kg/m^2) who reported higher PCS scores, thus indicating better quality of life.[42] Similarly, Elsenbruch *et al.*[41] also determined that BMI was a predictor of PCS on the SF-36. In addition, McCook *et al.*[30] found that BMI was significantly and negatively correlated with the weight domain of the PCOSQ ($P=0.001$), and a simple linear regression established that weight scale scores were predicted by BMI. Trent *et al.*[36] concluded that elevated BMI contributed significantly to the differences in quality of life observed between adolescents with PCOS and those in an age-matched control group, particularly on the domains of general health perceptions, physical functioning and family activities as measured on the CHQ-CF87.

However, the results from other studies suggest no relationship between BMI status and HRQoL in women with PCOS. For example, even when significant differences in BMI exist between two ethnicities, HRQoL weight scores (as measured on the PCOSQ) have been found to be similar.[57] In addition, in studies that have controlled for BMI in their analysis of PCOSQ weight scores, it has been found that women with PCOS who have a 'normal weight' still report problems with their weight.[28] As also suggested by Coffey *et al*,[28] the findings from this research suggest that all women with PCOS, regardless of their BMI measurement, have weight concerns and therefore relying on this clinical measurement alone as an indicator of poor quality of life would overlook the difficulties experienced by women with PCOS who have a normal weight. One potential explanation for this is that women with PCOS with a normal BMI struggle to maintain their weight at this level, although further research would be needed to explore this issue further.

The complex relationship between BMI measurement and self-reported quality of life weight scores is also evident in relation to other domains of HRQoL. For example, McCook *et al.*[30] found that, although BMI was a predictor of weight domain scores, no such relationship existed between BMI and the other domain scores on the PCOSQ. However, Hashimoto *et al.*[57] reported a significant association between weight status and body hair scores on the PCOSQ in Brazilian participants. Finally, controlling for an elevated BMI has been found to have no impact on psychosocial wellbeing and sexual satisfaction, thus leading the authors to conclude that obesity is not the only determinant of a poor HRQoL.[40]

Problems with proxy assessments of HRQoL

The lack of correlation between other clinical scores and HRQoL has been found for other areas of PCOS. For example, most adolescents with PCOS who had a clinical severity score of moderate to severe based on a Ferriman–Gallwey hirsutism score above 8, a Global Acne rating of more than 0 and a BMI above 30 kg/m^2 only perceived the impact of PCOS on their HRQoL as mild.[34] There is also now considerable evidence that the assessments that patients themselves make about their health status differ from the reports that healthcare professionals make about them.[58] In a study of menorrhagia, symptoms were classed as severe by the patient but the GP only rated the patients' symptoms as moderate. Similarly, patients who considered their symptoms to be only mild or moderate were rated as suffering from severe symptoms by their GP.[12]

Similar problems have occurred in the measurement of HRQoL for other non-gynaecological diseases. The assessment of quality of life has been found to differ between the primary caregivers of cardiac patients, that is, their staff and families, and the patients themselves.[59] Similarly, in relation to malignant disease, Present[60] found that estimates of quality of life given by patients with cancer differ greatly to those given by their carers. These findings and the results from other areas of medicine have led to the view that HRQoL assessment is only reliable if given by the patients themselves.[59,61]

Impact of PCOS-associated infertility and sexual functioning on HRQoL

There is currently no specific instrument that solely measures the impact of PCOS-associated infertility on HRQoL. Most of the information on the impact of infertility for women with this condition has derived from the infertility domain of the PCOSQ[23] (which consists of four items and measures: 'during the last two weeks how much of the time have you felt "concerned with infertility", "afraid of not being able to have children", "a lack of control over the situation with PCOS", "sad because of infertility problems"') or the use of *ad hoc* questions/questionnaires on this symptom.

The results of the infertility domain in studies that have used the PCOSQ are overall consistent: while it is not the area of HRQoL most negatively affected by the condition (as mentioned above, in studies that have used the PCOSQ, weight appears to be the worst area of HRQoL affected),[29] it is still a concern for women with PCOS and more so than when compared with healthy women of reproductive age.[28] However, there is one exception to this finding. In a comparison of the HRQoL of 35 Austrian women with 14 Muslim women (the Muslim participants were reported to originate predominantly from Turkey and the Near East), infertility caused the most concern for both the Muslim and Austrian women as measured on the PCOSQ but it was rated as more severe for the Muslim women.[62]

Several factors have been identified that may predict the impact of PCOS-associated infertility on HRQoL, particularly reproductive history and, more specifically, the birth of a viable infant. For example, McCook *et al.*[30] found that women with PCOS who had been pregnant but had experienced miscarriage(s) (no viable infants) reported the lowest scores on the infertility domain (and thus had a worse HRQoL), exceeding those of women who had been unsuccessful in establishing pregnancy. Both of these groups exhibited poorer functioning in this domain than the groups of fertile women who had given birth to at least one viable infant ($P=0.001$).

It appears that concerns about possible infertility are present in adolescent girls diagnosed with PCOS. For example, in one of the most comprehensive analyses of fertility and sexual concerns, carried out by Trent *et al*,[35] adolescents with PCOS (mean age 16.9 years) were 3.4 times more likely than their healthy counterparts (mean age 17.0 years) to be concerned about their ability to conceive in the future. In addition, participants with PCOS who were worried about their ability to have children in the future scored significantly lower on ten of the 12 subscales of the generic CHQ-CF87, including all domains with the exception of physical functioning and change in health in the last year.

This concern also appears to translate into adulthood when *ad hoc* questionnaires are used to obtain information about the impact of PCOS-associated infertility on HRQoL. For example, Elsenbruch *et al.*[40] found that, in their comparison of 50 women with PCOS with 50 age-matched healthy women, the women in the PCOS group had a significantly higher unfulfilled wish to conceive than those in the control group ($P<0.001$). However, this may be because 30% of the PCOS participants in the study were referred from their gynaecologist owing to 'infertility' problems, thus introducing the possibility of selection bias. This finding was supported in a study by Hahn *et al.*[42] that found that the proportion of women with PCOS wishing to conceive was significantly higher than that of women in the control group.

Quality of life issues surrounding sexual functioning have also been investigated, with the finding that sexual self-worth and satisfaction are diminished for women with PCOS,[63] even though partner status and the frequency of sexual intercourse was no different when compared with a control group.[40] This is perhaps not surprising, given that depression, poor body image and low self-esteem are often reported by this group of women. Interdisciplinary treatments, such as those covering PCOS-related symptoms together with psychological counselling, have been suggested as helpful in improving life satisfaction and coping of affected women.[63]

Treatments for PCOS that have measured associated changes to HRQoL

Despite the array of treatments available to symptomatic women with PCOS, there is surprisingly only very limited research available on the impact of these on HRQoL. For example, there are numerous treatments to assist with PCOS-associated infertility, including clomifene citrate, metformin and laparoscopic ovarian diathermy. While there have been many papers published on the clinical outcomes of these treatments, only one study incorporated an HRQoL questionnaire that specially focused on fertility treatment. In 2004, van Wely *et al.*[64] carried out a multicentre RCT in the Netherlands in which 168 women with PCOS were randomised to receive either laparoscopic electrocautery of the ovaries ($n=83$) or recombinant follicle-stimulating hormone (rFSH) ($n = 85$). HRQoL was assessed by means of the SF-36, the Rotterdam Symptom Checklist (RSCL) and the Centre for Epidemiological Studies Depression scale (CES-D), which were administered to the women before randomisation and 2, 12 and 24 weeks thereafter.

The results of the SF-36 indicated that baseline values were comparable with values from the reference population, thus reflecting the relatively healthy status of the participants. Intention-to-treat analysis comparing the electrocautery and rFSH strategies revealed no statistically significant treatment effects on any of the SF-36 domains. Two weeks after diagnostic laparoscopy, women on both treatment arms reported significantly more limitations in physical functioning, social functioning, vitality, bodily pain and role limitations due to physical problems, but these limitations had disappeared by weeks 12 and 24. The occurrence of a continuing pregnancy resulted in significantly more role limitations due to physical problems, but fewer role limitations due to emotional problems and improved mental health. When the analysis was limited to females without a continuing pregnancy, there were no significant differences in either treatment or time effect.

A second RCT was carried out by Clayton *et al.*[37] in the UK to evaluate the impact of laser treatment on the severity of facial hirsutism and on psychological morbidity in women with PCOS. Eighty-eight women with PCOS were recruited and randomised to receive either five high-fluence treatments (intervention group $n = 51$) or five low-fluence treatments (control group $n = 37$) performed over a 6-month period. HRQoL was measured using the WHOQOL-BREF. Anxiety and depression and self-esteem were also measured using the HADS and the Rosenberg Self-Esteem scale, respectively.

Although the study participants were generally white, well educated, of high social class and employed, and thus may not be representative of the overall PCOS population, laser treatment had a positive impact on HRQoL. Significantly greater change scores were found in the intervention group compared with the control group over the 6-month study period for self-reported severity of hirsutism, self-reported time spent on hair removal and mean HADS depression and anxiety score. The WHOQOL-BREF mean scores in the psychological domain increased from 49.6 at baseline to 61.2 at 6 months for the intervention group and from 50.1 to 51.5 for the control group. This difference between the groups was statistically significant on ANCOVA testing ($P < 0.05$). There were no significant differences between the groups with regard to the change in self-esteem scores, or the quality of life scores for the environmental, social and physical domains as measured on the WHOQOL-BREF.

Hahn *et al.*[43] completed a prospective observational study in Germany with 64 adult women with PCOS (mean age 29.3 years) to analyse the effects of metformin treatment on HRQoL, emotional wellbeing and sexuality. All participants received monotherapy with metformin, with dosages titrated in accordance with weight status. At baseline, and again at 1 month and 6 months after starting treatment, clinical, metabolic and endocrine parameters were assessed and women were asked to complete the SF-36 and SCL-90-R questionnaires, to evaluate HRQoL and psychological distress, respectively.

Before starting treatment, the women demonstrated significant reductions in quality of life compared with the normative population, particularly with regard to the psychological domains of the SF-36. Lower scores were also recognised in some physical aspects of HRQoL, although the PCS score was not significantly lower for women with PCOS compared with healthy counterparts. In response to treatment, the authors found that HRQoL improved after metformin treatment. Significant time effects indicative of improvements were found in the domains of role limitations due to physical problems, general health perceptions, energy and vitality, social functioning, and MCS scores. Overall, treatment effects were observed to be clearly larger for psychological aspects of quality of life than physical. However, despite a number of significant improvements after 6 months, when the results were compared with data from the German normative population, HRQoL remained significantly reduced in women with PCOS.

In 2010, Harris-Glocker *et al.*[65] measured the impact of metformin versus placebo in a lifestyle modification programme combined with oral contraceptives using the PCOSQ in 36 obese adolescent women with PCOS. HRQoL was measured using the PCOSQ. A similar improvement in scores in both the placebo and the metformin groups was found, leading the authors to conclude that the addition of metformin did not add an improvement in quality of life above those found with lifestyle modification and oral contraceptive treatment.

Conclusion

Overall, PCOS has a profound negative impact on a woman's HRQoL, and this appears to be worse than when compared with other gynaecological conditions and common chronic illnesses. The psychological impact is particularly adverse, both in terms of self-reported anxiety and depression and observed psychiatric morbidity (social phobias, eating disorders and suicide attempts). When measured using the PCOSQ, weight is the area that contributes most to a poor HRQoL. Considering the array of treatments available to offer symptomatic relief to women with PCOS, more studies observing the impact of treatment on HRQoL would be beneficial to provide guidance in clinical decision making to prescribing physicians. What appears to offer most promise for improving HRQoL is multidisciplinary management that combines clinical symptomatic treatment with psychological therapies.

To measure HRQoL outcomes, the PCOSQ appears to be a reliable and valid instrument. The responsiveness of the instrument is yet to be confirmed and more work is needed to confirm this property of the questionnaire. It has been recommended that the questionnaire should be supplemented with an acne domain, as this is the area of HRQoL most notably missing from the instrument.[24] Indeed, in 2007, a paper was published that incorporated such an acne domain into the questionnaire[32] and we would recommend future researchers to do this as well. More qualitative studies to explore the subjective meanings, opinions and experiences of women with PCOS are required. To date, only two qualitative studies focusing on HRQoL in adult women with PCOS have been published. Complementary studies and qualitative studies exploring HRQoL in adolescents with PCOS would provide beneficial contributions to the existing literature.

Finally, more quantitative studies are required to explore the HRQoL of adolescents with PCOS as this has been identified as an area in which limited research currently exists. The PCOSQ, the disease-specific HRQoL instrument for PCOS, has yet to be applied to an adolescent population and would provide a more specific insight into the domains of HRQoL affected in this patient group. In addition, this would provide a basis for comparative studies to elicit the differences in HRQoL between adults and adolescents with PCOS. A greater comprehension of HRQoL in adolescents with PCOS may aid in clinical decision making with regard to the management, treatment and supportive interventions implemented. Early and effective management of PCOS may result in the improvement of HRQoL in adolescence and the transition to adulthood.

Summary of key points

- HRQoL is an assessment generated by a patient's responses that encompasses physical, emotional and social aspects in relation to a specific disease or its treatment.
- HRQoL can be measured either qualitatively or quantitatively. Quantitative approaches are favoured for large-scale studies and use standard questionnaires. These questionnaires can be generic or more specific to the disease or condition.
- There is a disease-specific questionnaire instrument for PCOS that is both reliable and validated, although most studies have used generic questionnaires (usually either the SF-36 or CF-87).
- Evidence overwhelmingly shows a detrimental impact of PCOS on HRQoL. PCOS has a more negative impact than other gynaecological disorders investigated, and yields particularly lower mental health and psychological HRQoL scores than other common non-gynaecological illnesses. Physical functioning is less affected, especially when this outcome is measured using the SF-36.
- Although hirsutism and acne are recognised as detrimental symptoms, studies have consistently shown weight issues to be the most negative HRQoL dimension in women with PCOS, with the tendency to weight gain contributing to poor body image and low self-esteem.
- Infertility is consistently identified as another negative HRQoL factor and, for a few specific subgroups, has been found to have a more negative impact than weight.
- There is surprisingly little evidence on the efficacy of PCOS treatments to improve HRQoL. Existing studies generally show no or only limited improvements in the HRQoL domains.

References

1. Hart R, Hickey M, Franks S. Definitions, prevalence and symptoms of polycystic ovaries and polycystic ovary syndrome. *Best Pract Res Clin Obstet Gynaecol* 2004;18:671–83.
2. Homberg R. What is polycystic ovarian syndrome? A proposal for a consensus on the definition and diagnosis of polycystic ovarian syndrome. *Hum Reprod* 2002;17:2495–9.
3. Balen A, Michelmore K. What is polycystic ovary syndrome? Are national views important? *Hum Reprod* 2002;17:2219–27.
4. Fratantonio E, Vicari E, Pafumi C, Calogero AE. Genetics of polycystic ovarian syndrome. *Reprod Biomed Online* 2005;10:713–20.
5. Barth JH, Catalan J, Cherry CA, Day A. Psychological morbidity in women referred for treatment of hirsutism. *J Psychosom Res* 1993;37:615–19.
6. Mallon E, Newton JN, Klassen A, Stewart-Brown SL, Ryan TJ, Finlay AY. The quality of life in acne: a comparison with general medical conditions using generic questionnaires. *Br J Dermatol* 1999;140:676.
7. Sonino N, Fava GA, Mani E, Belluardo P, Boscaro M. Quality of life of hirsute women. *Postgrad Med J* 1993;69:186–9.
8. Downey J, Yingling S, McKinney M, Husami N, Jewelewicz R, Maidman J. Mood disorders, psychiatric symptoms, and distress in women presenting for infertility evaluation. *Fertil Steril* 1989;52:425–32.
9. Paulson JD, Haarmann BS, Salerno RL, Asmar P. An investigation of the relationship between emotional maladjustment and infertility. *Fertil Steril* 1988;49:258–62.
10. Colwell HH, Mathias SD, Pasta DJ, Henning JM, Steege JF. A health-related quality-of-life instruments for symptomatic patients with endometriosis: a validation study. *Am J Obstet Gynecol* 2007;179:47–55.

11. Jones GL, Kennedy SH, Jenkinson C. Health-related quality of life measurement in women with common benign gynecologic conditions: a systematic review. *Am J Obstet Gynecol* 2002;187:501–11.
12. Coulter A, Peto V, Jenkinson C. Quality of life and patient satisfaction following treatment for menorrhagia. *Fam Pract* 1994;11:394–401.
13. Guyatt GH, Feeny DH, Patrick DL. Measuring health-related quality of life. *Ann Intern Med* 1993;118:622–9.
14. Britten N. Qualitative interviews in medical research. *BMJ* 1995;311:251–3.
15. Mays N, Pope C. Assessing quality in qualitative research. *BMJ* 2000;50–2.
16. Kitzinger C, Willmott J. "The thief of womanhood": women's experience of polycystic ovarian syndrome. *Soc Sci Med* 2002;54:361.
17. Snyder BS. The lived experience of women diagnosed with polycystic ovary syndrome. *J Obstet Gynecol Neonatal Nurs* 2006;35:385–92.
18. Jenkinson C. *Assessment and Evaluation of Health and Medical Care: a Methods Text.* Buckingham: Open University Press; 1997.
19. Jenkinson C, McGee H. Patient assessed outcomes: measuring health status and quality of life. In: Jenkinson C, editor. *Assessment and Evaluation of Health and Medical Care: a Methods Text.* Buckingham: Open University Press; 1997. p. 64–84.
20. Streiner, DL, Norman G. *Health Measurement Scales: A Practical Guide to their Development and Use.* 2nd ed. Oxford: Oxford University Press; 1995.
21. Fayers PM, Machin D. *Quality of Life: Assessment, Analysis and Interpretation.* Chichester: John Wiley & Sons; 2000.
22. Nunally JC. *Psychometric Theory.* New Delhi: Tate McGraw Hill; 1978.
23. Cronin L, Guyatt G, Griffith L, Wong E, Azziz R, Futterweit W, *et al.* Development of a health-related quality-of-life questionnaire (PCOSQ) for women with polycystic ovary syndrome (PCOS). *J Clin Endocrinol Metab* 1998;83:1976–87.
24. Jones GL, Benes K, Clark TL, Denham R, Holder MG, Haynes TJ, *et al.* The Polycystic Ovary Syndrome Health-Related Quality of Life Questionnaire (PCOSQ): a validation. *Hum Reprod* 2004;19:371–7.
25. Guyatt G, Weaver B, Cronin L, Dooley JA, Azziz R. Health-related quality of life in women with polycystic ovary syndrome, a self-administered questionnaire, was validated. *J Clin Epidemiol* 2004;57:1279–87.
26. Jedel E, Kowalski J, Stener-Victorin E. Assessment of health-related quality of life: Swedish version of polycystic ovary syndrome questionnaire. *Acta Obstet Gynecol Scand* 2008;87:1329–35.
27. Kazis LE, Anderson JJ, Meenan RF. Effect sizes for interpreting changes in health status. *Med Care* 1989;27:S178–89.
28. Coffey S, Bano G, Mason HD. Health-related quality of life in women with polycystic ovary syndrome: a comparison with the general population using the Polycystic Ovary Syndrome Questionnaire (PCOSQ) and the Short Form-36 (SF-36). *Gynecol Endocrinol* 2006;22:80–6.
29. Jones GL, Hall JM, Balen AH, Ledger WL. Health-related quality of life measurement in women with polycystic ovary syndrome: a systematic review. *Hum Reprod Update* 2008;14:15–25.
30. McCook JG, Reame NE, Thatcher SS. Health-related quality of life issues in women with polycystic ovary syndrome. *J Obstet Gynecol Neonatal Nurs* 2005;34:12–20.
31. Ching HL, Burke V, Stuckey BG. Quality of life and psychological morbidity in women with polycystic ovary syndrome: body mass index, age and the provision of patient information are significant modifiers. *Clin Endocrinol (Oxf)* 2007;66:373–9.
32. Barnard L, Ferriday D, Guenther N, Strauss B, Balen AH, Dye L. Quality of life and psychological well being in polycystic ovary syndrome. *Hum Reprod* 2007;22:2279–86.
33. Ware JE, Sherbourne EC. The MOS 36-Item Short Form Health Survey 1: conceptual framework and item selection. *Med Care* 1992;30:473–83.
34. Trent ME, Rich M, Austin SB, Gordon CM. Quality of life in adolescent girls with polycystic ovary syndrome. *Arch Pediatr Adolesc Med* 2002;156:556–60.
35. Trent ME, Rich M, Austin SB, Gordon CM. Fertility concerns and sexual behavior in adolescent girls with polycystic ovary syndrome: implications for quality of life. *J Pediatr Adolesc Gynecol* 2003;16:33–7.

36. Trent M, Austin SB, Rich M, Gordon CM. Overweight status of adolescent girls with polycystic ovary syndrome: body mass index as mediator of quality of life. *Ambul Pediatr* 2005;5:107–11.
37. Clayton WJ, Lipton M, Elford J, Rustin M, Sherr L. A randomized controlled trial of laser treatment among hirsute women with polycystic ovary syndrome. *Br J Dermatol* 2005;152:986–92.
38. Lipton MG, Sherr L, Elford J, Rustin MH, Clayton WJ. Women living with facial hair: the psychological and behavioral burden. *J Psychosom Res* 2006;61:161–8.
39. Wong E, Cronin L, Griffith L, Irvine EJ, Guyatt GH. Problems of HRQL assessment: how much is too much? *J Clin Epidemiol* 2001;54:1081–5.
40. Elsenbruch S, Hahn S, Kowalsky D, Offner AH, Schedlowski M, Mann K, *et al.* Quality of life, psychosocial well-being, and sexual satisfaction in women with polycystic ovary syndrome. *J Clin Endocrinol Metab* 2003;88:5801–7.
41. Elsenbruch S, Benson S, Hahn S, Tan S, Mann K, Pleger K, *et al.* Determinants of emotional distress in women with polycystic ovary syndrome. *Hum Reprod* 2006;21:1092–9.
42. Hahn S, Janssen OE, Tan S, Pleger K, Mann K, Schedlowski M, *et al.* Clinical and psychological correlates of quality-of-life in polycystic ovary syndrome. *Eur J Endocrinol* 2005;153:853–60.
43. Hahn S, Benson S, Elsenbruch S, Pleger K, Tan S, Mann K, *et al.* Metformin treatment of polycystic ovary syndrome improves health related quality-of-life, emotional distress and sexuality. *Hum Reprod* 2006;21:1925–34.
44. Kosinski M, Keller SD, Ware JE Jr, Hatoum HT, Kong SX. The SF-36 Health Survey as a generic outcome measure in clinical trials of patients with osteoarthritis and rheumatoid arthritis: relative validity of scales in relation to clinical measures of arthritis severity. *Med Care* 1999;37(5 Suppl):MS23–39.
45. Bodner C, Garratt AM, Ratcliffe J, Macdonald LM, Penney, GC. Measuring health-related quality of life outcomes in women with endometriosis: results of the gynaecology audit project in Scotland. *Health Bull (Edinb)* 1997;55:109–17.
46. Jones G, Jenkinson C, Kennedy S. Evaluating the responsiveness of the Endometriosis Health Profile Questionnaire: the EHP-30. *Qual Life Res* 2004;13:705–13.
47. Benson S, Hahn S, Tan S, Mann K, Janssen OE, Schedlowski M, *et al.* Prevalence and implications of anxiety in polycystic ovary syndrome: results of an internet-based survey in Germany. *Hum Reprod* 2009;24:1446–51.
48. Mansson M, Holte J, Landin-Wilhelmsen K, Dahlgren E, Johansson A, Landen M. Women with polycystic ovary syndrome are often depressed or anxious – a case control study. *Psychoneuroendocrinology* 2008;33:1132–8.
49. Sundararaman PG, Shweta, Sridhar GR. Psychosocial aspects of women with polycystic ovary syndrome from south India. *J Assoc Physicians India* 2008;56:945–8.
50. Hoeger KM. Role of lifestyle modification in the management of polycystic ovary syndrome. *Best Pract Res Clin Endocrinol Metab* 2006;20:293–310.
51. Norman RJ, Noakes M, Wu R, Davies MJ, Moran L, Wanf JX. Improving reproductive performance in overweight/obese women with effective weight management. *Hum Reprod Update* 2004;10:267–80.
52. Brown PJ. Culture and evolution of obesity. *Hum Nat* 1991;2:57.
53. Deurenberg P, Deurenberg-Yap M, Guricci S. Asians are different from Caucasians and from each other in their body mass index/body fat per cent relationship. *Obes Rev* 2002;3:141–6.
54. Dramusic V, Goh VH, Rajan U, Wong YC, Ratnam SS. Clinical, endocrinologic, and ultrasonographic features of polycystic ovary syndrome in Singaporean adolescents. *J Pediatr Adolesc Gynecol* 1997;10:125–32.
55. Michelmore KF, Balen AH, Dunger DB. Polycystic ovaries and eating disorders: Are they related? *Hum Reprod* 2001;16:765–9.
56. Morgan JF, McCluskey SE, Brunton JN, Hubert Lacey J. Polycystic ovarian morphology and bulimia nervosa: a 9-year follow-up study. *Fertil Steril* 2002;77:928–31.
57. Hashimoto DM, Schmid J, Martins FM, Fonseca AM, Andrade LH, Kirchengast S, *et al.* The impact of the weight status on subjective symptomatology of the polycystic ovary syndrome: a cross-cultural comparison between Brazilian and Austrian women. *Anthropol Anz* 2003;61:297–310.

58. Fitzpatrick R. Applications of health status measures. In: Jenkinson C, editor. *Measuring Health and Medical Outcomes*. London: UCL Press; 1994. p. 27–41.
59. Woodend AK, Nair RC, Tang, AS. Definition of life quality from a patient versus health care professional perspective. *Int J Rehabil Res* 1997;20:71–80.
60. Present CA. Quality of life in cancer patients: who measures what? *Am J Clin Oncol* 1991;7:571–3.
61. Slevin ML, Plant H, Lynch D, Drinkwater J, Gregory WM. Who should measure quality of life, the doctor or the patient? *Br J Cancer* 1988;57:109–12.
62. Schmid J, Kirchengast S, Vytiska-Binstorfer E, Huber J. Infertility caused by PCOS – health-related quality of life among Austrian and Moslem immigrant women in Austria. *Hum Reprod* 2004;19:2251–7.
63. Janssen OE, Hahn S, Tan S, Benson S, Elsenbruch S. Mood and sexual function in polycystic ovary syndrome. *Semin Reprod Med* 2008;26:45–52.
64. van Wely M, Bayram N, Bossuyt PM, van der Veen F. Laparoscopic electrocautery of the ovaries versus recombinant FSH in clomiphene citrate-resistant polycystic ovary syndrome. Impact on women's health-related quality of life. *Hum Reprod* 2004;19:2244–50.
65. Harris-Glocker M, Davidson K, Kochman L, Guzick D, Hoeger K. Improvement in quality-of-life questionnaire measures in obese adolescent females with polycystic ovary syndrome treated with lifestyle changes and oral contraceptives, with or without metformin. *Fertil Steril* 2010;93:1016–19.

Chapter 5

Insulin resistance, the metabolic syndrome and polycystic ovary syndrome

Gerard Conway

Introduction

The first reports of a link between insulin and polycystic ovary syndrome (PCOS) appeared in the 1980s. First there was the demonstration of a link between hyperinsulinism and hyperandrogenism[1] and then, soon after, the demonstration that non-obese women with PCOS were insulin resistant.[2] These two seminal papers opened up a whole new field of investigation exploring the relationship between what was later to be called the metabolic syndrome and PCOS.[3]

Much of the initial work in this area focused on the correlation between insulin and androgens in the circulation, with a debate surrounding the direction of causation in this relationship. A consensus view gradually emerged supporting the role of insulin as a co-gonadotrophin amplifying the effect of luteinising hormone (LH) on theca cell testosterone production.[4] Recently, the opposing view that androgens might induce a state of insulin resistance has gained attention again.[5]

Recognition that insulin has a pathogenic role in PCOS has led to several new treatment strategies and branches of research:

- Addressing insulin resistance by any means has become routine in the management of PCOS.
- Elements of the insulin-signalling pathway have been explored as candidates for the inheritance of PCOS.
- The importance of PCOS in identifying individuals and family members at risk of developing type 2 diabetes has become an important part of preventive medicine.

Definitions and diagnosis

In clinical practice, the diagnosis of PCOS is relatively straightforward according to European guidelines. A more contentious area is the assessment of the metabolic syndrome in PCOS. Most clinical guidelines agree that an assessment of insulin status in individuals suspected of having the metabolic syndrome is not required in routine practice. If one is concerned, however, not to miss an opportunity to prevent transition to type 2 diabetes later in life, then metabolic status has to be addressed.

The various learned societies have developed criteria for the diagnosis of the metabolic syndrome. In addition, there are many parameters that correlate with insulin resistance that can be used as markers of the metabolic syndrome. A list of the cardinal features of the metabolic syndrome is presented in Box 5.1.

The gold standard for measuring insulin resistance is the euglycaemic hyperinsulinaemic clamp. As this is a laborious procedure, several other markers have been used, including the glucose/insulin ratio, homeostatic model assessment (HOMA) and the quantitative insulin sensitivity check index (QUICKI). These assessments of insulin sensitivity have their place only in research.

For practical purposes in the clinic setting, a simplified approach can be taken. At a random clinic visit in the non-fasting state, a measurement of waist circumference, body mass index and sex hormone-binding globulin and a family history of gestational or type 2 diabetes would allow important stratification for further investigation of the metabolic syndrome. Those identified as being at risk could then be recalled for a fasting lipoprotein profile, glucose and insulin concentration and perhaps an oral glucose tolerance test for a full assessment of metabolic status. The cost effectiveness of each element of this screening strategy will depend on the clinical setting, the ethnicity profile and the prevalence of obesity in the clinic population.

Mechanism of insulin resistance in PCOS

Various pathogenic mechanisms have been identified in the insulin signalling pathway to explain insulin resistance in women with PCOS.[6,7] It is generally accepted that the number of insulin receptors and their affinity for the ligand is normal in both adipocytes and fibroblasts.[8] On the intracellular aspect, abnormalities of phosphorylation of both serine and tyrosine residues of the insulin receptor have been identified. Further down the signalling pathway, reduced phophorylation of insulin receptor substrate 1 (*IRS1*) and reduced glucose transporter 4 (*GLUT4*) expression have also been demonstrated. Further details on this topic are provided in a 2006 review.[7]

Box 5.1 Summary of defining criteria for the metabolic syndrome based on World Health Organization, European Group for the Study of Insulin Resistance and American Heart Association guidelines; example cut-off points are presented but these differ according to each definition

Cardinal features – three of the following:

- central obesity; waist circumference > 85 cm
- raised triglycerides > 1.7 mmol/litre
- reduced high-density lipoprotein (HDL) cholesterol < 1.0 mmol/litre
- raised blood pressure > 140/85 mmHg
- fasting hyperglycaemia > 5.6 mmol/litre

Associated features:

- raised fasting insulin
- glucose intolerance on an oral glucose tolerance test
- hyperuricaemia
- microalbuminuria; albumin : creatinine ratio > 30 mg/g
- raised high-sensitivity C-reactive protein and other inflammatory markers
- raised liver enzyme (fatty liver)
- reduced plasminogen activator inhibitor 1 (PAI-1)
- reduced sex hormone-binding globulin (SHBG)

Interactions between the metabolic syndrome and ovarian function

Insulin as a co-gonadotrophin

Whether hyperandrogenism results from the hyperinsulinaemia of insulin resistance or vice versa has been debated since the correlation between them was first demonstrated.[9] Most of the evidence supports hyperinsulinaemia as the primary factor, especially the experiments in which decreasing the hyperandrogenaemia by bilateral oophorectomy or the administration of a gonadotrophin-releasing hormone (GnRH) agonist did not result in improved insulin sensitivity in women with PCOS.[10]

Insulin may act directly to stimulate ovarian androgen production by acting as a co-gonadotrophin augmenting LH activity. This action may be mediated through stimulation of ovarian insulin receptors or receptors for insulin-like growth factors.[11] Insulin may also act indirectly at the level of the pituitary by enhancing the amplitude of serum LH pulses.

Insulin appears to drive ovarian androgen production through the insulin receptor as opposed to cross-over stimulation of the insulin-like growth factor I (IGF-I) receptor.[12] Evidence of signalling through the IGF-I pathway is provided by *in vitro* studies of both granulosa and theca cells.[11] In this way, the concept has gained favour that the ovary remains sensitive to insulin when other compartments such as liver and muscle are relatively resistant to the action of insulin (hence the development of hyperinsulinaemia).[13,14]

Inflammation and the ovary

In recent years, altered inflammatory markers as part of the metabolic syndrome have highlighted an alternative pathway that may be relevant to the pathogenesis of PCOS.[15–17]

Obesity is increasingly thought of as a chronic inflammatory state characterised by abnormal cytokine production, increased acute-phase reactants and activation of inflammatory signalling pathways. Adipose tissue synthesises an array of inflammatory cytokines, including interleukin 6 (IL-6), IL-18, tumour necrosis factor α (TNF-α), adiponectin, leptin, C-reactive protein, plasminogen activator inhibitor 1 (PAI-1) and monocyte chemoattractant protein-1 (MCP1). Most of these have now been explored in women with PCOS and their association with obesity rather than PCOS status is the predominant factor.[15,17–19]

Leptin is particularly interesting because of its signalling to hypothalamic GnRH neurones but this connection is thought to be most important for states of undernutrition rather than obesity.[20]

In the context of PCOS, there is some debate as to whether altered circulating adipokine concentrations are accounted for completely by obesity or whether some of these changes are specific to PCOS. Given the overwhelming influence of adiposity on the secretion of these cytokines and their circulating concentrations, the cautious view is that inflammatory markers are unlikely to be specific to PCOS.

PCOS as a marker for type 2 diabetes

The relationship between PCOS and diabetes has been assessed in two ways. Many studies have recorded the prevalence of impaired glucose tolerance and diabetes using the oral glucose tolerance test as a screening method for cohorts of women with PCOS. The prevalence of impaired glucose tolerance in women with PCOS varies between 10% and 30% depending on the degree of obesity in the study group.[21–24] Similarly, the prevalence of type 2 diabetes in women with PCOS varies between 2% and 10%. The conversion rate from normal to impaired glucose tolerance has been estimated at 16% per year and from impaired glucose tolerance to diabetes the conversion rate is 2% per year.[25] With regard to gestational diabetes, women with PCOS have approximately a three-fold excess risk compared with women without PCOS.[26]

Reversing this process, women with type 2 diabetes or gestational diabetes have been assessed using ultrasonography for the prevalence of polycystic ovaries, which was found to be 82%[27] and 52%,[28] respectively, compared with the expected population prevalence of 22%.

In a historic cohort predating the obesity epidemic, the odds ratio for diabetes contributing to a cause of death was found to be 3.6 (95% CI 1.5–8.4) in women with PCOS compared with population reference data.[29]

PCOS and type 2 diabetes are therefore closely related, leading to the concept that PCOS is a 'prediabetic' state. This relationship is exaggerated by the epidemic of obesity, with a greater proportion of women gradually developing type 2 diabetes over time. Recognition of the risk of type 2 diabetes in young women with PCOS provides an opportunity for early education for diabetes prevention with lifestyle measures.

PCOS as a marker for cardiovascular disease

As part of the metabolic syndrome, women with PCOS have an array of adverse cardiovascular risk markers, including abnormal lipid profiles,[3] increased carotid artery intima–media thickness, endothelial dysfunction[30,31] and carotid artery calcification.[32] Some of these studies show that PCOS status is associated with adverse cardiovascular risk independently of obesity but in many cases this correction is performed by statistical adjustment or *post hoc* weight-matched subgroups rather than by pretest weight matching. It is as yet unclear to what degree obesity alone accounts for the adverse cardiovascular risk in women with PCOS compared with PCOS status *per se*.

It must be emphasised that all of these studies recorded adverse surrogate markers for cardiovascular disease and so far there is little evidence for an excess of cardiovascular events. One reason for this discrepancy is that most young women presenting with PCOS have a low absolute risk of heart disease simply because of their age. The studies that attempt to undertake long-term follow-up into an age group with a sufficient number of cardiovascular events to make a meaningful assessment are necessarily looking back at a time (between the 1930s and 1970s) when lifestyle patterns were very different. One study reported in several papers failed to indentify an excess of cardiovascular events in women with PCOS at follow-up over 30 years later.[29,33] It is therefore difficult to judge how the negative data on cardiovascular events relate to risk profile today. When using a different strategy of recording the experience of mothers of women with PCOS, it has been reported that they had a five-fold excess risk of cardiovascular events compared with mothers of women without PCOS.[34]

In conclusion, although women with PCOS exhibit a wide spectrum of adverse risk factors for cardiovascular disease, it is uncertain how these relate to cardiovascular events as today's women grow older.

PCOS and non-alcoholic steatohepatitis

Obesity and insulin resistance are also risk factors for non-alcoholic fatty liver disease (non-alcoholic steatohepatitis). Women with features of PCOS also show evidence of fatty liver disease, both by abnormal aminotransferase activity[35] and by markers of hepatic apoptosis.[36] As the obesity epidemic continues, these findings raise the possibility that chronic liver disease such as cirrhosis may be a late manifestation of the metabolic syndrome related to PCOS.

PCOS and implications for family members

One of the major areas of research over the past decade has been the genetic basis for PCOS. Much of the impetus for this research arises from the observation that the polycystic ovarian morphology is strongly inherited. Candidate genes for this pattern of inheritance include not only genes for various enzymes in the testosterone biosynthetic pathway but also genes that code for factors influencing insulin action. It is likely that PCOS is a multigenic disorder and it is possible that ovarian status and the metabolic syndrome are inherited separately.

From a practical point of view, it would be important to establish whether the inheritance of the metabolic syndrome leads to the identification of pedigrees at increased risk of cardiovascular disease or type 2 diabetes. Reports from various cohorts have now shown that markers of the metabolic syndrome can be found in first-degree relatives of index cases presenting with PCOS.[37] To a large extent, markers of the metabolic syndrome are accounted for by the inheritance pattern of obesity and in only a few instances has it been reported that PCOS is an important factor independently of obesity. These first-degree relatives include fathers, mothers, siblings and children of women with PCOS.[38–41]

Of particular interest is a 2008 report of excess cardiovascular events in mothers of women with PCOS.[34] This finding, taken together with the excess risk of the metabolic syndrome in fathers and brothers of women with PCOS, raises the importance of preventive medical approaches for families when PCOS is diagnosed. For instance, the detection of even modest changes in metabolic markers for a young woman with PCOS may lead to the identification of first-degree relatives with a greater absolute risk of heart disease or type 2 diabetes by virtue of their being male or in an older age group compared with the index woman with PCOS.

Treatment of PCOS and the metabolic syndrome

With the dominant influence of obesity in determining the manifestations of PCOS, it is not surprising that weight loss is at the top of the list for every treatment programme for the condition. No matter how weight loss is achieved, be it through lifestyle, pharmaceutical or surgical methods, the clinical features of PCOS improve.[42] With regard to diet, it has been suggested that carbohydrate restriction should be the mainstay of a dietary approach to weight loss because of the focus on insulin resistance. So far, the benefit of targeting one specific component of dietary intake has not been shown to have a benefit over caloric restriction in general.[43]

Metformin is included in the management plan for both PCOS and the metabolic syndrome. The place of metformin in the management of PCOS has been a point of considerable debate after the initial trials showing major benefit were followed by larger randomised controlled trials showing no benefit. The most comprehensive assessment of this area is a Cochrane Collaboration review[44] which concluded that metformin is of benefit in improving clinical pregnancy and ovulation rates, but which noted that there is no evidence of improvement in live birth rates either when used alone or in combination with clomifene citrate. The overall conclusion was that metformin has a limited place in improving reproductive outcomes in PCOS.

With regard to the metabolic syndrome, metformin is effective in preventing progression to type 2 diabetes but a greater preventive effect can be obtained from lifestyle measures.[45] It seems prudent, therefore, to emphasise diet and exercise for the prevention of type 2 diabetes rather than relying on long-term use of metformin for this purpose in young women.

It is not yet clear whether targeting of the inflammation pathway will be useful in PCOS or the metabolic syndrome. An intriguing early report on the use of atorvastatin in PCOS showed not only a reduction in total and low-density lipoprotein (LDL) cholesterol but also a reduction in C-reactive protein and testosterone in women with PCOS.[46] The changes in testosterone correlated significantly with insulin parameters but not with lipid changes, suggesting that an indirect pathway via inflammation might be the route of benefit. As new tools become available to manipulate inflammatory pathways, we can expect new insights into the pathogenesis of androgen excess in PCOS.

Conclusion

The metabolic syndrome is more prevalent than expected in women with PCOS and in their first-degree relatives. Metabolic status should be assessed to some degree in all women presenting with PCOS and those with risk markers of the metabolic syndrome should be informed of the importance of lifestyle measures to prevent progression to diabetes later in life. In addition, a family history should be taken to identify first-degree relatives who may also benefit from a metabolic assessment and education.

References

1. Burghen GA, Givens JR, Kitabchi AE. Correlation of hyperandrogenism with hyperinsulinism in polycystic ovarian disease. *J Clin Endocrinol Metab* 1980;50:113–16.
2. Chang RJ, Nakamura RM, Judd HL, Kaplan SA. Insulin resistance in nonobese patients with polycystic ovarian disease. *J Clin Endocrinol Metab* 1983;57:356–9.
3. Conway GS, Agrawal R, Betteridge DJ, Jacobs HS. Risk factors for coronary artery disease in lean and obese women with the polycystic ovary syndrome. *Clin Endocrinol (Oxf)* 1992;37:119–25.
4. Nisenblat V, Norman RJ. Androgens and polycystic ovary syndrome. *Curr Opin Endocrinol Diabetes Obes* 2009;16:224–31.
5. Corbould A. Effects of androgens on insulin action in women: is androgen excess a component of female metabolic syndrome? *Diabetes Metab Res Rev* 2008;24:520–32.
6. Dunaif A. Insulin resistance in women with polycystic ovary syndrome. *Fertil Steril* 2006;86 Suppl 1:S13–14.
7. Diamanti-Kandarakis E. Insulin resistance in PCOS. *Endocrine* 2006;30:13–17.
8. Dunaif A, Xia J, Book CB, Schenker E, Tang Z. Excessive insulin receptor serine phosphorylation in cultured fibroblasts and in skeletal muscle. A potential mechanism for insulin resistance in the polycystic ovary syndrome. *J Clin Invest* 1995;96:801–10.
9. Conway GS, Jacobs HS, Holly JM, Wass JA. Effects of luteinizing hormone, insulin, insulin-like growth factor-I and insulin-like growth factor small binding protein 1 in the polycystic ovary syndrome. *Clin Endocrinol (Oxf)* 1990;33:593–603.
10. Conway GS, Jacobs HS. Clinical implications of hyperinsulinaemia in women. *Clin Endocrinol (Oxf)* 1993;39:623–32.
11. Franks S, Gilling-Smith C, Watson H, Willis D. Insulin action in the normal and polycystic ovary. *Endocrinol Metab Clin North Am* 1999;28:361–78.
12. Poretsky L, Grigorescu F, Seibel M, Moses AC, Flier JS. Distribution and characterization of insulin and insulin-like growth factor I receptors in normal human ovary. *J Clin Endocrinol Metab* 1985;61:728–34.
13. Book CB, Dunaif A. Selective insulin resistance in the polycystic ovary syndrome. *J Clin Endocrinol Metab* 1999;84:3110–16.

14. Poretsky L. Commentary: Polycystic ovary syndrome – increased or preserved ovarian sensitivity to insulin? *J Clin Endocrinol Metab* 2006;91:2859–60.
15. Knebel B, Janssen OE, Hahn S, Jacob S, Gleich J, Kotzka J, *et al.* Increased low grade inflammatory serum markers in patients with polycystic ovary syndrome (PCOS) and their relationship to PPARgamma gene variants. *Exp Clin Endocrinol Diabetes* 2008;116:481–6.
16. Tsilchorozidou T, Mohamed-Ali V, Conway GS. Determinants of interleukin-6 and C-reactive protein vary in polycystic ovary syndrome, as do effects of short- and long-term metformin therapy. *Horm Res* 2009;71:148–54.
17. Gonzalez F, Rote NS, Minium J, Kirwan JP. Evidence of proatherogenic inflammation in polycystic ovary syndrome. *Metabolism* 2009;58:954–62.
18. Toulis KA, Goulis DG, Farmakiotis D, Georgopoulos NA, Katsikis I, Tarlatzis BC, *et al.* Adiponectin levels in women with polycystic ovary syndrome: a systematic review and a meta-analysis. *Hum Reprod Update* 2009;15:297–307.
19. Samy N, Hashim M, Sayed M, Said M. Clinical significance of inflammatory markers in polycystic ovary syndrome: their relationship to insulin resistance and body mass index. *Dis Markers* 2009;26:163–70.
20. Jacobs HS, Conway GS. Leptin, polycystic ovaries and polycystic ovary syndrome. *Hum Reprod Update* 1999;5:166–71.
21. Legro RS, Kunselman AR, Dodson WC, Dunaif A. Prevalence and predictors of risk for type 2 diabetes mellitus and impaired glucose tolerance in polycystic ovary syndrome: a prospective, controlled study in 254 affected women. *J Clin Endocrinol Metab* 1999;84:165–9.
22. Ehrmann DA, Barnes RB, Rosenfield RL, Cavaghan MK, Imperial J. Prevalence of impaired glucose tolerance and diabetes in women with polycystic ovary syndrome. *Diabetes Care* 1999;22:141–6.
23. Dabadghao P, Roberts BJ, Wang J, Davies MJ, Norman RJ. Glucose tolerance abnormalities in Australian women with polycystic ovary syndrome. *Med J Aust* 2007;187:328–31.
24. Espinos-Gomez JJ, Corcoy R, Calaf J. Prevalence and predictors of abnormal glucose metabolism in Mediterranean women with polycystic ovary syndrome. *Gynecol Endocrinol* 2009;25:199–204.
25. Legro RS, Gnatuk CL, Kunselman AR, Dunaif A. Changes in glucose tolerance over time in women with polycystic ovary syndrome: a controlled study. *J Clin Endocrinol Metab* 2005;90:3236–42.
26. Toulis KA, Goulis DG, Kolibianakis EM, Venetis CA, Tarlatzis BC, Papadimas I. Risk of gestational diabetes mellitus in women with polycystic ovary syndrome: a systematic review and a meta-analysis. *Fertil Steril* 2009;92:667–77.
27. Conn JJ, Jacobs HS, Conway GS. The prevalence of polycystic ovaries in women with type 2 diabetes mellitus. *Clin Endocrinol (Oxf)* 2000;52:81–6.
28. Kousta E, Cela E, Lawrence N, Penny A, Millauer B, White D, *et al.* The prevalence of polycystic ovaries in women with a history of gestational diabetes. *Clin Endocrinol (Oxf)* 2000;53:501–7.
29. Pierpoint T, McKeigue PM, Isaacs AJ, Wild SH, Jacobs HS. Mortality of women with polycystic ovary syndrome at long-term follow-up. *J Clin Epidemiol* 1998;51:581–6.
30. Tarkun I, Arslan BC, Canturk Z, Turemen E, Sahin T, Duman C. Endothelial dysfunction in young women with polycystic ovary syndrome: relationship with insulin resistance and low-grade chronic inflammation. *J Clin Endocrinol Metab* 2004;89:5592–6.
31. Heutling D, Schulz H, Nickel I, Kleinstein J, Kaltwasser P, Westphal S, *et al.* Asymmetrical dimethylarginine, inflammatory and metabolic parameters in women with polycystic ovary syndrome before and after metformin treatment. *J Clin Endocrinol Metab* 2008;93:82–90.
32. Christian RC, Dumesic DA, Behrenbeck T, Oberg AL, Sheedy PF 2nd, Fitzpatrick LA. Prevalence and predictors of coronary artery calcification in women with polycystic ovary syndrome. *J Clin Endocrinol Metab* 2003;88:2562–8.
33. Wild S, Pierpoint T, McKeigue P, Jacobs H. Cardiovascular disease in women with polycystic ovary syndrome at long-term follow-up: a retrospective cohort study. *Clin Endocrinol (Oxf)* 2000;52:595–600.
34. Cheang KI, Nestler JE, Futterweit W. Risk of cardiovascular events in mothers of women with polycystic ovary syndrome. *Endocr Pract* 2008;14:1084–94.

35. Setji TL, Holland ND, Sanders LL, Pereira KC, Diehl AM, Brown AJ. Nonalcoholic steatohepatitis and nonalcoholic fatty liver disease in young women with polycystic ovary syndrome. *J Clin Endocrinol Metab* 2006;91:1741–7.
36. Tan S, Bechmann LP, Benson S, Dietz T, Eichner S, Hahn S, *et al.* Apoptotic markers indicate nonalcoholic steatohepatitis in polycystic ovary syndrome. *J Clin Endocrinol Metab* 2010;95:343–8.
37. Kahsar-Miller MD, Nixon C, Boots LR, Go RC, Azziz R. Prevalence of polycystic ovary syndrome (PCOS) in first-degree relatives of patients with PCOS. *Fertil Steril* 2001;75:53–8.
38. Diamanti-Kandarakis E, Alexandraki K, Bergiele A, Kandarakis H, Mastorakos G, Aessopos A. Presence of metabolic risk factors in non-obese PCOS sisters: evidence of heritability of insulin resistance. *J Endocrinol Invest* 2004;27:931–6.
39. Sam S, Legro RS, Bentley-Lewis R, Dunaif A. Dyslipidemia and metabolic syndrome in the sisters of women with polycystic ovary syndrome. *J Clin Endocrinol Metab* 2005;90:4797–802.
40. Sam S, Coviello AD, Sung YA, Legro RS, Dunaif A. Metabolic phenotype in the brothers of women with polycystic ovary syndrome. *Diabetes Care* 2008;31:1237–41.
41. Coviello AD, Sam S, Legro RS, Dunaif A. High prevalence of metabolic syndrome in first-degree male relatives of women with polycystic ovary syndrome is related to high rates of obesity. *J Clin Endocrinol Metab* 2009;94:4361–6.
42. Norman RJ, Noakes M, Wu R, Davies MJ, Moran L, Wang JX. Improving reproductive performance in overweight/obese women with effective weight management. *Hum Reprod Update* 2004;10:267–80.
43. Stamets K, Taylor DS, Kunselman A, Demers LM, Pelkman CL, Legro RS. A randomized trial of the effects of two types of short-term hypocaloric diets on weight loss in women with polycystic ovary syndrome. *Fertil Steril* 2004;81:630–7.
44. Tang T, Lord JM, Norman RJ, Yasmin E, Balen AH. Insulin-sensitising drugs (metformin, rosiglitazone, pioglitazone, D-chiro-inositol) for women with polycystic ovary syndrome, oligo amenorrhoea and subfertility. *Cochrane Database Syst Rev* 2009;(4):CD003053.
45. Knowler WC, Fowler SE, Hamman RF, Christophi CA, Hoffman HJ, Brenneman AT, *et al.* 10-year follow-up of diabetes incidence and weight loss in the Diabetes Prevention Program Outcomes Study. *Lancet* 2009;374:1677–86.
46. Sathyapalan T, Kilpatrick ES, Coady AM, Atkin SL. The effect of atorvastatin in patients with polycystic ovary syndrome: a randomized double-blind placebo-controlled study. *J Clin Endocrinol Metab* 2009;94:103–8.

6

Chapter 6

Management of polycystic ovary syndrome through puberty and adolescence

Rachel Williams and David Dunger

Introduction

While polycystic ovary syndrome (PCOS) is a well-established condition in adulthood, there is also evidence that the clinical and biochemical features of PCOS may manifest during puberty and in the immediate years post menarche. In 1980, Yen[1] postulated that the development of PCOS begins during puberty, and proposed that it is linked to increasing insulin resistance and weight gain. Some years later, Siegberg *et al.*[2] reported oligomenorrhoea in adolescent girls with or without hirsutism associated with increased concentrations of luteinising hormone (LH), testosterone and androstenedione, and others observed associations in adolescents of menstrual irregularities, increased LH, testosterone and androstenedione with multicystic ovaries of increased volume.[3,4] In the early 1990s, Ibañez and colleagues[5] proposed that PCOS may have its origin during early development and may initially manifest as precocious pubarche even before the onset of pubertal development. While it is clear that PCOS is a real entity in the adolescent population, there is still no clear consensus on diagnostic criteria or management options. In this review, we discuss the issues around the diagnosis and management of PCOS through puberty and adolescence, focusing on specific diagnostic and therapeutic challenges.

Diagnosis

Even in adult women, there has been debate[6] about the interpretation and application of the 2003 Rotterdam diagnostic criteria, which are two out of the following three:[7,8]

- oligo-ovulation and/or anovulation
- hyperandrogenism
- polycystic ovaries.

There are particular difficulties with their extrapolation to the adolescent population and there are currently no alternative criteria. The characteristics of the menstrual cycle in healthy girls in the years immediately following menarche, together with the inappropriateness of certain investigations, result in particular problems pertaining to adolescence. These will now be discussed in more detail.

The menstrual cycle during adolescence

It is important to be familiar with what is considered normal for the adolescent female population when considering features of the menstrual cycle as a diagnostic criterion for PCOS.[9,10] Particularly in the first 2 years from menarche, anovulation and irregular cycles are common.[11] Three years post menarche, 59% of cycles may remain anovulatory, with regular cycles being established more quickly (about 3 years) in those girls who experience an earlier rather than a later menarche.[12] Features of the menstrual cycle in the first 2 years from menarche from US[9] and UK[10] authors are similar and are summarised in Table 6.1. By the third year post menarche, cycle length will fall to between 21 and 34 days in the majority of girls.[10] Thus, in the evaluation of the menstrual cycle of girls up to 24 months from menarche, an irregular cycle with a long intermenstrual interval is not necessarily abnormal.

Although irregular menses may be considered a normal variant, in a longitudinal cohort study of Dutch adolescents aged between 15 and 18 years from within the general population, 50% of those who were oligomenorrhoeic at age 15 remained so at age 18.[13] In the same cohort, increased body mass index (BMI), androgen and LH concentrations and polycystic ovaries but not fasting insulin to glucose ratio were associated with the persistence of oligomenorrhoea at age 18.[13] Thus it is important to consider other features of PCOS, such as hyperandrogenism, obesity and insulin resistance, when evaluating an adolescent who presents soon after menarche with oligomenorrhoea.

Ovarian appearance on ultrasound

Transvaginal ultrasound is inappropriate in the adolescent population and the imaging of polycystic ovaries may present technical difficulties, particularly in those who are obese. While the use of rectal ultrasound may get around this problem, it is not in common use and is equally inappropriate in this age group. Imaging should be undertaken by skilled and experienced personnel. When adequate imaging of the ovaries is achieved, the appearance of multiple ovarian follicles during adolescence is common, with 26% of ovaries at age 15 having a multicystic appearance that reflects normal pubertal maturation.[14,15] Increased ovarian volume in addition to a multicystic appearance is more supportive of a diagnosis of PCOS in the adult population.[16] However, there are only limited normative data during adolescence. In 40 normal premenarchal girls up to the age of 14, ovarian volume was approximately 2 cm^3.[17] In the adult population, an ovarian volume of greater than 10 cm^3 is considered abnormal, but there are no equivalent guidelines for adolescents. The data that are available are often retrospective and from girls who already have a diagnosis of PCOS. One such study reported increased ovarian volume (defined as more than 10 cm^3) in

Table 6.1 Features of the menstrual cycle in healthy girls in the first 2 years post menarche

Feature	Study	
	American Academy of Pediatrics/Diaz *et al.* (1996)[9]	Hickey and Balen (2003)[10]
Age at menarche	12.4 years	12–13 years
Menstrual cycle interval	21–45 days	21–45 days
95th centile for cycle interval	90 days	90 days
Menstrual flow length	<7 days	2–7 days
Blood flow	3–6 pads or tampons per day	3–6 pads per day

43% of girls (aged 10–18 years) with a diagnosis of PCOS.[18] Increased ovarian volume in the daughters of women with PCOS in comparison with daughters of women without PCOS has also been reported.[19] Interestingly, it is not until the girls reach Tanner stage 5 that their ovarian volume is abnormal by adult standards (mean volume 13.9 cm^3 [SD 4.4 cm^3] versus 6.9 cm^3 [SD 3.9 cm^3] in the girls in the control group), suggesting that earlier in puberty a cut-off ovarian volume of lower than this may be appropriate.[19] Further robust normative data within the adolescent population, recording the number and size of ovarian follicles and ovarian volume in conjunction with features of the menstrual cycle, would be helpful.

Hormonal changes during puberty

Pubertal development is associated with rapid changes in pituitary gonadal and adrenal hormones and there is a paucity of robust normative data. Data collected longitudinally from a cohort of British girls are given in Table 6.2 and demonstrate the steady rise in androgen concentrations coupled with a fall in sex hormone-binding globulin (SHBG) with progression through puberty.

Puberty is also associated with a physiological increase in insulin resistance with compensatory hyperinsulinaemia.[20] The interpretation of indices of insulin resistance such as fasting insulin may be difficult as an apparent elevation in fasting insulin concentration may reflect a physiological rather than pathological insulin resistance.[20]

In addition to biochemical hyperandrogenaemia, the determination of serum antiMüllerian hormone (AMH), released by the ovarian granulosa cells, has been proposed as a marker for follicle count and PCOS in adult women.[21] Elevated concentrations of AMH in comparison with girls in a control group have been demonstrated in girls born to mothers with PCOS, both in infancy and prepubertally (4–7 years),[22] which may suggest that follicular development is altered in this population as early as infancy. Before recommending this as part of the biochemical work-up for PCOS in the adolescent population, adequate longitudinal reference data throughout childhood and puberty in healthy girls not born to mothers with PCOS will be required.

Clinical presentation

The presenting symptoms in adolescents with PCOS are likely to differ from those in their adult counterparts, with concerns about hirsutism, weight and irregular menses, rather than infertility, being more common. A study of young women with PCOS

Table 6.2 Longitudinal concentrations of androgens and sex hormone-binding globulin (SHBG) in healthy British girls (*n*= 27) by puberty (Tanner) stage; data are expressed as median and interquartile range; reproduced with permission from Ahmed[75]

Tanner stage	Age (years)	Testosterone (nmol/litre)	SHBG (nmol/litre)	DHEAS (micromol/ litre)	A4 (nmol/litre)
1	10.2 (9.6–10.7)	0.3 (0.3–0.5)	66 (56–94)	3.5 (2.4–5.2)	3.3 (2.7–4.0)
2	11.4 (10.5–11.9)	0.3 (0.3–0.8)	57 (48–69)	5.1 (2.4–7.5)	4.2 (3.4–4.8)
3	12.2 (11.6–12.8)	0.8 (0.5–1.1)	57 (40–71)	6.8 (4.5–9.6)	5.8 (5.1–7.9)
4	13.2 (12.6–13.8)	1.1 (0.8–1.5)	45 (34–66)	7.0 (4.6–10.0)	6.1 (5.7–7.5)
5	14.9 (14.2–15.2)	1.4 (1.1–1.6)	43 (33–61)	12.1 (9.0–17.7)	8.7 (7.4–11.3)

A4 = androstenedione; DHEAS = dehydroepiandrosterone sulfate aged 9–17.5 years reported that 30% presented with menstrual irregularities and 60% with features of androgen excess including hirsutism, acne and hair thinning.[23] More recently, the characteristics of 70 adolescents referred to a multidisciplinary clinic in Wisconsin, USA, for evaluation of PCOS have been reported. The mean age was 16.2 years (range 13–22 years), 84% were overweight (BMI above the 85th centile) and 70% were obese (BMI above the 95th centile). Forty-three percent had oligomenorrhoea, 21% had secondary amenorrhoea and 21% were experiencing regular menses. Clinical evidence of androgen excess manifested as acne in 70% and hirsutism in 60%. There was impaired glucose tolerance (detectable by an oral glucose tolerance test) in 6% and frank type 2 diabetes in 3%.[24]

The frequency of overweight in this cohort is striking and one that is consistent in both adult and adolescent populations. Weight gain due to increased fat mass is common in girls post menarche[25] and it has been suggested that this may accentuate the normal insulin resistance of puberty, leading to functional hyperandrogenism.[26] Indeed, PCOS is more often reported in obese rather than lean adolescents and there has been a concern that the increasing rates of adolescent obesity may precipitate PCOS in those with a genetic or developmental predisposition.[5]

The physical characteristics of PCOS such as overweight, hirsutism and acne are completely the opposite of those desired by the adolescent population and the psychological effects of the PCOS phenotype should not be underestimated. Increased anxiety and depression has been reported in adolescents with PCOS in comparison with healthy adolescents.[27] A pilot study exploring the use of a cognitive behavioural strategy in obese adolescents with depression and PCOS led to improvements in depression scores and also reductions in weight.[28] Improvements in quality of life scores following treatment with lifestyle modification and the oral contraceptive pill (OCP) has also been reported in obese adolescents with PCOS.[28] Thus the psychological impact of PCOS and the possibility of a positive response to psychological intervention should not be discounted at this critical time of neurodevelopmental maturation.

Developmental origins of PCOS

Ibañez and de Zegher and colleagues,[5] through detailed study of Spanish populations living around Barcelona, have identified what they refer to as the 'precocious pubarche' (PP) sequence. PP is defined by the onset of pubic hair under the age of 8 years and is often associated with bone age advance and raised dehydroepiandrosterone (DHEA) and dehydroepiandrosterone sulfate (DHEAS) concentrations. Ibañez noted that, in girls presenting in this fashion, low birth weight and rapid postnatal weight gain increased the risk for progression to functional ovarian hyperandrogenism and PCOS.[5,29] In less selected populations, there are unlikely to be simple associations with birth weight and findings from other populations have differed.[26,30–33] Nevertheless, the data from the Ibañez group are consistent with animal and human studies suggesting that fetal growth restraint followed by rapid postnatal weight gain can increase risk of obesity[34] and be associated with increased adrenal androgens at age 8.[29] These associations seem to be driven by the early development of insulin resistance and increased central adiposity.[35] Presentation with PP appears to have an increased prevalence in Spain and other Mediterranean countries and in different ethnic groups.[36,37] It has been proposed that the clinical presentation with PP may relate to genetic diversity within these populations, including polymorphic variation within the androgen receptor[38] and the aromatase gene.[39,40] In other populations, the same sequence of early weight gain, obesity and height, and adrenal androgens, although not presenting with precocious pubarche, may still manifest as a longer term risk for the development of ovarian hyperandrogenism and PCOS. Indeed, in a study of populations selected by birth weight, it was found that the same sequence of early weight gain and insulin resistance could indeed progress to PCOS and could be reversed with the insulin sensitiser metformin in combination with flutamide and an OCP.[41] Thus early identification of risk and early intervention in susceptible individuals may be an option, but currently insufficient data are available to substantiate these recommendations in more diverse ethnic groups.

Differential diagnosis

The diagnosis of PCOS may be made incidentally in girls undergoing investigation for severe obesity or prospectively in young women being investigated for irregular periods, acne or hirsutism. There may be a family history of PCOS or infertility and, although the classic biochemical features and ovarian ultrasound appearances may be not be evident immediately, diagnosis unravels over time. PCOS should be a diagnosis of exclusion and, where there is evidence of severe virilisation, a diagnosis of cryptogenic congenital adrenal hyperplasia must be excluded using a combination of basal and stimulated (using tetracosactide) 17-hydroxyprogesterone (17OHP) concentrations and, in the case of borderline results, genetic testing.[42] In non-obese patients in whom there is evidence of severe insulin resistance, including acanthosis nigricans, an underlying type A insulin resistance secondary to mutations in the insulin receptor should be considered.[43] There is a growing consensus that an oral glucose tolerance test with the determination of insulin concentrations may be important in the complete evaluation of an adolescent with possible PCOS in view of the potential risk for type 2 diabetes and the metabolic syndrome.[44]

Treatment

In those who are obese, lifestyle and dietary modifications are the first line of treatment. Data from the Finnish Diabetes Prevention Study suggest that even modest weight reduction can reduce cardiovascular risk and risk for type 2 diabetes.[45] It is likely that the same may be true for the sequelae of PCOS if the diagnosis and intervention are made at an early stage, yet the data are scant. Furthermore, success at achieving weight loss with lifestyle and dietary intervention in adolescents is poor, with many gaining weight again very rapidly.[46] In one study, a control arm comprising lifestyle modification alone (diet and exercise) resulted in reductions in biochemical hyperandrogenism in adolescents with PCOS.[47] However, in the longer term, the success of such interventions has been disappointing owing to poor compliance and they are likely only to be a realistic long-term strategy in girls who are highly motivated.[48] Symptomatic treatment focused on the restoration of regular menses is the most common starting point and the OCPs have been the mainstay of pharmacological therapy for PCOS for many decades.

Oral contraceptive pills

As well as stabilising the menstrual cycle, some classes of OCP may improve the other symptoms of PCOS. The reported effects of OCPs on insulin resistance are variable, which probably reflects the lack of reliable standardisation either of insulin assays across centres or of the plethora of derived indices of insulin sensitivity that are available. In non-hyperandrogenic women, even OCPs containing low-dose estrogens (20–35 micrograms) and less androgenic progestins may adversely affect insulin resistance and glucose tolerance.[49] Drospirenone-containing oral contraceptive preparations have been shown to reduce hyperandrogenism but worsen indices of insulin resistance and central adiposity in lean adolescents with PCOS.[50] In a randomised study of obese (mean BMI 39 kg/m^2) hyperinsulinaemic girls with PCOS, comparing treatment with metformin or the OCP, the OCP alone resulted in weight loss, reductions in concentrations of androgens and increased insulin sensitivity but it was difficult to distinguish between a direct effect of the OCP or a secondary effect of the associated weight loss.[51]

OCPs containing the antiandrogen cyproterone acetate are commonly used in the UK but there has been little formal evaluation of their efficacy. There are three studies, all from the same group, evaluating the effects of cyproterone acetate in the adolescent PCOS population. The first compared 12 months of treatment with OCPs containing either desogestrel or cyproterone acetate both combined with ethinylestradiol in 24 young women (aged 14–19 years) with PCOS. Both agents resulted in the restoration of normal menses and a reduction in hirsutism score, with decreases in both total and low-density lipoprotein (LDL) cholesterol. However, in the group receiving cyproterone acetate, there was an increase in triglyceride and the high-density lipoprotein (HDL) cholesterol fraction.[52] The second study was of similar design, with very similar results including an increase in triglyceride concentrations in the cyproterone acetate group,[53] and the third study reported increases in derived indices of insulin resistance in the cyproterone acetate group.[54] The authors recommended that OCPs containing cyproterone acetate are effective in treating the symptoms of PCOS but should be avoided in the adolescent population owing to undesirable effects on lipid metabolism and insulin sensitivity.[52–54]

There is a low risk of liver toxicity with cyproterone acetate and liver function tests should be monitored 6-monthly when it is used.[55] In general, OCP preparations should be avoided in women at high risk of thromboembolism and some have argued that there is an increased risk of thromboembolism in women taking cyproterone acetate preparations over and above that of those taking preparations containing levonorgestrel or norethisterone.[56,57] Reports from large data sets such as the UK general practice database are more reassuring and the results from early smaller studies may have been confounded.[58,59]

Importantly, in the UK, combined pill preparations containing cyproterone acetate are licensed for the treatment of androgen excess but not for contraception (although they do function as reliable contraceptive agents) and thus their use should be limited to those in whom hyperandrogenism is a predominant feature.

Metformin

The effects of metformin administration in adolescent girls with PCOS has been assessed in both obese and non-obese populations. In obese girls with PCOS with impaired glucose tolerance, metformin administration (850 mg twice daily for 3 months) improved glucose tolerance and insulin sensitivity and effectively reduced androgen concentrations and the adrenal sterogenic response to adrenocorticotrophic hormone (ACTH).[60] In another study, metformin with lifestyle modifications and dietary advice led to modest weight loss, with improvements in insulin resistance and lipid variables leading to resumption of regular menses.[61]

A randomised double-blind placebo-controlled trial conducted in 22 adolescent girls (aged 13–18 years) with PCOS that compared metformin (750 mg twice daily) with placebo over 12 weeks in conjunction with healthy lifestyle counselling demonstrated that metformin was more effective than placebo in the reduction of androgen concentrations and the restoration of regular menses. HDL cholesterol also increased in the girls treated with metformin but there were no significant effects on parameters of insulin sensitivity assessed using an oral glucose tolerance test.[62]

Ibañez and de Zegher and colleagues have conducted a series of studies demonstrating that treatment with metformin leads to improvement in insulin sensitivity, improvement of hirsutism, the establishment of regular menses and improvement in dyslipidaemia in Catalan girls presenting with PP who later progress to PCOS.[63]

Thiazolidinediones

The thiazolidinediones (TDZs) are a relatively new class of insulin-sensitising drugs that bind the orphan peroxisome proliferator-activated receptor (PPAR) gamma receptor. There are limited data from the adult PCOS population that indicate that the use of TDZs in women with PCOS leads to the establishment of regular menses together with clinical and biochemical reductions in hyperandrogenism.[64–67] However, TDZs are contraindicated in pregnancy and therefore should not be used where pregnancy is the desired outcome or if accidental pregnancy is a possibility. Ibañez *et al.*[68–70] have published the results of up to 24 months of treatment with pioglitazone in non-obese young women (mean age 19.6 years) with evidence of hyperandrogenism exploring the effects of combination therapy with a TDZ, flutamide, metformin and a transdermal combined contraceptive preparation. They reported improvements in insulin sensitivity and cardiovascular risk factors such as visceral fat and intima–media thickness.

Antiandrogens

In addition to cyproterone acetate, which is widely used within a combined oral contraceptive preparation, other antiandrogens have been studied in adolescent girls with PCOS. Spironolactone, which has several antiandrogenic properties including effects on 5α-reductase and inhibition of enzymes associated with androgen biosynthesis, has been used in the treatment of hirsutism associated with PCOS. In adolescents and young women (mean age 22 years) with PCOS, spironolactone administration for 6 months at a dose of 50 mg per day was shown to improve glucose tolerance to the same extent as metformin (1000 mg per day) in addition to reducing hyperandrogenaemia.[71] In this open-label study, spironolactone appeared to have comparable clinical efficacy, with fewer adverse events than metformin. Effects on dyslipidaemia were not reported.

Flutamide is a nonsteroidal androgen receptor blocker mainly used to treat prostate cancer.[72] In adolescent young women with PCOS, short-term (4 weeks) administration of flutamide at a dose of 250 mg per day led to reductions in hirsutism score, free androgen index, testosterone and androstenedione concentrations with concomitant increases in concentrations of SHBG, but with less impressive effects on the menstrual cycle and metabolic parameters.[73] There have been concerns that flutamide may be potentially hepatotoxic but this appears to be dose dependent, having been predominantly described in men being treated at higher doses (total daily dose of 750 mg) for prostate cancer.[55] Ibañez *et al.*[74] reported 190 individuals treated with what they describe as low- and ultralow-dose (250 to 62.5 mg per day) flutamide for a mean duration of 19 months. Liver enzymes were monitored 3-monthly during the first year of treatment and annually thereafter. There were no reported incidents of elevation in liver enzymes or hepatotoxicity using low doses of flutamide in an adolescent population.[74]

Recommendations

Clinical evaluation

When PCOS is suspected during puberty or adolescence, a detailed history should be taken, including birth weight, age of onset and pattern of pubertal development, age at menarche and details of the menstrual cycle. A family history of PCOS should be sought. It should be considered that it may be embarrassing for girls to discuss intimate matters with doctors, and it may be more appropriate for more personal questions to be put by a specialist nurse, with whom they have had a chance to develop a relationship, as part of a team assessment. The examination should record height, weight, BMI and population-referenced standard deviation scores. Blood pressure and waist circumference are helpful in the evaluation of cardiovascular risk. Acanthosis nigricans and degree and details of hyperandrogenism also should be recorded, including acne and hirsutism.

Investigations

As a starting point, blood should be taken for testosterone, SHBG, 17OHP, DHEAS and androstenedione in addition to liver function tests and lipids. Consider the results in the light of clinical findings and bear in mind that laboratory reference ranges for androgens and SHBG are almost certainly for adult women rather than pubertal or adolescent females. Where there is virilisation, post-ACTH concentrations of 17OHP and testosterone should be determined. If there is clinical evidence of insulin resistance or if obesity is a striking feature, consider undertaking an oral glucose tolerance test determining insulin and C-peptide in addition to glucose. If insulin concentrations are very high (above 500 pmol/litre post glucose), consider an underlying insulin receptor mutation.

Transabdominal ultrasound should be performed by experienced personnel and follicle size and count recorded in addition to ovarian volume.

Where there is clinical evidence of hyperandrogenism (remembering that acne but not hirsutism is a feature of normal puberty), a history of abnormal menses in conjunction with increased ovarian volume (in the absence of adequate data in younger women, the currently accepted adult cut-off of 10 cm^3 can be used) and multicystic ovaries (remembering that at age 15 approximately 25% of normal girls will have this), especially in an obese individual, the diagnosis is relatively easy to make. In its milder form, or where there is a clear clinical picture without supportive ultrasound or biochemical features, the diagnosis may be more difficult. Likewise, girls who do not have the clinical phenotype but who are found to have polycystic ovaries on ultrasound should not be labelled as having PCOS.

Treatment

As well as lifestyle advice, diet and exercise in obese individuals, most clinicians take a rather symptomatic approach to the treatment of PCOS during adolescence. Irregular periods are treated with OCPs with or without the inclusion of cyproterone acetate depending on the extent of hirsutism and acne. Metformin is often reserved as a second-line therapy for those with acanthosis nigricans or impaired glucose tolerance and flutamide and other antiandrogens are only used if hirsutism and acne become intractable. Although such an approach to therapy may be effective, it is probably important to determine at an early stage the degree to which there are associated problems with glucose tolerance and risk of cardiovascular disease. Individuals with impaired glucose tolerance and increased cardiovascular risk probably warrant more aggressive therapy and close monitoring.

When considering treatment alternatives, it is important to consider each girl as an individual. Where contraception is required, a pragmatic approach should be adopted. As symptoms will be alleviated by a combined pill preparation and, for most girls of this age, fertility is not a concern, it is reasonable to use a combined preparation of ethinylestradiol and desogestrel first line. Given the concerns regarding worsening metabolic risk with agents containing drospirenone or cyproterone acetate, these should only be used second line in those girls where hyperandrogenism is a prominent phenotypic feature, until the safety and efficacy profiles have been more thoroughly evaluated in the adolescent population. Spironolactone and flutamide could also be considered as second- and third-line agents in cases where hirsutism is a predominant feature.

As insulin resistance is a primary feature of the PCOS phenotype and it is likely to be exacerbated by physiological increases in insulin resistance and increases in fat mass during puberty, it would seem intuitive to treat first line with insulin-sensitising agents, particularly where obesity is a feature. However, the patient's wishes must be taken into consideration to optimise concordance. In addition, it is important to bear in mind that treatment with metformin, with a subsequent restoration of ovulatory cycles, may increase rates of unplanned pregnancy in this population. Therefore, metformin should be used first line in those girls with more prominent features of insulin resistance such as acanthosis nigricans and could be used in addition to an OCP if there is a risk of pregnancy. To minimise gastrointestinal adverse effects, a dose of 500 mg once a day should be started and titrated upwards slowly to 750 mg twice a day as a maintenance dose.

Monitoring

Given the comorbidities associated with PCOS, namely infertility, cardiovascular risk and gestational and type 2 diabetes, and given that girls who develop the phenotype early in life are likely to have a longer exposure than their adult counterparts, girls in whom there is a diagnosis of PCOS should be followed up annually in a clinic that ideally includes an adolescent gynaecologist, an endocrinologist, a specialist nurse, a dietician and, if at all possible, a psychologist. Annual assessment of cardiovascular risk should at the very least include documentation of waist circumference, blood pressure, lipids and fasting insulin and glucose (with oral glucose tolerance tests in those with features of insulin resistance). Treatment of comorbidities such as hypertension should be instigated early and aggressively by appropriate personnel.

Conclusion

Overall, this review indicates that great strides have been made in trying to understand the pathophysiology of PCOS and how it relates to early life events. However, although there is considerable experience of the use of some drugs for the treatment of established PCOS in adolescence, there remains a paucity of robust data to inform us of the most appropriate management and surveillance strategies in adolescents with PCOS.

References

1. Yen SS, The polycystic ovary syndrome. *Clin Endocrinol (Oxf)* 1980;12:177–207.
2. Siegberg R, Nilsson CG, Stenman UH, Widholm O. Endocrinologic features of oligomenorrheic adolescent girls. *Fertil Steril* 1986;46:852–7.
3. Venturoli S, Porcu E, Fabbri R, Magrini O, Paradisi R, Pallotti G, *et al.* Postmenarchal evolution of endocrine pattern and ovarian aspects in adolescents with menstrual irregularities. *Fertil Steril* 1987;48:78–85.
4. Apter D, Bützow T, Laughlin GA, Yen SS. Accelerated 24-hour luteinizing hormone pulsatile activity in adolescent girls with ovarian hyperandrogenism: relevance to the developmental phase of polycystic ovarian syndrome. *J Clin Endocrinol Metab* 1994;79:119–25.
5. Ibañez L, Potau N, Virdis R, Zampolli M, Terzi C, Gussinyé M, *et al.* Postpubertal outcome in girls diagnosed of premature pubarche during childhood: increased frequency of functional ovarian hyperandrogenism. *J Clin Endocrinol Metab* 1993;76:1599–603.
6. Balen AH, Homberg R, Franks S. Defining polycystic ovary syndrome. *BMJ* 2009;338:a2968.
7. Rotterdam ESHRE/ASRM-Sponsored PCOS Consensus Workshop Group. Revised 2003 consensus on diagnostic criteria and long-term health risks related to polycystic ovary syndrome. *Fertil Steril* 2004;81:19–25.
8. Fauser B, Tarlatzis B, Chang J, Azziz R, Legro R, Dewailly D, *et al*; The Rotterdam ESHRE/ASRM-sponsored PCOS consensus workshop group. Revised 2003 consensus on diagnostic criteria and long-term health risks related to polycystic ovary syndrome (PCOS). *Hum Reprod* 2004;19:41–7.
9. American Academy of Pediatrics Committee on Adolescence; American College of Obstetricians and Gynecologists Committee on Adolescent Health Care, Diaz A, Laufer MR, Breech LL. Menstruation in girls and adolescents: using the menstrual cycle as a vital sign. *Pediatrics* 2006;118:2245–50.
10. Hickey M, Balen A. Menstrual disorders in adolescence: investigation and management. *Hum Reprod* Update 2003;9:493–504.
11. Apter D, Vihko R. Premenarcheal endocrine changes in relation to age at menarche. *Clin Endocrinol (Oxf)* 1985;22:753–60.
12. Vihko R, Apter D. Endocrine characteristics of adolescent menstrual cycles: impact of early menarche. *J Steroid Biochem* 1984;20:231–6.
13. van Hooff MH, Voorhorst FJ, Kaptein MB, Hirasing RA, Koppenaal C, Schoemaker J. Predictive value of menstrual cycle pattern, body mass index, hormone levels and polycystic ovaries at age 15 years for oligo-amenorrhoea at age 18 years. *Hum Reprod* 2004;19:383–92.
14. Bridges NA, Cooke A, Healy MJ, Hindmarsh PC, Brook CG. Standards for ovarian volume in childhood and puberty. *Fertil Steril* 1993;60:456–60.
15. Venturoli S, Porcu E, Fabbri R, Pluchinotta V, Ruggeri S, Macrelli S, *et al.* Longitudinal change of sonographic ovarian aspects and endocrine parameters in irregular cycles of adolescence. *Pediatr Res* 1995;38:974–80.
16. Jonard S, Robert Y, Dewailly D. Revisiting the ovarian volume as a diagnostic criterion for polycystic ovaries. *Hum Reprod* 2005;20:2893–8.
17. Stanhope R, Adams J, Jacobs HS, Brook CG. Ovarian ultrasound assessment in normal children, idiopathic precocious puberty, and during low dose pulsatile gonadotrophin releasing hormone treatment of hypogonadotrophic hypogonadism. *Arch Dis Child* 1985;60:116–9.
18. Shah B, Parnell L, Milla S, Kessler M, David R. Endometrial thickness, uterine, and ovarian ultrasonographic features in adolescents with polycystic ovarian syndrome. *J Pediatr Adolesc Gynecol* 2010;23:146–52.
19. Sir-Petermann T, Codner E, Pérez V, Echiburú B, Maliqueo M, Ladrón de Guevara A, *et al.* Metabolic and reproductive features before and during puberty in daughters of women with polycystic ovary syndrome. *J Clin Endocrinol Metab* 2009;94:1923–30.
20. Caprio S, Plewe G, Diamond MP, Simonson DC, Boulware SD, Sherwin RS, *et al.* Increased insulin secretion in puberty: a compensatory response to reductions in insulin sensitivity. *J Pediatr* 1989;114:963–7.
21. La Marca A, Pati M, Orvieto R, Stabile G, Carducci Artenisio A, *et al.* Serum anti-mullerian hormone levels in women with secondary amenorrhea. *Fertil Steril* 2006;85:1547–9.

22. Sir-Petermann T, Codner E, Maliqueo M, Echiburú B, Hitschfeld C, Crisosto N, *et al.* Increased anti- Müllerian hormone serum concentrations in prepubertal daughters of women with polycystic ovary syndrome. *J Clin Endocrinol Metab* 2006;91:3105–9.
23. Rosenfield RL, Ghai K, Ehrmann DA, Barnes RB. Diagnosis of the polycystic ovary syndrome in adolescence: comparison of adolescent and adult hyperandrogenism. *J Pediatr Endocrinol Metab* 2000;13 Suppl 5:1285–9.
24. Bekx MT, Connor EC, Allen DB. Characteristics of adolescents presenting to a multidisciplinary clinic for polycystic ovarian syndrome. *J Pediatr Adolesc Gynecol* 2010;23:7–10.
25. Ahmed ML, Ong KK, Morrell DJ, Cox L, Drayer N, Perry L, *et al.* Longitudinal study of leptin concentrations during puberty: sex differences and relationship to changes in body composition. *J Clin Endocrinol Metab* 1999;84:899–905.
26. Lewy VD, Danadian K, Witchel SF, Arslanian S. Early metabolic abnormalities in adolescent girls with polycystic ovarian syndrome. *J Pediatr* 2001;138:38–44.
27. Laggari V, Diareme S, Christogiorgos S, Deligeoroglou E, Christopoulos P, Tsiantis J, *et al.* Anxiety and depression in adolescents with polycystic ovary syndrome and Mayer-Rokitansky-Küster-Hauser syndrome. *J Psychosom Obstet Gynaecol* 2009;30:83–8.
28. Rofey DL, Szigethy EM, Noll RB, Dahl RE, Lobst E, Arslanian SA. Cognitive-behavioral therapy for physical and emotional disturbances in adolescents with polycystic ovary syndrome: a pilot study. *J Pediatr Psychol* 2009;34:156–63.
29. Ong KK, Potau N, Petry CJ, Jones R, Ness AR, Honour JW, *et al*; Avon Longitudinal Study of Parents and Children Study Team. Opposing influences of prenatal and postnatal weight gain on adrenarche in normal boys and girls. *J Clin Endocrinol Metab* 2004;89:2647–51.
30. Apter D, Bützow T, Laughlin GA, Yen SS. Metabolic features of polycystic ovary syndrome are found in adolescent girls with hyperandrogenism. *J Clin Endocrinol Metab* 1995;80:2966–73.
31. Jaquet D, Leger J, Chevenne D, Czernichow P, Levy-Marchal C. Intrauterine growth retardation predisposes to insulin resistance but not to hyperandrogenism in young women. *J Clin Endocrinol Metab* 1999;84:3945–9.
32. Laitinen J, Taponen S, Martikainen H, Pouta A, Millwood I, Hartikainen AL, *et al.* Body size from birth to adulthood as a predictor of self-reported polycystic ovary syndrome symptoms. *Int J Obes Relat Metab Disord* 2003;27:710–5.
33. Jabbar M, Pugliese M, Fort P, Recker B, Lifshitz F. Excess weight and precocious pubarche in children: alterations of the adrenocortical hormones. *J Am Coll Nutr* 1991;10:289–96.
34. Ong KK, Ahmed ML, Emmett PM, Preece MA, Dunger DB. Association between postnatal catch-up growth and obesity in childhood: prospective cohort study. *BMJ* 2000;320(7240):967–71.
35. Ong KK, Petry CJ, Emmett PM, Sandhu MS, Kiess W, Hales CN, *et al*; ALSPAC study team. Insulin sensitivity and secretion in normal children related to size at birth, postnatal growth, and plasma insulin-like growth factor-I levels. *Diabetologia* 2004;47:1064–70.
36. Oberfield SE, Mayes DM, Levine LS, Adrenal steroidogenic function in a black and Hispanic population with precocious pubarche. *J Clin Endocrinol Metab* 1990;70:76–82.
37. Siklar Z, Oçal G, Adiyaman P, Ergur A, Berberoglu M. Functional ovarian hyperandrogenism and polycystic ovary syndrome in prepubertal girls with obesity and/or premature pubarche. *J Pediatr Endocrinol Metab* 2007;20:475–81.
38. Ong KK, de Zegher F, López-Bermejo A, Dunger DB, Ibáñez L. Flutamide metformin for post-menarcheal girls with preclinical ovarian androgen excess: evidence for differential response by androgen receptor genotype. *Eur J Endocrinol* 2007;157:661–8.
39. Petry CJ, Ong KK, Michelmore KF, Artigas S, Wingate DL, Balen AH, *et al.* Association of aromatase (CYP 19) gene variation with features of hyperandrogenism in two populations of young women. *Hum Reprod* 2005;20:1837–43.
40. Petry CJ, Ong KK, Michelmore KF, Artigas S, Wingate DL, Balen AH, *et al.* Associations between common variation in the aromatase gene promoter region and testosterone concentrations in two young female populations. *J Steroid Biochem Mol Biol* 2006;98(4–5):199–206.
41. Ibáñez L, de Zegher F. Low-dose combination of flutamide, metformin and an oral contraceptive for non-obese, young women with polycystic ovary syndrome. *Hum Reprod* 2003;18:57–60.
42. Rumsby G, Avey CJ, Conway GS, Honour JW. Genotype–phenotype analysis in late onset 21-hydroxylase deficiency in comparison to the classical forms. *Clin Endocrinol (Oxf)* 1998;48:707–11.

43. Savage DB, Semple RK, Chatterjee VK, Wales JK, Ross RJ, O'Rahilly S. A clinical approach to severe insulin resistance. *Endocr Dev* 2007;11:122–32.
44. Arslanian SA, Lewy VD, Danadian K. Glucose intolerance in obese adolescents with polycystic ovary syndrome: roles of insulin resistance and beta-cell dysfunction and risk of cardiovascular disease. *J Clin Endocrinol Metab* 2001;86:66–71.
45. Uusitupa M, Louheranta A, Lindström J, Valle T, Sundvall J, Eriksson J, *et al.* The Finnish Diabetes Prevention Study. *Br J Nutr* 2000;83 Suppl 1:S137–42.
46. Tang T, Lord JM, Norman RJ, Yasmin E, Balen AH. Insulin-sensitising drugs (metformin, rosiglitazone, pioglitazone, D-chiro-inositol) for women with polycystic ovary syndrome, oligo amenorrhoea and subfertility. *Cochrane Database Syst Rev* 2009;(4):CD003053.
47. Hoeger K, Davidson K, Kochman L, Cherry T, Kopin L, Guzick DS. The impact of metformin, oral contraceptives, and lifestyle modification on polycystic ovary syndrome in obese adolescent women in two randomized, placebo-controlled clinical trials. *J Clin Endocrinol Metab* 2008;93:4299–306.
48. Reinehr T, Widhalm K, l'Allemand D, Wiegand S, Wabitsch M, Holl RW; APV-Wiss Study Group and German Competence Net Obesity. Two-year follow-up in 21,784 overweight children and adolescents with lifestyle intervention. *Obesity (Silver Spring)* 2009;17:1196–9.
49. Teede HJ, Meyer C, Hutchison SK, Zoungas S, McGrath BP, Moran LJ. Endothelial function and insulin resistance in polycystic ovary syndrome: the effects of medical therapy. *Fertil Steril* 2010;93:184–91.
50. Ibáñez L, de Zegher F. Ethinylestradiol-drospirenone, flutamide-metformin, or both for adolescents and women with hyperinsulinemic hyperandrogenism: opposite effects on adipocytokines and body adiposity. *J Clin Endocrinol Metab* 2004;89:1592–7.
51. Allen HF, Mazzoni C, Heptulla RA, Murray MA, Miller N, Koenigs L, *et al.* Randomized controlled trial evaluating response to metformin versus standard therapy in the treatment of adolescents with polycystic ovary syndrome. *J Pediatr Endocrinol Metab* 2005;18:761–8.
52. Creatsas G, Koliopoulos C, Mastorakos G. Combined oral contraceptive treatment of adolescent girls with polycystic ovary syndrome. Lipid profile. *Ann N Y Acad Sci* 2000;900:245–52.
53. Mastorakos G, Koliopoulos C, Creatsas G. Androgen and lipid profiles in adolescents with polycystic ovary syndrome who were treated with two forms of combined oral contraceptives. *Fertil Steril* 2002;77:919–27.
54. Mastorakos G, Koliopoulos C, Deligeoroglou E, Diamanti-Kandarakis E, Creatsas G. Effects of two forms of combined oral contraceptives on carbohydrate metabolism in adolescents with polycystic ovary syndrome. *Fertil Steril* 2006;85:420–7.
55. Thole Z, Manso G, Salgueiro E, Revuelta P, Hidalgo A. Hepatotoxicity induced by antiandrogens: a review of the literature. *Urol Int* 2004;73:289–95.
56. Martínez F, Avecilla A. Combined hormonal contraception and venous thromboembolism. *Eur J Contracept Reprod Health Care* 2007;12:97–106.
57. Seaman HE, de Vries CS, Farmer RD. The risk of venous thromboembolism in women prescribed cyproterone acetate in combination with ethinyl estradiol: a nested cohort analysis and case–control study. *Hum Reprod* 2003;18:522–6.
58. Franks S, Layton A, Glasier A. Cyproterone acetate/ethinyl estradiol for acne and hirsutism: time to revise prescribing policy. *Hum Reprod* 2008;23:231–2.
59. Seaman HE, de Vries CS, Farmer RD. Venous thromboembolism associated with cyproterone acetate in combination with ethinyloestradiol (Dianette): observational studies using the UK General Practice Research Database. *Pharmacoepidemiol Drug Saf* 2004;13:427–36.
60. Arslanian SA, Lewy V, Danadian K, Saad R. Metformin therapy in obese adolescents with polycystic ovary syndrome and impaired glucose tolerance: amelioration of exaggerated adrenal response to adrenocorticotropin with reduction of insulinemia/insulin resistance. *J Clin Endocrinol Metab* 2002;87:1555–9.
61. Glueck CJ, Morrison JA, Friedman LA, Goldenberg N, Stroop DM, Wang P. Obesity, free testosterone, and cardiovascular risk factors in adolescents with polycystic ovary syndrome and regularly cycling adolescents. *Metabolism* 2006;55:508–14.
62. Bridger T, MacDonald S, Baltzer F, Rodd C. Randomized placebo-controlled trial of metformin for adolescents with polycystic ovary syndrome. *Arch Pediatr Adolesc Med* 2006;160:241–6.

63. Ibáñez L, Valls C, Potau N, Marcos MV, de Zegher F. Sensitization to insulin in adolescent girls to normalize hirsutism, hyperandrogenism, oligomenorrhea, dyslipidemia, and hyperinsulinism after precocious pubarche. *J Clin Endocrinol Metab* 2000;85:3526–30.
64. Azziz R, Ehrmann DA, Legro RS, Fereshetian AG, O'Keefe M, Ghazzi MN; PCOS/Troglitazone Study Group. Troglitazone decreases adrenal androgen levels in women with polycystic ovary syndrome. *Fertil Steril* 2003;79:932–7.
65. Rautio K, Tapanainen JS, Ruokonen A, Morin-Papunen LC. Endocrine and metabolic effects of rosiglitazone in overweight women with PCOS: a randomized placebo-controlled study. *Hum Reprod* 2006;21:1400–7.
66. Garmes HM, Tambascia MA, Zantut-Wittmann DE. Endocrine-metabolic effects of the treatment with pioglitazone in obese patients with polycystic ovary syndrome. *Gynecol Endocrinol* 2005;21:317–23.
67. Dunaif A, Scott D, Finegood D, Quintana B, Whitcomb R. The insulin-sensitizing agent troglitazone improves metabolic and reproductive abnormalities in the polycystic ovary syndrome. *J Clin Endocrinol Metab* 1996;81:3299–306.
68. Ibáñez L, López-Bermejo A, del Rio L, Enríquez G, Valls C, de Zegher F. Combined low-dose pioglitazone, flutamide, and metformin for women with androgen excess. *J Clin Endocrinol Metab* 2007;92:1710–14.
69. Ibáñez L, López-Bermejo A, Díaz M, Enríquez G, del Río L, de Zegher F. Low-dose pioglitazone and low-dose flutamide added to metformin and oestro-progestagens for hyperinsulinaemic women with androgen excess: add-on benefits disclosed by a randomized double-placebo study over 24 months. *Clin Endocrinol (Oxf)* 2009;71:351–7.
70. Ibáñez L, López-Bermejo A, Díaz M, Enríquez G, Valls C, de Zegher F. Pioglitazone (7.5 mg/day) added to flutamide-metformin in women with androgen excess: additional increments of visfatin and high molecular weight adiponectin. *Clin Endocrinol (Oxf)* 2008;68:317–20.
71. Ganie MA, Khurana ML, Eunice M, Gupta N, Gulati M, Dwivedi SN, *et al.* Comparison of efficacy of spironolactone with metformin in the management of polycystic ovary syndrome: an open-labeled study. *J Clin Endocrinol Metab* 2004;89:2756–62.
72. Sciarra A, Cardi a, Di Silverio F. Antiandrogen monotherapy: recommendations for the treatment of prostate cancer. *Urol Int* 2004;72:91–8.
73. Ibáñez L, Potau N, Marcos MV, de Zegher F. Treatment of hirsutism, hyperandrogenism, oligomenorrhea, dyslipidemia, and hyperinsulinism in nonobese, adolescent girls: effect of flutamide. *J Clin Endocrinol Metab* 2000;85:3251–5.
74. Ibáñez L, Jaramillo A, Ferrer A, de Zegher F. Absence of hepatotoxicity after long-term, low-dose flutamide in hyperandrogenic girls and young women. *Hum Reprod* 2005;20:1833–6.
75. Ahmed ML. Endocrine changes during puberty. In: *Pubertal Growth in Diabetic Children*. PhD thesis, The Open University; 2008.

7

Chapter 7

Long-term health risks of polycystic ovary syndrome

Didier Dewailly

Polycystic ovary syndrome (PCOS) is a lifelong disease. It is most often diagnosed in adolescents and young women who present with symptoms of hyperandrogenism and/or disorders of ovulation.[1] From that moment, the individuals and their doctors must be aware that PCOS carries various long-term health risks owing to its intrinsic hormonal derangement and also to the associated metabolic disorders such as obesity, hyperinsulinism and insulin resistance, hyperlipidaemia and pancreatic β-cell dysfunction. The pubertal onset of PCOS thus provides a unique opportunity to detect these risks early and to engage preventive measures.

Although many intermediary risk factors are present in most women with PCOS, the risks for the occurrence of clinical events are difficult to quantify precisely in the absence of large-scale prospective studies. The few available epidemiological studies are difficult to compare with each other and are not conclusive because different definitions for PCOS have been used, series were sometimes small and some included individuals who were too young to be exposed to the events predicted by the risk factors.

Increased cardiovascular risk

The increased cardiovascular risk in women with PCOS has been extensively discussed in the recent literature, as reviewed by Rizzo *et al.*[2] While there is no doubt that many cardiovascular risk factors are present to various degrees in women with PCOS, a clear-cut demonstration of an increased prevalence of cardiovascular events in comparison with age-matched women without PCOS is still awaited.

An early report suggested a seven-fold increased risk of myocardial infarction in women with PCOS but this was estimated from a theoretical calculation, not from case records.[3] Conversely, two studies from the UK were negative[4,5] but the cohorts were relatively young and the diagnosis of PCOS was established only on past ovarian wedge resection data that might have modified the disease evolution. In addition, there were no age-matched control cohorts. Other studies have been controversial.[2] A 2008 study that prospectively evaluated the cardiovascular outcomes 6 years after positive angiographic coronary data in women aged 63 ± 10 years found an association between past clinical features of PCOS and the prevalence of coronary abnormalities, with shorter cardiovascular event-free survival.[6] Although the data are still scarce, it is becoming more and more evident that the cardiovascular risk factors found in many young women with PCOS will translate into more cardiovascular events at a later age.

Surrogates for cardiovascular disease

Traditional measures and the metabolic syndrome

Many abnormalities found in young women with PCOS suggest that they are at risk for cardiovascular disease. The more commonly used parameters are the traditional measures of family history, body mass index (BMI), waist circumference, blood pressure and standard biochemical indices including fasting glycaemia, total cholesterol, high-density lipoprotein (HDL) cholesterol and triglycerides. These routine markers have been gathered together to build metabolic scores defining the well-known metabolic syndrome. Various classifications have been proposed by organisations such as the National Cholesterol Education Program Adult Treatment Panel (ATP III), the European Group for the Study of Insulin Resistance (EGIR) and the World Health Organization (WHO). In 2006, a consensus definition was proposed by the International Diabetes Federation (IDF) that stipulated that increased waist circumference is a prerequisite to which at least two other items must be added to qualify a patient as having the metabolic syndrome (Box 7.1).[7]

The presence of the metabolic syndrome in a given patient certainly predicts a cardiovascular risk but it has been emphasised that it is not more powerful in predicting cardiovascular events than a single risk factor such as hypertension or smoking.[8] Also, because the prevalence of the metabolic syndrome increases with age, it might not be a sensitive enough parameter to detect the cardiovascular risk in young populations early. Indeed, some complications such as hypertension and abnormal glycaemic control occur relatively late, except in cases of a strong family history.

New markers

There is a need for more sensitive and earlier markers of cardiovascular risk and many have been proposed. They can be schematically subdivided into markers of hyperinsulinaemia and insulin resistance, central adiposity, hyperlipidaemia, oxidative stress, low-grade inflammation, endothelial dysfunction and subclinical atherosclerosis. All these factors overlap with each other in terms of risk prediction and many are redundant. It is also unclear how much useful information they add to that given by the traditional measures. Indices of subclinical atherosclerosis, such as intima–media thickness[9] and coronary arterial calcifications,[10] are more closely associated with later cardiovascular events but they become positive much too late. The markers of endothelial dysfunction seem more interesting[11] but studying artery vasodilator response is not easy to perform in the routine clinical set-up. Biochemical markers such as homocysteine or endothelin 1 seem promising but they have not been fully investigated as risk predictors in the young.[12] The same is true of C-reactive protein (CRP) and other markers of inflammation.[13] In older women, however, one study[7]

Box 7.1 Definition of the metabolic syndrome according to the International Diabetes Federation (IDF) criteria[7]

Waist circumference > 80 cm, plus any two of the following:

- raised tryglycerides > 1.5 g/litre
- reduced high-density lipoprotein (HDL) cholesterol < 0.5 g/litre
- raised systolic blood pressure > 130 mmHg (and/or diastolic blood pressure > 85 mmHg)
- raised fasting glucose > 1 g/litre or previously diagnosed diabetes

has shown that past PCOS associated with increased high-sensitivity CRP (above 3.0 mg/dl) is associated with a 12.2-fold higher risk of death from cardiovascular disease than in women without PCOS and with normal CRP.

Waist circumference and HDL cholesterol

Numerous studies have shown that waist circumference is the variable that correlates most closely with visceral adiposity. It is currently viewed as the main abnormality predicting cardiovascular risk, even in young obese women. Waist circumference is able to identify children susceptible to developing cardiovascular diseases in adulthood.[14] It is therefore the single best anthropometric indicator of visceral adipose tissue and it is a predictor of incidental chronic disease and premature mortality.

In addition, it must be emphasised that a low serum level of HDL cholesterol has independent and strong predictive value, irrespective of the presence or absence of the metabolic syndrome. In people with a history of cardiovascular events, HDL cholesterol has been shown to accurately indicate the 'residual' cardiovascular risk (that is, the remaining risk once targets for control of hypertension, elevated total cholesterol and/or hyperglycaemia have been reached).[15] In our experience, increased waist circumference and decreased HDL cholesterol are the most frequent metabolic abnormalities found in young women (aged 16–20 years) with PCOS (Table 7.1).[16] It must be emphasised, however, that the adult threshold for a decreased HDL cholesterol (less than 0.5 g/litre in women) does not seem appropriate in those younger than 20 years. Lowering this threshold to 0.4 g/litre, as for children, would seem more judicious but this awaits confirmation.[16]

PCOS as a risk factor on its own

Hyperandrogenism by itself seems to correlate closely with cardiovascular risk.[7] However, studies using the free androgen index (FAI) as a marker of androgenicity should be viewed with some caution. FAI is calculated from the total testosterone (TT) and sex hormone-binding globulin (SHBG) serum levels according to the formula (TT/SHBG) × 100. Hyperinsulinaemia is well known to strongly reduce hepatic production of SHBG and to lower its serum level.[17] This effect therefore induces a rise in the TT/SHBG ratio independently of androgen production.

Table 7.1 Frequency of markers of the metabolic syndrome in women with polycystic ovary syndrome; data from Dewailly *et al.*[16]

Marker	Frequency by age subgroup (years)			P (χ^2 test)
	16–20 (n=55)	20–30 (n=548)	30–40 (n=238)	
Waist circumference > 80 cm	50.9%	59.7%	65.7%	0.07
Systolic blood pressure > 130 mmHg and/or diastolic blood pressure > 85 mmHg	10.9%	10.2%	13%	0.61
High-density lipoprotein (HDL) cholesterol < 0.5 g/litre (or < 0.4 g/litre)	60.0% (27.0%)	42.3%	43.3%	0.04 (0.05)
Triglycerides > 1.5 g/litre	9.1%	10.9%	14.2%	0.32
Hyperglycaemia[a]	1.8%	6.8%	12.7%	0.004

[a] Hyperglycaemia was defined as the presence of either fasting hyperglycaemia (≥ 1 g/litre) or previously diagnosed diabetes

Diagnosis of PCOS itself might serve as an indicator of cardiovascular risk. PCOS defined by the National Institutes of Health (NIH) classification[18] is associated with a more adverse metabolic profile including greater total and abdominal obesity, insulin resistance and risk factors for cardiovascular disease and type 2 diabetes than non-NIH phenotypes.[19] Accordingly, among the phenotypes yielded by the Rotterdam classification,[20] there is a gradation in metabolic and cardiovascular risk factors, worsening according to the extent and severity of symptoms of PCOS.[21–24]

Recommendations

There are currently no consensus guidelines regarding screening for cardiovascular disease in women with PCOS. Fasting lipid profiles and glucose examinations should be performed regularly. For some authors, carotid intima–media thickness examinations should begin at age 30 years and coronary calcium screening should begin at age 45 years. Treatment of the associated cardiovascular risk factors, including insulin resistance, hypertension, smoking and dyslipidaemia, should be incorporated into routine PCOS follow-up. Multidisciplinary programmes, including dietary and educational counselling, exercise training, stress management and psychosocial support, are needed for adequate reduction of cardiovascular risk in young women with PCOS. There is no solid evidence that the combined oral contraceptive pill (OCP) or progestin treatments worsen this risk, provided that classical contraindications are respected. However, more studies are needed to resolve controversies regarding the safety of long-term OCP use in women with PCOS as the available studies are still few and conflicting.[25]

Risk for type 2 diabetes and impaired glucose tolerance

In contrast to the controversy about cardiovascular risk, the risk for type 2 diabetes has been well validated in a number of PCOS populations worldwide. The overall risk is increased 3 to 7 times. It varies in absolute value from one country to another. In the USA, the predicted prevalence of type 2 diabetes in women with PCOS has been estimated to be as high as 10% when the WHO criteria are used in women aged 20–45 years.[26] In some European populations, it is 'only' 2.5%.

Obviously, obesity has a great impact on the prevalence of type 2 diabetes but the risk persists in non-obese women with PCOS. Other risk factors are family history of type 2 diabetes, central adiposity, past gestational diabetes, hyperandrogenism and oligomenorrhoea. Typically, the onset of type 2 diabetes occurs in the fourth or fifth decade, which is earlier than in the normal population. In many cases but not all, it is preceded by impaired glucose tolerance (IGT) that occurs at a much higher rate in women with PCOS than in the normal population: 30–40% versus 8% in US populations.[27] Not all women with IGT will become diabetic, however. The rate of conversion from IGT to type 2 diabetes has been estimated as being about 50% in an Australian series after an average follow-up of 6.2 years.[28] It is noteworthy that about 10% of women in this series moved directly from normoglycaemia to type 2 diabetes. The mechanism driving the change from hyperinsulinaemia and insulin resistance to type 2 diabetes is impairment in pancreatic β-cell function, which is similar to what has been observed in other groups at risk for type 2 diabetes. This abnormality may be detected early by sophisticated testing. It is under strong genetic influence, as indicated by the clustering of first-degree relatives of people with type 2 diabetes.

All women with PCOS should thus be screened for the onset of IGT and type 2 diabetes. It is still debated, however, whether an oral glucose tolerance test should be performed in every woman with PCOS, only in those who are obese (BMI > 30 kg/m^2) or only in those with first-degree relatives with type 2 diabetes.[29] Glycaemia should be checked once a year. There is no consensus on the recommended frequency of performing an oral glucose tolerance test in women with initially normal glucose tolerance but an interval of 2 years seems reasonable.[29]

Complications of obesity

In addition to its major impact on cardiovascular and type 2 diabetes risks, obesity can be complicated by obstructive sleep apnoea, the prevalence of which is increased in women with PCOS and the severity of which is strongly correlated with insulin levels and measures of glucose intolerance.[30]

Obesity in PCOS is also associated with poor self-image and depression. While the symptoms of hyperandrogenism and infertility also negatively affect quality of life, weight concerns seem to have the most effect in this regard.[31] Obesity also carries severe obstetrical risks.

Gynaecological malignancies

Endometrial hyperplasia and cancer

Chronic anovulation and thus the prolonged exposure to unopposed estrogen can lead to endometrial hyperplasia, which can progress to carcinoma. It is estimated that 18% of cases of adenomatous hyperplasia will progress to cancer in the following 2–10 years. The risk factors for endometrial carcinoma include obesity, hypertension, type 2 diabetes, unopposed estrogen and nulliparity. These are all conditions that may be associated with PCOS. There is therefore a possible link between PCOS and endometrial carcinoma but it is very difficult to identify the true risk because the numbers of women in the published studies have been relatively small. A meta-analysis published in 2009[32] showed that the odds of developing endometrial cancer are nearly three times higher (OR 2.70; 95% CI 1.00–7.29) in women with PCOS compared with women without PCOS.

The Royal College of Obstetricians and Gynaecologists has advised that women with PCOS should have regular induction of withdrawal bleeding to prevent endometrial hyperplasia. From epidemiological studies, it is clear that current or previous use of the OCP provides a strong preventive benefit against endometrial cancer.[33]

Breast cancer

Women with PCOS do not appear to be more likely to develop breast cancer. In the meta-analysis by Chittenden *et al*,[32] aggregated data showed that the combined odds ratio of having breast cancer in women with PCOS was 0.88 (95% CI 0.44–1.77) compared with women without PCOS.

Ovarian cancer

Only one study[34] has looked at the association between PCOS and ovarian cancer. The authors compared women who had been diagnosed with epithelial ovarian cancer with a randomly selected age-matched population. From these data, women with PCOS were found to be twice as likely to develop ovarian cancer as those without the condition. However, the authors advised caution in interpreting their data because the number of women with ovarian cancer in the study was small.

Conclusion

Every risk discussed in this chapter can be attenuated provided that the doctors and patients are aware of them. Information and education are crucial but they are currently insufficiently developed. Although hyperandrogenism and infertility may be less of a problem in older women with PCOS, patients should be warned that the metabolic problems will remain and may even worsen with age. The most rational approach is a change in diet and lifestyle habits that should be encouraged as early as possible, with the help of appropriate coaching. This has a cost but it must be realised that the largest part of the economic burden of PCOS is due to its long-term health risks. In an economic evaluation that did not take into account cardiovascular disease, PCOS-associated diabetes represented 40% of the total annual cost of PCOS.[35] Public health authorities should be more sensitive to the fact that PCOS is not just a cosmetic or a fertility problem.

References

1. Norman RJ, Dewailly D, Legros RS, Hickey TE. Polycystic ovary syndrome. *Lancet* 2007;370:685–97.
2. Rizzo M, Berneis K, Spinas G, Rini GB, Carmina E. Long-term consequences of polycystic ovary syndrome on cardiovascular risk. *Fertil Steril* 2009;91(4 Suppl):1563–7.
3. Dahlgren E, Janson PO, Johansson S, Lapidus L, Oden A. Polycystic ovary syndrome and risk for myocardial infarction. Evaluated from a risk factor model based on a prospective population study of women. *Acta Obstet Gynecol Scand* 1992;71:599–604.
4. Pierpoint T, McKeigue PM, Isaacs AJ, Wild SH, Jacobs HS. Mortality of women with polycystic ovary syndrome at long-term follow-up. *J Clin Epidemiol* 1998;51:581–6.
5. Wild S, Pierpoint T, McKeigue P, Jacobs H. Cardiovascular disease in women with polycystic ovary syndrome at long-term follow-up: a retrospective cohort study. *Clin Endocrinol (Oxf)* 2000;52:595–600.
6. Shaw LJ, Bairey Merz CN, Azziz R, Stanczyk FZ, Sopko G, Braunstein GD, *et al.* Postmenopausal women with a history of irregular menses and elevated androgen measurements at high risk for worsening cardiovascular event-free survival: results from the National Institutes of Health – National Heart, Lung, and Blood Institute (NHLBI)-sponsored Women's Ischemia Syndrome Evaluation (WISE). *J Clin Endocrinol Metab* 2008;93:1276–84.
7. Alberti KG, Zimmet P, Shaw J. Metabolic syndrome-a new world-wide definition. A consensus statement from the International Diabetes Federation. *Diabet Med* 2006;23:469–80.
8. Nilsson PM. Cardiovascular risk in the metabolic syndrome: fact or fiction? *Curr Cardiol Rep* 2007;9:479–85.
9. Talbott EO, Guzick DS, Sutton-Tyrrell K, McHugh-Pemu KP, Zborowski JV, Remsberg KE, *et al.* Evidence for association between polycystic ovary syndrome and premature carotid atherosclerosis in middle-aged women. *Arterioscler Thromb Vasc Biol* 2000;20:2414–21.
10. Talbott EO, Zborowski JV, Rager JR, Boudreaux MY, Edmundowicz DA, Guzick DS. Evidence for an association between metabolic cardiovascular syndrome and coronary and aortic calcification among women with polycystic ovary syndrome. *J Clin Endocrinol Metab* 2004;89:5454–61.
11. Orio F Jr, Palomba S, Cascella T, De Simone B, Di Biase S, Russo T, *et al.* Early impairment of endothelial structure and function in in young normal-weight women with polycystic ovary syndrome. *J Clin Endocrinol Metab* 2004;89:4588–93.
12. Diamanti-Kandarakis E, Alexandraki K, Piperi C, Protogerou A, Katsikis I, Paterakis T, *et al.* Inflammatory and endothelial markers in women with polycystic ovary syndrome. *Eur J Clin Invest* 2006;36:691–7.
13. Kelly CC, Lyall H, Petrie JR, Gould GW, Connell JM, Sattar N. Low-grade chronic inflammation in women with polycystic ovarian syndrome. *J Clin Endocrinol Metab* 2001;86:2453–5.
14. Botton J, Heude B, Kettaneh A, Borys JM, Lommez A, Bresson JL, *et al.* Cardiovascular risk factor levels and their relationships with overweight and fat distribution in children: the Fleurbaix Laventie Ville Santé II study. *Metabolism* 2007;56:614–22.

15. Sazonov V, Beetsch J, Phatak H, Wentworth C, Evans M. Association between dyslipidemia and vascular events in patients treated with statins: report from the UK General Practice Research Database. *Atherosclerosis* 2010;208:210–16.
16. Dewailly D, Contestin M, Gallo C, Catteau-Jonard S. Metabolic syndrome in young women with the polycystic ovary syndrome: revisiting the threshold for an abnormally decreased high-density lipoprotein cholesterol serum level. *BJOG* 2010;117:175–80.
17. Pugeat M, Crave JC, Elmidani M, Nicolas MH, Garoscio-Cholet M, Lejeune H, *et al.* Pathophysiology of sex hormone binding globulin (SHBG): relation to insulin. *J Steroid Biochem Mol Biol* 1991;40:841–9.
18. Zawadzki JK, Dunaif A. Diagnostic criteria for polycystic ovary syndrome: towards a rational approach. In: Dunaif A, Givens JR, Haseltine F, editors. *Polycystic Ovary Syndrome.* Boston: Blackwell Scientific 1992. p. 377–84.
19. Carmina E, Longo RA, Rini GB, Lobo RA. Phenotypic variation in hyperandrogenic women influences the findings of abnormal metabolic and cardiovascular risk parameters. *J Clin Endocrinol Metab* 2005;90:2545–9.
20. Rotterdam ESHRE/ASRM-Sponsored PCOS Consensus Workshop Group. Revised 2003 consensus on diagnostic criteria and long-term health risks related to polycystic ovary syndrome. *Fertil Steril* 2004;81:19–25.
21. Moran L, Teede H. Metabolic features of the reproductive phenotypes of polycystic ovary syndrome. *Hum Reprod Update* 2009;15:477–88.
22. Dewailly D, Catteau-Jonard S, Reyss AC, Leroy M, Pigny P. Oligo-anovulation with polycystic ovaries (PCO) but not overt hyperandrogenism. *J Clin Endocrinol Metab* 2006;91:3922–7.
23. Welt CK, Gudmundsson JA, Arason G, Adams J, Palsdottir H, Gudlaugsdottir G, *et al.* Characterizing discrete subsets of polycystic ovary syndrome as defined by the Rotterdam criteria: the impact of weight on phenotype and metabolic features. *J Clin Endocrinol Metab* 2006;91:3842–8.
24. Barber TM, Wass JA, McCarthy MI, Franks S. Metabolic characteristics of women with polycystic ovaries and oligo-amenorrhoea but normal androgen levels: implications for the management of polycystic ovary syndrome. *Clin Endocrinol (Oxf)* 2007;66:513–17.
25. Yildiz BO. Oral contraceptives in polycystic ovary syndrome: risk–benefit assessment. *Semin Reprod Med* 2008;26:111–20.
26. Legro RS, Kunselman AR, Dodson WC, Dunaif A. Prevalence and predictors of risk for type 2 diabetes mellitus and impaired glucose tolerance in polycystic ovary syndrome: a prospective, controlled study in 254 affected women. *J Clin Endocrinol Metab* 1999;84:165–9.
27. Ehrmann D, Barnes R, Rosenfield R, Cavaghan M, Imperial J. Prevalence of impaired glucose tolerance and diabetes in women with polycystic ovary syndrome. *Diabetes Care* 1999;22:141–6.
28. Norman RJ, Masters L, Milner CR, Wang JX, Davies MJ. Relative risk of conversion from normoglycaemia to impaired glucose tolerance or non-insulin dependent diabetes mellitus in polycystic ovarian syndrome. *Hum Reprod* 2001;16:1995–8.
29. Salley KE, Wickham EP, Cheang KI, Essah PA, Karjane NW, Nestler JE. Glucose intolerance in polycystic ovary syndrome – a position statement of the Androgen Excess Society. *J Clin Endocrinol Metab* 2007;92:4546–56.
30. Tasali E, Van Cauter E, Ehrmann DA. Polycystic ovary syndrome and obstructive sleep apnea. *Sleep Med Clin* 2008;3:37–46.
31. Jones GL, Hall JM, Balen AH, Ledger WL. Health-related quality of life measurement in women with polycystic ovary syndrome: a systematic review. *Hum Reprod Update* 2008;14:15–25.
32. Chittenden BG, Fullerton G, Maheshwari A, Bhattacharya S. Polycystic ovary syndrome and the risk of gynaecological cancer: a systematic review. *Reprod Biomed Online* 2009;19:398–405.
33. Grimes DA, Economy KE. Primary prevention of gynecologic cancers. *Am J Obstet Gynecol* 1995;172:227–35.
34. Schildkraut JM, Schwingl PJ, Bastos E, Evanoff A, Hughes C. Epithelial ovarian cancer risk among women with polycystic ovary syndrome. *Obstet Gynecol* 1996;88:554–9.
35. Azziz R, Marin C, Hoq L, Badamgarav E, Song P. Health care-related economic burden of the polycystic ovary syndrome during the reproductive life span. *J Clin Endocrinol Metab* 2005;90:4650–8.

Chapter 8

Approaches to lifestyle management in polycystic ovary syndrome

Renato Pasquali and Alessandra Gambineri

Introduction

Polycystic ovary syndrome (PCOS), one of the most common hyperandrogenic disorders, affects 4–7% of women.[1] The definition of PCOS is currently based on the presence of hyperandrogenism (either clinical [hirsutism] and/or biochemical [increased testosterone blood levels]), chronic oligo-ovulation/anovulation and polycystic morphology of the ovaries at ultrasound, with the exclusion of other causes of hyperandrogenism such as adult-onset congenital adrenal hyperplasia, hyperprolactinaemia and androgen-secreting neoplasms.[2] Insulin resistance and associated hyperinsulinaemia are also now recognised as important pathogenetic factors in determining hyperandrogenaemia in most women with PCOS, particularly when obesity is present.[3,4]

Although significant progress has been made towards the development of universally accepted diagnostic criteria for PCOS,[1,2] the optimal treatment for women with PCOS has not yet been defined. In general, treatment should aim to improve:

- the overall PCOS phenotype
- hyperandrogenism and hyperandrogenaemia
- menstrual abnormalities such as anovulation
- infertility
- obesity
- insulin resistance and/or associated metabolic disturbances
- cardiovascular risk factors.

Treatment should also aim to prevent long-term metabolic (such as type 2 diabetes), neoplastic (such as endometrial cancer) and cardiovascular diseases.

The available interventions include lifestyle modifications, administration of pharmaceutical agents (such as antiandrogens and estro-progestin compounds, clomifene citrate, insulin-sensitising agents, gonadotrophins and gonadotrophin-releasing hormone analogues), the use of laparoscopic ovarian diathermy and the application of assisted reproductive technology (ART).

Recognition of the controversies surrounding the treatment of this enigmatic syndrome led to a second international workshop endorsed by the European Society of Human Reproduction and Embryology (ESHRE) and the American Society for Reproductive Medicine (ASRM). The workshop was held in Thessaloniki, Greece, in 2007 to address the therapeutic challenges of treating women with infertility and PCOS and to answer important questions regarding the efficacy and safety of the various treatments available for these women.[5] The consensus conference dedicated considerable time to the impact of lifestyle interventions to improve the fertility problems of PCOS. This is consistent with the fact that women with PCOS are often overweight or obese and the evidence that excess fat may play an independent pathophysiological role in the development of androgen excess, infertility and metabolic disturbances.[6,7] In addition, there is consistent evidence that excess body weight renders women with PCOS more susceptible to developing type 2 diabetes[8] and increases the risk of developing cardiovascular diseases.[9] We support the concept that, in the presence of excess weight and particularly of obesity, the primary aim should be weight loss, since all available studies published so far have documented that this tends to improve all features of PCOS, often regardless of the actual number of kilograms lost.[10]

If we accept this simple concept, we should also accept that treatment of obesity *per se* should not be substantially different in the presence of PCOS and that simply adopting the World Health Organization recommendations for the treatment of obesity[11] is probably the best way to achieve successful results, even if this is not so easy to achieve. In a 2009 review[12] of the efficacy of commonly used procedures to treat obesity in women with PCOS, including lifestyle intervention (namely low dietary intake and structured physical activity, anti-obesity drugs and bariatric surgery), we found that important benefits can be achieved regarding hormonal derangements, menstrual abnormalities and infertility and metabolic alterations. In another review,[13] we supported the concept that weight loss probably represents the major insulin sensitiser therapy in obese women with PCOS, even if insulin-sensitising agents are added to weight-loss regimens.

The aim of this chapter is to briefly review the role of obesity in the pathophysiology of PCOS, to summarise all major aspects of lifestyle intervention and to discuss the available methodological approaches.

Prevalence of obesity and PCOS

The increasing epidemic of obesity and related disorders is a worldwide public health emergency.[14] The problem of excess weight and obesity has achieved global recognition only in the last 10–15 years. Most importantly, evidence is emerging that excess weight is increasing not only in adults but in children too, particularly in western countries.[14] It is thus possible that the increasing epidemic of obesity may be a factor in the worldwide increased incidence of young women attending endocrinological or gynaecological clinics because of menstrual irregularities, clinical hyperandrogenism and infertility problems, which are features that suggest a PCOS phenotype.

The prevalence of obesity in PCOS appears to be much greater than that expected in the general population, ranging from 30% to 70% depending on ethnicity, geographical areas, environmental factors, genetic susceptibility and other still unknown factors.[3] Across the entire spectrum of body mass index (BMI), the prevalence of abdominal fatness can probably be explained by excess exposure to higher than normal total and free testosterone, which in women specifically tends to enlarge visceral fat depots.[15,16]

Despite this association, it is unclear whether the increase in population obesity has altered the prevalence of PCOS or whether the presence of obesity in PCOS simply reflects the increasing prevalence of obesity worldwide. A Spanish study reported a four-fold higher prevalence rate of PCOS among more than 100 overweight or obese women attending an endocrinology clinic compared with the general population.[17] Another study performed in the USA[18] found that, although the prevalence of PCOS tended to increase with increasing BMI, prevalence rates tended to parallel those of obesity in the general population, which suggests that obesity in PCOS may reflect environmental factors to a great extent. Unfortunately, both cross-sectional and prospective epidemiological studies are still lacking.

Evidence that early weight gain favours the development of PCOS

The concept that early weight gain may be responsible for the development of PCOS was developed in around 1980 by Samuel Yen.[19] Infertility is associated with earlier onset obesity, and menstrual disorders are frequent with the onset of excess weight during puberty.[20] Moreover, excess body weight during adolescence may be associated with menstrual and ovulatory disorders.[21] Adolescent girls may develop transient anovulation with high luteinising hormone (LH) levels and mild hyperandrogenaemia,[22] and peripubertal obesity by itself is associated with hyperandrogenaemia and hyperinsulinaemia throughout puberty, being especially marked shortly before and during early puberty.[23] However, some of these girls may normalise androgen levels and LH secretion, whereas many others may develop permanent hyperandrogenism and the PCOS phenotype.[24] Excess adiposity may subsequently play a role in the worsening of hyperandrogenism and other clinical features of PCOS after adolescence.[21,25]

A number of studies have provided evidence supporting the hypothesis that the natural course of PCOS may in fact originate in fetal life and that factors in the intrauterine environment may play a role in the early pathogenesis of the syndrome. In a pioneering study, Cresswell *et al.*[26] found that, of 235 women aged 40–42 years who were born in 1952–53 in Sheffield, 21% had features of PCOS. They were divided into two groups, corresponding to the more common clinical phenotypes, with one group comprising obese hirsute women with higher levels of plasma LH and testosterone (these women had above-average birth weight and had been born to overweight mothers), and the other group comprising normal-weight women with high plasma LH but normal testosterone concentrations (these women had been born after term). According to the authors' hypothesis, these two groups of women with PCOS may have had different origins in intrauterine life, with one associated with maternal obesity and the other characterised by altered hypothalamic control of LH release resulting from prolonged gestation.

Animal studies have given scientific support to an intrauterine or perinatal origin of PCOS. Nilsson *et al.*[27] found that neonatal testosterone imprinting of female rats was followed by insulin resistance, enlargement of visceral fat and increased muscle mass, without elevation of circulating testosterone, in adult age. Further studies performed in various animal models have provided compelling evidence that both early and late androgenisation *in utero* may favour the development of the PCOS phenotype later in life when these animals enter the post-pubertal adult age.[28] Two animal models have been particularly investigated: rhesus monkeys and sheep.[28,29] Collectively, these studies provide evidence that the intrauterine hormonal environment (higher than normal testosterone levels) may programme target tissue differentiation, supporting the hypothesis that even mild excess androgen exposure in human fetal development promotes PCOS in adulthood.[28,29] One consequence of premature androgenisation is an enlargement of visceral adipose tissue, which further emphasises the important role of adiposity in determining metabolic alterations often associated with PCOS.[29,30]

Pathophysiological aspects of adipose tissue in PCOS

In normal-weight women, in the presence of normal insulin sensitivity, adipocytes release limited amounts of free fatty acids (FFAs) and regular amounts of lipoprotein lipase (LPL). In addition, normal testosterone supports insulin in suppressing FFA release from adipocytes. In contrast, obese women are characterised by increased production of FFA and inhibition of LPL secretion because of the presence of high insulin due to the insulin-resistant state. In addition, increased androgens aggravate the detrimental effects of insulin resistance on FFA release from adipocytes. Increased expression of androgen receptors has been found in women with abdominal obesity and PCOS.[15] The androgen receptors in female adipose tissue seem to have the same characteristics as those found in male adipose tissue; however, estrogens downregulate the density of these receptors, which can explain the opposite effects of testosterone in males and females.[15] Testosterone may thus cause accumulation of visceral adipose tissue in women, which is consistent with the important role of hyperandrogenaemia in determining the high prevalence of the abdominal fat distribution pattern in hyperandrogenised women with PCOS.

In these women, intravisceral adipocytes behave in an abnormal way in terms of their effects on the metabolic and hormonal profile, which is associated with defective insulin activity.[31] The adipocytes also have an effect on steroid metabolism, specifically on androgen metabolism.[15] There is no defect in the process by which insulin binds to its receptor in women with PCOS;[4,31] instead, visceral adipocytes are believed to express defects in insulin intracellular signalling. The β-subunits of the insulin receptor increase serine phosphorylation, which inhibits the intracellular transmission of the insulin message in the adipocytes and decreases tyrosine phosphorylation. This defect, in turn, translates into decreased activity of the phosphoinositide3-kinase (PI3K) enzyme, which is the key enzyme for recruitment of glucose transporter 4 (GLUT4), finally decreasing cellular glucose uptake.[32] The visceral adipocytes also show increased sensitivity to lipolysis, which is in keeping with insulin resistance.[33] The mechanism is believed to reflect the fact that the complex formed by protein kinase A and hormone-sensitive lipase is overactivated in women with PCOS.

The role of adipocytes in steroid hormonal metabolism in PCOS is also important, since they favour the conversion of Δ4-androstenedione to testosterone via the 17β-hydroxydehydrogenase enzyme. Locally produced androgens may lead to increased visceral adiposity.[18] In turn, visceral adipocytes are able to convert inactive cortisone to metabolically active cortisol, via the 11β-hydroxydehydrogenase type 1 enzyme located in the liver and visceral adipose tissue, which may favour a decrease in insulin sensitivity.[34] These combined metabolically active steroids may therefore play a crucial role in the development of visceral obesity and insulin resistance in women with PCOS.

Obesity worsens the PCOS phenotype and associated metabolic alterations

Obesity has profound effects on the clinical, hormonal and metabolic features of PCOS, which largely depend on the degree of excess body fat and on the pattern of fat distribution. This topic has been extensively reviewed.[7] Briefly, obese women with PCOS are characterised by significantly lower sex hormone-binding globulin (SHBG) plasma levels[1] and more hyperandrogenaemia (particularly total and free testosterone and Δ4-androstenedione) than their normal-weight counterparts.[7] Moreover, a higher proportion of obese women with PCOS complain of hirsutism and other androgen-dependent disorders, such as acne and androgenic alopecia, than normal-weight women with PCOS. The androgen profile can, in turn, be further negatively affected in women with PCOS with the abdominal obesity phenotype,[7,8] regardless of BMI values.

Menstrual abnormalities are more frequent in obese than normal-weight women with PCOS.[10,35] In the presence of obesity, the incidence of pregnancy is also significantly reduced, and blunted responsiveness to pharmacological treatments or after ART has been reported.[10] All available studies on this topic have clearly demonstrated that obesity has a negative impact on spontaneous fertility[36] and ART[37] in women with PCOS.

As expected, obesity exacerbates the metabolic abnormalities associated with PCOS. Insulin resistance is almost always present in obese women with PCOS, although it may occur even in those with normal weight.[4] Accordingly, both fasting and glucose-stimulated insulin concentrations are usually significantly higher in women with PCOS.[4] In the presence of obesity, early insulin secretion may also be significantly decreased in PCOS, thereby favouring the development of glucose intolerance states.[4] In any case, it has been shown that worsened insulin resistance in the long term may represent an important factor in the development of impaired glucose tolerance (IGT) and type 2 diabetes and that this may occur only in the presence of obesity.[38] This is confirmed by the finding that, at the first examination, IGT is present in as many as 20–40% of obese women with PCOS, while it is very uncommon in those presenting with normal weight.[4] In addition, abdominal obesity is associated with a greater prevalence of the metabolic syndrome in PCOS, and obesity *per se* plays a major role in distinguishing those with and without the metabolic syndrome.[39]

It is noteworthy that the available data indicate that women with PCOS have a significantly greater and earlier tendency to develop type 2 diabetes than the general population, but this appears to occur mainly in the presence of obesity and rarely in normal-weight women.[40] Unpublished preliminary data from our study group investigating more than 300 women with PCOS followed up for an average period of 20 years indicate that the incidence of type 2 diabetes is approximately 20% and that the presence of obesity and insulin resistance at the first examination are the most important predictive factors.

Finally, as reported above, there is a great debate as to whether women with PCOS are at a significantly higher risk for cardiovascular diseases and whether this is influenced by excess weight or obesity.[8]

Treatment of obesity improves PCOS

The treatment of PCOS must take into account hyperandrogenism and reproductive, metabolic and psychological features. In a systematic review,[12] we reported that:

- with regard to reproductive features, reducing biochemical and clinical hyperandrogenism, regulating menstrual cycles, restoring ovulation and reproductive function and improving reproductive outcomes are important
- from a metabolic perspective, addressing insulin resistance and the metabolic syndrome are important in reducing long-term metabolic morbidity
- from a psychological perspective, addressing factors including self-esteem and dysthymia is critical to improving motivation for effective lifestyle change.

Importantly, we also clarified that, in the presence of obesity and insulin resistance, lifestyle intervention should be adopted as a primary initial treatment strategy, either alone or in combination with anti-obesity pharmacological options. Unfortunately, this is not the most common therapeutic strategy worldwide. This can be explained by the fact that any treatment of obesity requires experienced professionals, that the well-known negative experience worldwide may be discouraging and that, being a chronic condition, obesity often requires long-term management, possibly involving GPs and social support. Nevertheless, many studies have provided evidence that, even in the short term and when women have been adequately motivated to achieve 'measurable' outcomes such as pregnancy[41] or relevant improvements in health, this is not a utopian target.

Lifestyle management

The fundamental therapy of obesity is changing dietary habits and reducing energy intake. This makes it possible to reduce body weight and improve weight maintenance over the long term, thus helping to prevent further weight gain.[41] In the general population, guidelines for obesity management in women recommend an initial weight loss of at least 5–10% for reduction of obesity-related risk factors, with a long-term goal of achieving and maintaining a reduction in weight and/or waist circumference to close to normal values for women.[42,43] The success of a weight-loss strategy can be further increased by incorporating additional measures such as regular physical activity and attention to psychological adjustment, including behaviour modification and stress-management strategies.[42,43] These strategies can be implemented through the use of lifestyle modification techniques. These consist of a multifaceted approach of dietary, exercise and behaviour therapy, and aim to teach principles and techniques for achieving dietary and exercise goals for long-term weight management.[44]

Evidence on the effectiveness of dietary interventions without exercise or behavioural advice in obese women with PCOS comes from a multitude of uncontrolled intervention studies on weight reduction for women with PCOS, with patient numbers ranging from six to 143 and durations ranging from 1 week to over 1 year.[41] Most of these studies have employed various forms of dietary restriction with resultant weight reductions ranging from less than 5% to more than 15%. Following diet-induced weight loss, the following benefits have been described:

- a reduction in either total or free testosterone and androstenedione and, sometimes, adrenal androgens
- an increase, in the long term, in SHBG blood levels
- some clinically measurable improvements in hirsutism, particularly in long-term studies
- an improvement in menses and ovulation in all the studies reporting this endpoint
- the occurrence of spontaneous pregnancies, when investigated
- a significant metabolic improvement and some benefit in cardiovascular risk factors, including markers of low-grade inflammation.

Structured exercise as a fundamental lifestyle component can improve the efficacy, feasibility and sustainability of lifestyle treatment in women with PCOS[45,46] and can add benefits to the metabolic background regardless of weight loss and dietary advice.[47–49] However, very few studies have focused specifically on exercise. Two recent studies found a significant improvement in body weight and metabolic derangements and suggested that exercise alone may significantly improve insulin resistance and clinical outcomes in PCOS.[45,46]

Evidence of the effects of behavioural modification added to hypocaloric dieting and/or physical exercise are consistent with the same results, although this has not been widely investigated.[41]

There are currently controversies regarding lifestyle treatment of PCOS, particularly with respect to dietary macronutrient composition. We suggest that this may be irrelevant, since the same controversies have been raised over the past three decades about the treatment of obesity *per se*. The few available short-term studies on PCOS have failed to show any significant specific effect of different diets containing different amounts of carbohydrates, proteins and lipids. Generally speaking, it seems that energy restriction rather than diet composition is associated with some benefit, thus confirming the majority of studies performed in obesity in the past few decades.

Lifestyle treatment of PCOS can be combined with pharmacological anti-obesity treatment. Unfortunately, this has been performed in very few studies, in spite of the potential additional benefit achievable by anti-obesity agents, particularly in the long term. The available anti-obesity drugs are orlistat and sibutramine.[50] Over the past 15 years, a series of trials have shown that both drugs can produce a significantly higher and independent benefit compared with placebo in reducing body weight and waist circumference and in improving metabolic abnormalities, including those defining the metabolic syndrome.[50] Most importantly, they have also been shown to maintain weight loss and metabolic benefits in the long term in obese people both with and without diabetes.[50] The studies performed in overweight or obese women with PCOS substantially confirm what has been reported in simple obesity, although they have all been short-term studies. An additional and specific benefit achieved in some of these studies was a significant decrease in androgen blood concentrations.[41]

Metformin should not be considered a weight-loss compound, although its benefits in the treatment of PCOS have been clearly established. A comprehensive review by Palomba *et al.*[51] was published in 2009. Theoretically, it could be that long-term metformin use can even prevent further weight gain or the development of type 2 diabetes, as suggested by long-term trials performed in the general population.[52]

Given the disappointing results of diet-based approaches to the treatment of obesity, interest in bariatric surgery is increasing worldwide. A meta-analysis of the effects of bariatric surgery in more than 22 000 procedures found an average weight loss of more than 50%, associated with improvement or complete resolution of diabetes, hyperlipidaemia, hypertension and obstructive sleep apnoea in more than 60% of patients.[53] Most importantly, these data are supported by a large long-term prospective study confirming that weight loss and metabolic and cardiovascular benefits are achievable and that a significant decrease in all-cause mortality could be detected 10 years post-surgery.[54] An uncontrolled study assessing the effect of bariatric surgery in morbidly obese women with PCOS reported sustained weight loss and complete resolution of all features defining PCOS, including hirsutism, hyperandrogenism, menstrual irregularity, anovulation, insulin resistance and metabolic abnormalities.[55] In another small study examining gastric bypass in overweight women with PCOS, a 56.7% weight loss over 1 year improved menstrual cyclicity, hirsutism and natural conception.[56] This opens up new perspectives on the pathophysiological impact of obesity on PCOS.

Lifestyle modification and infertility

Preconceptional counselling in women with PCOS should identify risk factors for reproductive failure and correct them before initiation of treatment. Since obesity represents a potential negative factor for fertility, its treatment should always aim at improving the dysmetabolic–endocrine environment associated with PCOS, particularly when ART is planned. Weight loss is therefore recommended as the first-line therapy in obese women with PCOS seeking pregnancy. However, as reviewed by the 2007 Thessaloniki consensus conference,[5] there is a paucity of studies suggesting that weight loss before conception improves live birth rates in obese women with or without PCOS, although multiple observational studies have noted that weight loss is associated with improved spontaneous ovulation rates in women with PCOS, while pregnancies have been reported after losing as little as 5% of initial body weight.[5] To date, no properly designed studies to guide the choice of such interventions in overcoming infertility in women with PCOS have been carried out. In general, however, it is quite clear that lifestyle treatment, even in the short term, can significantly improve pregnancy rates and outcomes.

Any intervention with therapeutic lifestyle protocols (see previous paragraph) should be conducted before pregnancy, not concurrently with fertility treatment, until the risks and benefits of these therapies with respect to pregnancy are better understood. However, caution should be advised in conceiving during the use of unbalanced hypocaloric diets, excessive physical exertion or pharmacological intervention or during the period of rapid weight loss after bariatric surgery, since the effects of these interventions on the evolution of early pregnancy are not yet known.

Conclusion

PCOS is a highly prevalent endocrine disorder that is primarily characterised by a hyperandrogenic state and ovulatory disturbances and which is associated with multiple metabolic abnormalities and a high prevalence of excess weight or obesity, particularly of the abdominal phenotype. Recognition of the pathophysiological impact of obesity on PCOS offers a unique challenge from a therapeutic point of view; by treating obesity, the PCOS phenotype can be successfully improved and possibly eliminated.

Guidelines for the treatment of obesity can be applied, probably without any substantial specific changes, to the treatment of overweight and obese women with PCOS. Lifestyle intervention as a therapeutic approach for obesity associated with PCOS should be encouraged worldwide.

References

1. Azziz R, Carmina E, Dewailly D, Diamanti-Kandarakis E, Escobar-Morreale HF, Futterweit W, *et al*; Androgen Excess Society. Position statement: Criteria for defining polycystic ovary syndrome as a predominatly hyperandrogenic syndrome: an Androgen Excess Society guideline. *J Clin Endocrinol Metab* 2006;91:4237–45.
2. The Rotterdam ESHRE/ASRM-Sponsored PCOS consensus workshop group. Revised 2003 consensus on diagnostic criteria and long-term health risks related to polycystic ovary syndrome (PCOS). *Hum Reprod* 2004;19:41–7.
3. Ehrmann DA. Polycystic ovary syndrome. *N Engl J Med* 2005;352:1223–36.
4. Dunaif A. Insulin resistance and the polycystic ovary syndrome: mechanisms and implications for pathogenesis. *Endocr Rev* 1997;18:774–800.
5. Thessaloniki ESHRE/ASRM-Sponsored PCOS Consensus Workshop Group. Consensus on infertility treatment related to polycystic ovary syndrome. *Hum Reprod* 2008;23:462–77.
6. Norman RJ, Dewailly D, Legro RS, Hickey TE. Polycystic ovary syndrome. *Lancet* 2007;370:685–97.

7. Gambineri A, Pelusi C, Vicennati V, Pagotto, U, Pasquali R. Obesity and the polycystic ovary syndrome. *Int J Obes Rel Metab Dis* 2002;26:883–96.
8. Salley KE, Wickham EP, Cheang KI, Essah PA, Karjane NW, Nestler JE. Glucose intolerance in polycystic ovary syndrome – a position statement of the Androgen Excess Society. *J Clin Endocrinol Metab* 2007;92:4546–56.
9. Shaw LJ, Bairey, Merz CN, Stanczyk FZ, Sopko G, Braunstein GD, *et al.* Postmenopausal women with a history of irregular menses and elevated androgen measurements at high risk for worsening cardiovascular event-free survival: results from the National Institutes of Health–National Heart, Lung, and Blood Institute sponsored Women's Ischemia Syndrome Evaluation. *J Clin Endocrinol Metab* 2008;93:1276–84.
10. Pasquali R, Gambineri A, Pagotto U. The impact of obesity on reproduction in women with polycystic ovary syndrome. *BJOG* 2006;113:1148–59.
11. World Health Organization. *Obesity: Preventing and Managing the Global Epidemic.* Report on a WHO Consultation. Technical Report Series, No 894. Geneva: WHO/NUT/NCD; 1997.
12. Moran LJ, Pasquali R, Teede HJ, Hoeger KM, Norman RJ. Treatment of obesity in polycystic ovary syndrome: a position statement of the Androgen Excess and Polycystic Ovary Syndrome Society. *Fertil Steril* 2009;92:1966–82.
13. Pasquali R, Gambineri A. Targeting insulin sensitivity in the treatment of polycystic ovary syndrome. *Expert Opin Ther Targets* 2009;13:1205–26.
14. Haslan DW, James WP. Obesity. *Lancet* 2005;366:1197–209.
15. Pasquali R. Obesity and androgens: facts and perspectives. *Fertil Steril* 2006;85:1319–40.
16. Kirchengast S, Huber J. Body composition characteristics and body fat distribution in lean women with polycystic ovary syndrome. *Hum Reprod* 2001;16:1255–60.
17. Asuncion M, Calvo RM, San Millan JL, Sancho J, Avila S, Escobar-Morreale HF. A prospective study of the prevalence of the polycystic ovary syndrome in unselected Caucasian women from Spain. *J Clin Endocrinol Metab* 2000;85:2434–8.
18. Yildiz B, Krochenhauer ES, Azziz R. Impact of obesity on the risk for polycystic ovary syndrome. *J Clin Endocrinol Metab* 2007;93:162–8.
19. Yen SS. The polycystic ovary syndrome. *Clin Endocrinol (Oxf)* 1980;12:177–208.
20. Lake JK, Power C, Cole TJ. Women's reproductive health: the role of body mass index in early and adult life. *Int J Obes Rel Metab Dis* 1997;21:432–8.
21. Pasquali R, Gambineri A. Polycystic ovary syndrome: a multifaceted disease from adolescence to adult age. *Ann N Y Acad Sci* 2006;1092:158–74.
22. Apter D. Pubertal development in PCOS. In: Azziz R, Nestler JE, Dewailly D, editors. *Androgen Excess Disorders in Women.* Philadelphia: Lippincot-Raven; 1997. p. 327–38.
23. McCartney CR, Blank SK, Prendergast KA, Chhabra S, Eagleson CA, Helm KD, *et al.* Obesity and sex steroid changes across puberty: evidence for marked hyperandrogenemia in pre- and early pubertal obese girls. *J Clin Endocrinol Metab* 2007;92:430–6.
24. Venturoli S, Porcu E, Fabbri R, Magrini O, Gammi L, Paradisi R, *et al.* Longitudinal evaluation of the different gonadotropin pulsatile patterns in anovulatory cycles of young girls. *J Clin Endocrinol Metab* 1992;74:836–41.
25. Diamanti-Kandarakis E, Christakou C, Palioura E, Kandaraki E, Livadas S. Does polycystic ovary syndrome start in childhood? *Pediatr Endocrinol Rev* 2008;5:904–11.
26. Cresswell JL, Barker DJ, Osmond C, Egger P, Phillips DI, Fraser RB. Fetal growth, length of gestation, and polycystic ovaries in adult life. *Lancet* 1997;350:1131–5.
27. Nilsson C, Niklasson M, Eriksson E, Bjorntorp P, Holmang A. Imprinting of female offspring with testosterone results in insulin resistance and changes in body fat distribution of adult age in rats. *J Clin Invest* 1998;101:74–8.
28. Dumesic DA, Abbott DH, Padmanabhan V. Polycystic ovary syndrome and its developmental origins. *Rev Endocr Metab Disord* 2007;8:127–41.
29. Abbott DH, Tarantal AF, Dumesic DA. Fetal, infant, adolescent and adult phenotypes of polycystic ovary syndrome in prenatally androgenized female rhesus monkeys. *Am J Primatol* 2009;71:776–84.
30. de Zegher F, Lopez-Bermejo A, Ibáñez L. Adipose tissue expandability and the early origins of PCOS. *Trends Endocrinol Metab* 2009;20:418–23.

31. Poretsky L, Cataldo NA, Rosenwaks Z, Giudice LC. The insulin-related ovarian regulatory system in health and disease. *Endocr Rev* 1999;20:535–82.
32. Diamanti-Kandarakis E. Role of obesity and adiposity in polycystic ovary syndrome. *Int J Obes (Lond)* 2007;31 Suppl 2:S8–13.
33. Ek I, Arner P, Rydén M, Thörne A, Hoffstedt J, Wahrenberg H. A unique defect in the regulation of visceral fat cell lipolysis in the polycystic ovary syndrome as an early link to insulin resistance. *Diabetes* 2002;51:484–92.
34. Andrews RC, Walker BR. Glucocorticoids and insulin resistance: old hormones, new targets. *Clin Sci* 1999;51:513–23.
35. Pasquali R, Pelusi C, Genghini S, Cacciari M, Gambineri A. Obesity and reproductive disorders in women. *Hum Reprod Update* 2003;9:359–72.
36. Pasquali R, Patton L, Gambineri A. Obesity and infertility. *Curr Opin Endocrinol Diab Obes* 2007;14:482–7.
37. Tamer Erel C, Senturk LM. The impact of body mass index on assisted reproduction. *Curr Opin Obstet Gynecol* 2009;21:228–35.
38. Pasquali R, Gambineri A, Anconetani B, Vicennati V, Colitta D, Caramelli E, *et al.* The natural history of the metabolic syndrome in young women with the polycystic ovary syndrome and the long-term effect of oestrogen-progestagen treatment. *Clin Endocrinol (Oxf)* 1999;50:517–27.
39. Gambineri A, Repaci A, Patton L, Grassi I, Pocognoli P, Cognigni GE, *et al.* Prominent role of low HDL-cholesterol in explaining the high prevalence of the metabolic syndrome in polycystic ovary syndrome. *Nutr Metab Cardiovasc Dis* 2009:19:1–8.
40. Salley KE, Wickham EP, Cheang KI, Essah PA, Karjane NW, Nestler JE. Glucose intolerance in polycystic ovary syndrome – a position statement of the Androgen Excess Society. *J Clin Endocrinol Metab* 2007;92:4546–56.
41. Moran LJ, Brinkworth GD, Norman RJ. Dietary therapy in polycystic ovary syndrome. *Semin Reprod Med* 2008;26:85–92.
42. Clinical guidelines on the identification, evaluation, and treatment of overweight and obesity in adults: executive summary. Expert Panel on the Identification, Evaluation, and Treatment of Overweight in Adults. *Am J Clin Nutr* 1998;68:899–917.
43. National Health & Medical Research Council. *Clinical Practice Guidelines for the Management of Overweight and Obesity in Adults.* Canberra: Australian Government Publishing Service; 2003.
44. Wadden TA, Butryn ML. Behavioral treatment of obesity. *Endocrinol Metab Clin North Am* 2003;32:981–1003.
45. Vigorito C, Giallauria F, Palomba S, Cascella T, Manguso F, Lucci R, *et al.* Beneficial effects of a three-month structured exercise training program on cardiopulmonary functional capacity in young women with polycystic ovary syndrome. *J Clin Endocrinol Metab* 2007;92:1379–84.
46. Palomba S, Giallauria F, Falbo A, Russo T, Oppedisano R, Tolino A, *et al.* Structured exercise training programme versus hypocaloric hyperproteic diet in obese polycystic ovary syndrome patients with anovulatory infertility: a 24-week pilot study. *Hum Reprod* 2008;23:642–50.
47. Bruner B, Chad K, Chizen D. Effects of exercise and nutritional counseling in women with polycystic ovary syndrome. *Appl Physiol Nutr Metab* 2006;31:384–91.
48. Bruce CR, Kriketos AD, Cooney GJ, Hawley JA Disassociation of muscle triglyceride content and insulin sensitivity after exercise training in patients with type 2 diabetes. *Diabetologia* 2004;47:23–30.
49. O'Gorman DJ, Karlsson HK, McQuaid S, Yousif O, Rahman Y, Gasparro D, *et al.* Exercise training increases insulin-stimulated glucose disposal and GLUT4 (SLC2A4) protein content in patients with type 2 diabetes. *Diabetologia* 2006;49:2983–92.
50. Bray GA. Medical therapy for obesity – current status and future hopes. *Med Clin North Am* 2007;91:1225–53.
51. Palomba S, Falbo A, Zullo F, Orio F Jr. Evidence-based and potential benefits of metformin in the polycystic ovary syndrome: a comprehensive review. *Endocr Rev* 2009;30:1–50.
52. Knowler WC, Barrett-Connor E, Fowler SE, Hamman RF, Lachin JM, Walker EA, *et al*; Diabetes Prevention Program Research Group. Reduction in the incidence of type 2 diabetes with lifestyle intervention or metformin. *N Engl J Med* 2002;346:393–403.

53. Buchwald H, Avidor Y, Braunwald E, Jensen MD, Pories W, Fahrbach K, *et al.* Bariatric surgery: a systematic review and meta-analysis. *JAMA* 2004;292:1724–37.
54. Sjostrom L, Narbro K, Sjostrom CD, Karason K, Larsson B, Wedel H, *et al.* Effects of bariatric surgery on mortality in Swedish obese subjects. *N Engl J Med* 2007;357:741–52.
55. Escobar-Morreale HF, Botella-Carretero JI, Alvarez-Blasco F, Sancho J, San Millan JL. The polycystic ovary syndrome associated with morbid obesity may resolve after weight loss induced by bariatric surgery. *J Clin Endocrinol Metab* 2005;90:6364–9.
56. Eid GM, Cottam DR, Velcu LM, Mattar SG, Korytkowski MT, Gosman G, *et al.* Effective treatment of polycystic ovarian syndrome with Roux-en-Y gastric bypass. *Surg Obes Rel Dis* 2005;1:77–80.

Chapter 9
Management of obesity in polycystic ovary syndrome, including anti-obesity drugs and bariatric surgery

Alexander D Miras and Carel W le Roux

Introduction

The interaction between excess adiposity and disturbed female fertility is best represented by polycystic ovary syndrome (PCOS). This syndrome has been studied by both gynaecologists and endocrinologists as the mechanisms leading to its diverse manifestations are complex. PCOS is very common in the developed world, with up to 10% of premenopausal women being affected.[1–4] Clinically, PCOS is characterised by the development of hirsutism, oligo-ovulation/anovulation and subfertility/infertility. The pathophysiology of the syndrome, even though not yet fully delineated, implicates insulin resistance as a central factor as it leads to hyperinsulinaemia and androgen excess. High circulating insulin levels inhibit the production of sex hormone-binding globulin (SHBG) from the liver and directly cause excess androgen production at the level of the ovary. These two processes lead to the aesthetically troublesome hirsutism and contribute to irregular menses or even cause secondary amenorrhoea. However, it is even more worrying that women with PCOS are at increased risk of cardiovascular mortality and morbidity[5–7] owing to their occult disturbed metabolism, which shares features of the metabolic syndrome. These include impaired glucose tolerance and type 2 diabetes, hypertension, dyslipidaemia and increased waist circumference.[8–15]

Approximately 40% of women living in the developed world are obese or overweight.[16] The prevalence of obesity in women with PCOS varies widely, from 10% to 70% of cases.[17–19] Modest weight loss can, however, reverse many of the features of the syndrome and lower the cardiometabolic risk profile.[20–27]

This review focuses on the treatment of obesity in the context of PCOS with anti-obesity medication and obesity (bariatric) surgery. Metformin and rimonabant are not reviewed here as the former is an insulin sensitiser and its effects on weight reduction in women with PCOS have been discouraging[28,29] and the latter has been withdrawn from the market.

Lifestyle modification

Clark *et al.*[23] studied obese women with infertility before and after dietary changes and an exercise programme. The intervention group lost an average of 10.2 kg over a 6-month period. Ninety percent of these anovulatory women started ovulating spontaneously even after a moderate weight loss of 6.5 kg, compared with none from the group that dropped out from the intervention. Seventy-seven percent of the intervention group successfully conceived (32.7% spontaneously) and 67% achieved a live birth owing to a much lower miscarriage rate. The study group also reported an improvement in various psychological parameters including self-esteem and depression.

Holte *et al.*[21] investigated obese women with PCOS before and after 6 months of weight loss. The mean weight loss achieved was 12.4 kg, which is equivalent to a reduction of 3.7 kg/m^2 in body mass index (BMI) terms. Weight reduction by diet caused preferential reduction of truncal fat and significantly reduced insulin resistance as measured by the euglycaemic hyperinsulinaemic clamp technique to the level of a BMI-matched control group of women without PCOS. This result is in opposition to the theory that women with PCOS have an obesity-independent inherent disorder of insulin action. The authors suggested that subcutaneous fat causes insulin resistance as a result of the increased flux of free fatty acids to the liver and adipose tissues.[21] On the contrary, the early exaggerated insulin secretory response to intravenous glucose in women with PCOS did not change after weight loss, leading to the hypothesis that this is a primary abnormality of the syndrome and leads to higher carbohydrate intake and consequent weight gain. The same investigators reported a statistically significant decrease in serum testosterone and increase in SHBG.

Very low calorie diets in women with PCOS can lead to improvement in reproductive function even after 4–6 weeks and may also reduce hirsutism.[24] A possible mechanism may involve insulin-like growth factor-binding protein 1 (IGFBP-1), which is increased by such diets and leads to lower serum levels of insulin-like growth factor I (IGF-I) and reduced androgen production through the P450c17n system.[30] Maintenance of weight loss by a high-protein isocaloric energy-restricted diet resulted in a minor increase in the levels of high-density lipoprotein (HDL) cholesterol, a decrease in the area under the curve for glucose after a test meal and a decrease in free androgen index (FAI). Overall, the authors suggested that maximum caloric restriction is preferential for achieving conception while a high-protein maintenance diet results in borderline improvements in endocrine and metabolic parameters.

These results are supported by Huber-Buchholz *et al.*[20] Lifestyle modification intervention that set 'realistic' weight-loss targets of 5% for obese women with PCOS was used as opposed to short-term low-calorie diets that are not sustainable in the long term. Mean weight loss of only 2–5% facilitated a significant reduction in central adiposity (11%), serum luteinising hormone (39%) and fasting insulin levels (33%), contributing to the re-establishment of ovulation of half of the previously anovulatory women. The levels of free testosterone and SHBG did not change significantly after lifestyle modification and the authors did not supply an explanation for this. Similar lifestyle modifications cause improvement in lipid parameters, with a reduction in total cholesterol of 29%, triglycerides of 31% and fasting glucose of 6%.[22]

Anti-obesity medication

Orlistat

Orlistat has been used in clinical practice for more than 10 years. It is a gastric and pancreatic lipase inhibitor and reduces the dietary lipid absorption. A Cochrane review[31] has extensively examined the studies in which it has been used for the treatment of obesity. In trials of obese patients, orlistat causes 2.9% more weight loss compared with diet and lifestyle changes alone. BMI is reduced by an average of 1.1 kg/m^2. Orlistat has beneficial cardiometabolic effects, with a reduction of systolic blood pressure of 1.5 mmHg and total cholesterol of 0.32 mmol/litre and a reduction in the incidence of type 2 diabetes from 9.2% to 6.2%. Over 80% of patients receiving orlistat experience at least one gastrointestinal adverse effect such as diarrhoea, with 5% of patients discontinuing treatment owing to these effects. Levels of fat-soluble vitamins A, D and E and β-carotene can be lowered by orlistat treatment but with no significant clinical consequences.

Only three studies have been published so far on the effects of orlistat in women with PCOS. The first examined the effects of orlistat versus metformin administration for 3 months in a group of obese women with PCOS.[32] Dietary advice was given and the women were prescribed a weight-maintenance diet. After 12 weeks, orlistat treatment resulted in a 4.7% weight loss compared with 1.0% in the metformin group. In both groups, total testosterone decreased to similar degrees after treatment but there was no significant change in SHBG, fasting glucose or insulin resistance as measured by the homeostatic model assessment (HOMA) method. The authors suggested that these results can be explained by the small study sample ($n=21$) and the large variability in HOMA insulin resistance in women with PCOS. Owing to the small number of participants, the effects of treatment on menstrual regularity, ovulation, pregnancy rates and hirsutism were not studied.

In another study, orlistat was administered to two groups, one comprising obese women with PCOS and the other obese women without PCOS.[33] The medication was given together with an energy-restricted diet in both groups for a total of 24 weeks. The effects of diet and orlistat were similar on BMI (reduction of 6 kg/m^2) and waist circumference (reduction of 14 cm) in both groups and reached statistical significance. Contrary to the earlier trial, insulin resistance decreased significantly in the first 12 weeks of treatment in both groups, but there was no difference between groups at the end of the study, possibly as a result of the high variability of HOMA insulin resistance. Total testosterone and FAI levels significantly decreased in the PCOS but not the control group and again the main changes were observed in the first trimester of intervention. SHBG levels increased only in the first trimester in the PCOS group compared with a consistent increase in the control group throughout the treatment period. It is hypothesised that women with PCOS have an inherent pathological ovarian dysfunction causing hyperandrogenaemia independently of weight changes. Again, markers of menstrual function and hirsutism were not studied in this trial.

The last study compared the effects of 12 weeks of metformin, orlistat and pioglitazone treatment on the biological variability of insulin resistance in obese women with PCOS.[34] This trial was performed as insulin resistance variability is very wide in women with PCOS. Overall, insulin resistance was reduced most markedly by pioglitazone, followed by orlistat and metformin, while insulin resistance variability was decreased more by orlistat, followed by pioglitazone and metformin. All treatments significantly reduced the FAI.

Sibutramine

Sibutramine is a centrally acting serotonin and noradrenaline re-uptake inhibitor that promotes weight loss by enhancing satiety. It was initially developed as an antidepressant agent but its effects on mood were disappointing. Based on a Cochrane meta-analysis,[31] patients on sibutramine lose on average 4.3% more weight compared with placebo. The BMI decrease is of the order of 1.5 kg/m^2 and the reduction in waist circumference 4.0 cm. The effects of sibutramine on glycaemia have been inconsistent and in most studies not dissimilar to those of placebo. Mild improvements in lipid parameters have been shown, with an increase in HDL cholesterol of 0.04 mmol/litre and a reduction in triglycerides of 0.18 mmol/litre. Sibutramine can lead to increases in blood pressure and heart rate in some patients before weight loss takes place. Patients on sibutramine should thus be monitored after initiation. However, it can be argued that this potential increase in blood pressure would be offset by the weight loss, which leads to impressive blood pressure reductions.[35–37] The most commonly reported adverse effects of the drug include insomnia, nausea and constipation.

Three studies have been published on the effects of sibutramine treatment on women with PCOS. The first, in 2003, recruited 40 obese women with PCOS and randomised them to sibutramine only, to ethinylestradiol and cyproterone acetate, and to a combination of all three medications for 6 months in addition to a 1200 kcal per day diet.[38] The sibutramine group exhibited significant improvements in weight with an impressive 14.4 kg loss and even reductions in diastolic blood pressure (3 mmHg) compared with baseline. Additionally, metabolic parameters improved, including serum triglycerides and area under the curve for both glucose and insulin following a standard oral glucose tolerance test. Hirsutism score improvement, free serum testosterone reduction and SHBG increases following 6 months of sibutramine were similar to those in the ethinylestradiol and cyproterone group. There were no major adverse metabolic effects in the oral contraceptive group, probably because all women were on a hypocaloric diet and lost weight. However, serum triglycerides were increased, a finding that is consistent with previous literature and warrants caution when using these agents. The combination of all three agents resulted in even greater improvements in hyperandrogenaemia and hirsutism but these did not reach statistical significance.

The second study recruited 84 obese women with PCOS and randomised them to a 600 kcal per day deficient diet and to sibutramine plus diet for 6 months.[39] At the end of the study, the percentage weight loss in the sibutramine and diet group was greater than that in the diet-only group (15.4% versus 11.1%). The combination of anti-obesity medication and diet resulted in greater improvements in hyperandrogenaemia (FAI reduction of 29.7% versus 2.7%) and insulin sensitivity (examined by the area under the curve of an oral glucose tolerance test) compared with diet alone. Again, reductions in blood pressure were noted in the sibutramine group compared with baseline, reinforcing the concept that weight loss may offset the possible rise in blood pressure. The authors suggested that the improvements in insulin sensitivity cannot be explained by weight loss alone and that reductions of FAI and serum triglycerides contribute via a separate mechanism.

The most recent study yielded similar results.[40] Forty-two women with PCOS were randomised to sibutramine 15 mg daily (a higher dose than previous studies, which used 10 mg) and placebo for 6 months. All participants received lifestyle modification advice, including reductions in dietary fat and an increase in physical activity monitored by a step counter. The sibutramine group lost significantly more weight compared with the placebo group (7.8 kg versus 2.8 kg) and exhibited significant reductions in serum triglycerides, FAI and cystatin C, which is a marker of glomerular filtration rate and cardiovascular disease. More importantly, menstrual frequency, an indirect measurement of ovulation, increased in both groups. Contrary to previous studies, sibutramine did not have beneficial effects on blood pressure or insulin sensitivity, even after weight loss, for reasons that are not clear. Even though no adverse effects on the fetus have been observed after sibutramine use in the first trimester,[41] it is recommended that effective contraception should be used as menstruation can resume unexpectedly even after minimal weight loss.

Bariatric surgery

Background

The traditional weight-reduction therapies involving hypocaloric diets and exercise are effective in the short term and can deliver a maximum of 7% weight loss.[42] Unfortunately, the vast majority of obese patients regain this weight within a year and only 20% of them can maintain the weight loss for longer periods.[43,44] The use of anti-obesity medication is of great assistance in these weight-reduction efforts but, should the drug be discontinued, weight is regained.[42,45] Lay people and even members of the medical profession perceive this failure of lifestyle modification to represent lack of 'moral fibre' in this group of patients, which leads to dismissal of their enormous efforts. Patients are told repeatedly to try harder and harder when this is exactly what they are doing.

Over the past few decades, researchers in the field of obesity have described gut hormones and central nervous system pathways that are activated in the presence of weight loss and resist it in an attempt to reach weight homeostasis in a traditional metabolic feedback loop mechanism. From a historical point of view, this mechanism has saved the human species during periods of famine and, being evolutionarily successful, has been robustly adopted by human physiology.

Bariatric surgery facilitates an average of 15–35% weight loss, depending on the procedure used.[46] It is the most successful weight-loss modality to date in terms of long-term efficacy, with the majority of the weight loss maintained for at least 15 years.[47,48] Immediately postoperatively, the common associated comorbidity of type 2 diabetes is impressively either cured or at least ameliorated, something that has led to the concept of 'metabolic surgery'. In the longer term, bariatric surgery results in improvements in hypertension, hyperlipidaemia and lung function, and reductions in cancer risk and overall mortality.[47,48]

Bariatric procedures were first developed in the mid-1950s[49–51] and over the past 6 decades have undergone numerous modifications, while new ones are being developed and perfected. The priority is to make them as safe as possible and less disruptive to human anatomy thus causing fewer postoperative nutritional deficiencies and complications while simultaneously achieving maximum weight loss.

Historically, and from a surgical point of view, these procedures were divided into restrictive, malabsorptive or combinative even though this classification does not correspond to the mechanism by which weight loss is facilitated.

Restrictive procedures include gastric banding, sleeve gastrectomy and horizontal or vertical banded gastroplasty. Banded gastroplasty is no longer performed. Gastric banding involves the creation of a small gastric pouch after placement of an adjustable silastic band below the cardia of the stomach that is attached to a subcutaneous port that allows for adjustments of its volume, thus creating pressure on the gastric tissue. Sleeve gastrectomy involves an 80% vertical gastric resection, leaving a stomach with a volume of 50–200 ml. It can be used as the first-stage surgical procedure before a biliopancreatic bypass in high-risk very obese patients or even as a single procedure with few adverse effects and significant weight-loss efficacy. The procedure is relatively recent and some authors have suggested caution until longer term data become available. The gastroplasties were used mainly in the 1990s and partitions of the stomach were formed after vertical or horizontal stapling. All these procedures can be performed laparoscopically with fewer perioperative complications and reduced inpatient stays than when performed by laparotomy.

The so-called purely malabsorptive or bypass procedures include the jejuno-ileal and duodenojejunal bypass and the biliopancreatic diversion. The jejuno-ileal bypass has largely been abandoned owing to the development of liver cirrhosis and nutritional complications. Biliopancreatic diversion was developed in the 1970s and consists of a partial gastrectomy and anastomosis of the gastric pouch with the distal small intestine. The bypassed small intestine is anastomosed to the alimentary limb 50 cm proximal to the ileocaecal valve. More recently, a modification has occurred as, following a sleeve gastrectomy with preservation of the antrum, pylorus and short segment of the duodenum, a 'duodenal switch-biliopancreatic diversion' can be performed. This kind of surgery attempts to decrease nutrient absorption by excluding food from various parts of the gastrointestinal tract.

Finally, the combinative procedure that is currently considered by many to be the gold standard in bariatric surgery is the Roux-en-Y gastric bypass. Via a laparoscopic approach, a gastric pouch of 30 ml is created and anastomosed to the jejunum. The excluded biliary limb is anastomosed to the alimentary limb at a distal segment of the jejunum to form a jejuno-jejunostomy.

The mechanism by which the bypass procedures cause weight loss and resolution of associated comorbidities is not yet fully understood but gastric restriction and malabsorption seem to play less of a role than initially thought. Alternative mechanisms include alteration in the levels of enteral hormones, changes in energy expenditure and even changes in food preferences and taste perception in the central nervous system.[52–59]

The National Institute for Health and Clinical Excellence (NICE) recommends that bariatric surgery is an option for patients with a BMI of more than 40 kg/m^2 or for patients with a BMI of more than 35 kg/m^2 with significant comorbidities in whom medical and drug treatment has failed. Similar criteria are used by other international societies and institutes.

Bariatric surgery and PCOS

The effects of bariatric surgery on the various aspects of PCOS have only been investigated in a handful of studies. In 1981, obese women who had undergone jejuno-ileal bypass between 1969 and 1976 were studied and the results were rather disappointing as libido was decreased in 60% of the women, probably as a result of electrolyte imbalance and depression postoperatively.[60] However, surgery increased the number of women with normal menstrual patterns from 25 preoperatively to 34 postoperatively, out of the 38 who took part in the trial. This led to increased rates of pregnancy but reduced mean weight and length of the infants compared with previous pregnancies. This was thought to be a risk factor for fetal outcomes even though these were not studied in the long term. Women were advised to delay pregnancy for at least 1–2 years, especially if they had electrolyte imbalance, malnutrition or vitamin deficiencies.

Another study, in 1988, investigated the effects of jejuno-ileal bypass and horizontal and vertical banded gastroplasty in 138 obese women without specifying their PCOS diagnosis.[61] Even though the results were not broken down by procedure, bariatric surgery normalised the menstrual cycles of 104 of the 109 premenopausal women. No change in hirsutism was observed. All nine women who tried to conceive after their surgery were successful and seven of them had nine normal births while the other two miscarried. The rates of gestational diabetes, pre-eclampsia and venous thromboembolism were reduced to 0% after surgery. All nine deliveries were vaginal, with none of the women requiring caesarean section. Overall, these results were very promising, although there was no mention of management of electrolyte imbalances or other complications following surgery.

Bastounis *et al.*[62] recruited 38 obese women in Greece. They all underwent vertical banded gastroplasty. Unfortunately, women with PCOS were excluded from the study. Following a mean weight loss of 70 ± 10 kg, the women exhibited statistically significant reductions in free testosterone, androstenedione, and fasting glucose and insulin. SHBG almost doubled postoperatively.

Only since 2005 have studies been performed exclusively in women with PCOS. The first study retrospectively studied 24 women with PCOS.[63] They had all undergone gastric bypass and were followed for at least 1 year. Their mean BMI decreased from 50 ± 7.5 kg/m^2 to 30 ± 4.5 kg/m^2 after surgery. This led to a 75% rate of moderate to complete resolution of hirsutism and 100% resolution of menstrual abnormalities within 3.4 ± 2.1 months of their surgery. The five women who wished to conceive were successful without any additional fertility treatment. Unfortunately, the authors did not obtain any hormonal data from these women. They also did not mention how hirsutism was quantified, explain the nature of the menstrual abnormalities or discuss any complication of surgery in terms of malabsorption/electrolyte disturbances. Even so, the results were very encouraging and were the first to provide evidence for the use of gastric bypass in the treatment of obesity and associated gynaecological disturbances in women with PCOS.

A more comprehensive trial prospectively studied obese women with and without a formal diagnosis of PCOS who underwent either biliopancreatic diversion or gastric bypass.[64] Menstrual cycles were restored postoperatively in all 12 of the women with PCOS and this was associated with serum progesterone concentrations above 4 ng/ml in the luteal phase, confirming ovulation. The mean weight loss of 41 ± 9 kg was paralleled by statistically significant reductions and normalisation of total and free testosterone, androstenedione and dehydroepiandrosterone sulfate and significant increases in SHBG. Hirsutism as measured by the modified Ferriman-Gallwey score was also significantly reduced. The authors concluded that the diagnosis of PCOS could no longer be sustained in all 12 women postoperatively. Additionally, insulin resistance measured by fasting insulin and HOMA values that was present only in the obese women with PCOS and not in the other obese female groups decreased to the reference range for the lean premenopausal population. However, it would have been helpful if the authors had provided the exact mean values and standard deviations of the measured parameters, both pre- and postoperatively.

These results were further supported by the data from a survey of women who underwent mainly gastric bypass surgery at the University of Pennsylvania.[65] Of the 195 responders, 98 reported having had abnormal menstrual cycles before their surgery. After surgery and a mean reduction in BMI of 40%, 70 of these women regained normal menstrual cycles while the other 28 continued to experience oligomenorrhoea/amenorrhoea. Impressively, menstruation restarted on average 1.6 months postoperatively, before maximal weight loss. This study, while useful because of the large number of responders, did not report hormone data and may also suffer from selection and recall bias, which are common pitfalls of survey-based research.

Pregnancy after bariatric surgery

It is important to guide women who undergo bariatric surgery for weight loss and fertility through a successful pregnancy, especially as ovulation is restored within just a few months postoperatively and often suddenly and unexpectedly. Three reviews have recently critically analysed the data from case–control and cohort studies of pregnancy after bariatric surgery.[66–68]

Even though no trials have assessed the efficacy of the oral contraceptive pill after bariatric surgery, there are concerns regarding its absorption. Women of reproductive age should thus be advised to use additional contraceptive methods to avoid an undesired conception.

The data from case–control and cohort studies suggest that, after bariatric surgery, women have a lower rate of pre-eclampsia, gestational diabetes and macrosomic babies after successful pregnancies. These benefits are counterbalanced by higher rates of intrauterine growth restriction and a persistently high risk of caesarean section. Even though the results are not consistent, there appears also to be a benefit with regard to neonatal complications, including preterm birth.

Monitoring for nutritional deficiencies is crucial. The available studies suggest that these are uncommon but could potentially lead to fetal complications including neonatal hypocalcaemia, mental developmental delay, neural tube defects, low birth weight and preterm birth. There are no commonly agreed guidelines for the management of nutrition during pregnancy in women after bariatric surgery. Most centres recommend monitoring of iron, vitamin B_{12}, folate, calcium and soluble vitamin levels and adequate replacement according to the type of bariatric surgery undergone previously.

Maternal complications such as bowel obstruction due to internal hernias, gastric ulceration and staple line stricture are rare but have been reported. In these cases, the bariatric surgeon is asked to work closely with the obstetrician and to have a low threshold for computed tomography imaging and surgical exploration, as bowel obstruction can lead to maternal and fetal morbidity and mortality.

The timing of conception after surgery is another controversial issue. Most centres recommend delaying this for at least 12–24 months after bariatric surgery. There are no robust data to support this recommendation. While the rates of miscarriage and preterm birth are higher in pregnancies within 1 year after surgery, there are numerous successful pregnancies within 1–2 years of surgery.

Larger randomised clinical trials (where possible) and prospective cohort studies are necessary to provide more robust evidence and to shape guidelines for the management of pregnancy in women who have previously undergone bariatric surgery. In the meantime, the chances for a safe pregnancy are increased in the hands of a multidisciplinary team with close cooperation between the bariatric surgeon, obstetrician, endocrinologist, dietician and midwife.

Conclusion

Obesity and its consequences for female health are clinically obvious in the context of PCOS. Treatment of the obesity *per se* can reverse the gynaecological comorbidities of the syndrome. Diet and increased levels of physical activity are crucial first steps in the management of obesity but are not sustainable in the long term. The use of anti-obesity medication as an adjunct to lifestyle modification has yielded reasonable results in terms of weight loss and improvement in hirsutism and infertility. The most effective treatment of obesity in women with PCOS, based on the limited data available, appears to be bariatric surgery, which results in resolution of all of the syndrome's parameters. Further studies should be conducted before PCOS in the context of obesity is introduced as a new indication for bariatric surgery. The management of pregnancies in women following bariatric surgery should be conducted by a specialist multidisciplinary team, and recommendations ought to be robust and based on more comprehensive trials focusing on nutritional support, timing of conception and the management of complications in this high-risk group of women.

References

1. Franks S. Polycystic ovary syndrome. *N Engl J Med* 1995;28;333:853–61.
2. Dunaif A. Insulin resistance and the polycystic ovary syndrome: mechanism and implications for pathogenesis. *Endocr Rev* 1997;18:774–800.
3. Knochenhauer ES, Key TJ, Kahsar-Miller M, Waggoner W, Boots LR, Azziz R. Prevalence of the polycystic ovary syndrome in unselected black and white women of the southeastern United States: a prospective study. *J Clin Endocrinol Metab* 1998;83:3078–82.
4. Asunción M, Calvo RM, San Millán JL, Sancho J, Avila S, Escobar-Morreale HF. A prospective study of the prevalence of the polycystic ovary syndrome in unselected Caucasian women from Spain. *J Clin Endocrinol Metab* 2000;85:2434–8.
5. Lakhani K, Constantinovici N, Purcell WM, Fernando R, Hardiman P. Internal carotid-artery response to 5% carbon dioxide in women with polycystic ovaries. *Lancet* 2000;30:356:1166–7.
6. Lakhani K, Seifalian AM, Hardiman P. Impaired carotid viscoelastic properties in women with polycystic ovaries. *Circulation* 2002;2:106:81–5.
7. Macut D, Micić D, Cvijović G, Sumarac M, Kendereski A, Zorić S, *et al.* Cardiovascular risk in adolescent and young adult obese females with polycystic ovary syndrome (PCOS). *J Pediatr Endocrinol Metab* 2001;14 Suppl 5:1353–9.
8. Dahlgren E, Johansson S, Lindstedt G, Knutsson F, Odén A, Janson PO, Mattson LA, *et al.* Women with polycystic ovary syndrome wedge resected in 1956 to 1965: a long-term follow-up focusing on natural history and circulating hormones. *Fertil Steril* 1992;57:505–13.
9. Ehrmann DA, Barnes RB, Rosenfield RL, Cavaghan MK, Imperial J. Prevalence of impaired glucose tolerance and diabetes in women with polycystic ovary syndrome. *Diabetes Care* 1999;22:141–6.
10. Legro RS, Kunselman AR, Dodson WC, Dunaif A. Prevalence and predictors of risk for type 2 diabetes mellitus and impaired glucose tolerance in polycystic ovary syndrome: a prospective, controlled study in 254 affected women. *J Clin Endocrinol Metab* 1999;84:165–9.
11. Pasquali R, Casimirri F. The impact of obesity on hyperandrogenism and polycystic ovary syndrome in premenopausal women. *Clin Endocrinol (Oxf)* 1993;39:1–16.
12. Holte J, Bergh T, Berne C, Lithell H. Serum lipoprotein lipid profile in women with the polycystic ovary syndrome: relation to anthropometric, endocrine and metabolic variables. *Clin Endocrinol (Oxf)* 1994;41:463–71.
13. Robinson S, Henderson AD, Gelding SV, Kiddy D, Niththyananthan R, Bush A, *et al.* Dyslipidaemia is associated with insulin resistance in women with polycystic ovaries. *Clin Endocrinol (Oxf)* 1996;44:277–84.
14. Wild RA, Painter PC, Coulson PB, Carruth KB, Ranney GB. Lipoprotein lipid concentrations and cardiovascular risk in women with polycystic ovary syndrome. *J Clin Endocrinol Metab* 1985;61:946–51.
15. Holte J, Gennarelli G, Berne C, Bergh T, Lithell H.Elevated ambulatory day-time blood pressure in women with polycystic ovary syndrome: a sign of a pre-hypertensive state? *Hum Reprod* 1996;11:23–8.
16. Wickelgren I. Obesity: how big a problem? *Science* 1998;280:1364–7.
17. Balen AH, Conway GS, Kaltsas G, Techatrasak K, Manning PJ, West C, *et al.* Polycystic ovary syndrome: the spectrum of the disorder in 1741 patients. *Hum Reprod* 1995;10:2107–11.
18. Legro RS. The genetics of obesity. Lessons for polycystic ovary syndrome. *Ann N Y Acad Sci* 2000;900:193–202.
19. Ehrmann DA. Polycystic ovary syndrome. *N Engl J Med* 2005;352:1223–36.
20. Huber-Buchholz MM, Carey DG, Norman RJ. Restoration of reproductive potential by lifestyle modification in obese polycystic ovary syndrome: role of insulin sensitivity and luteinizing hormone. *J Clin Endocrinol Metab* 1999;84:1470–4.

21. Holte J, Bergh T, Berne C, Wide L, Lithell H. Restored insulin sensitivity but persistently increased early insulin secretion after weight loss in obese women with polycystic ovary syndrome. *J Clin Endocrinol Metab* 1995;80:2586–93.
22. Andersen P, Seljeflot I, Abdelnoor M, Arnesen H, Dale PO, Løvik A, *et al.* Increased insulin sensitivity and fibrinolytic capacity after dietary intervention in obese women with polycystic ovary syndrome. *Metabolism* 1995;44:611–16.
23. Clark AM, Thornley B, Tomlinson L, Galletley C, Norman RJ. Weight loss in obese infertile women results in improvement in reproductive outcome for all forms of fertility treatment. *Hum Reprod* 1998;13:1502–5.
24. Moran LJ, Noakes M, Clifton PM, Tomlinson L, Galletly C, Norman RJ. Dietary composition in restoring reproductive and metabolic physiology in overweight women with polycystic ovary syndrome. *J Clin Endocrinol Metab* 2003;88:812–19.
25. Norman RJ, Davies MJ, Lord J, Moran LJ. The role of lifestyle modification in polycystic ovary syndrome. *Trends Endocrinol Metab* 2002;13:251–7.
26. Harlass FE, Plymate SR, Fariss BL, Belts RP. Weight loss is associated with correction of gonadotropin and sex steroid abnormalities in the obese anovulatory female. *Fertil Steril* 1984;42:649–52.
27. Kiddy DS, Hamilton-Fairley D, Bush A, Short F, Anyaoku V, Reed MJ, *et al.* Improvement in endocrine and ovarian function during dietary treatment of obese women with polycystic ovary syndrome. *Clin Endocrinol (Oxf)* 1992;36:105–11.
28. Tang T, Glanville J, Hayden CJ, White D, Barth JH, Balen AH. Combined lifestyle modification and metformin in obese patients with polycystic ovary syndrome. A randomized, placebo-controlled, double-blind multicentre study. *Hum Reprod* 2006;21:80–9.
29. Lord JM, Flight IH, Norman RJ. Insulin-sensitising drugs (metformin, troglitazone, rosiglitazone, pioglitazone, D-chiro-inositol) for polycystic ovary syndrome. *Cochrane Database Syst Rev* 2003;(3):CD003053.
30. Poretsky L, Cataldo NA, Rosenwaks Z, Giudice LC. The insulin-related ovarian regulatory system in health and disease. *Endocr Rev* 1999;20:535–82.
31. Padwal R, Li SK, Lau DC. Long-term pharmacotherapy for obesity and overweight. *Cochrane Database Syst Rev* 2004;(3):CD004094.
32. Jayagopal V, Kilpatrick ES, Holding S, Jennings PE, Atkin SL. Orlistat is as beneficial as metformin in the treatment of polycystic ovarian syndrome. *J Clin Endocrinol Metab* 2005;90:729–33.
33. Panidis D, Farmakiotis D, Rousso D, Kourtis A, Katsikis I, Krassas G. Obesity, weight loss, and the polycystic ovary syndrome: effect of treatment with diet and orlistat for 24 weeks on insulin resistance and androgen levels. *Fertil Steril* 2008;89:899–906.
34. Cho LW, Kilpatrick ES, Keevil BG, Coady AM, Atkin SL. Effect of metformin, orlistat and pioglitazone treatment on mean insulin resistance and its biological variability in polycystic ovary syndrome. *Clin Endocrinol (Oxf)* 2009;70:233–7.
35. Jordan J, Scholze J, Matiba B, Wirth A, Hauner H, Sharma AM. Influence of Sibutramine on blood pressure: evidence from placebo-controlled trials. *Int J Obes (Lond)* 2005;29:509–16.
36. Hazenberg BP. Randomized, double-blind, placebo-controlled, multicenter study of sibutramine in obese hypertensive patients. *Cardiology* 2000;94:152–8.
37. Kim SH, Lee YM, Jee SH, Nam CM. Effect of sibutramine on weight loss and blood pressure: a meta-analysis of controlled trials. *Obes Res* 2003;11:1116–23.
38. Sabuncu T, Harma M, Harma M, Nazligul Y, Kilic F. Sibutramine has a positive effect on clinical and metabolic parameters in obese patients with polycystic ovary syndrome. *Fertil Steril* 2003;80:1199–204.
39. Florakis D, Diamanti-Kandarakis E, Katsikis I, Nassis GP, Karkanaki A, Georgopoulos N, *et al.* Effect of hypocaloric diet plus sibutramine treatment on hormonal and metabolic features in overweight and obese women with polycystic ovary syndrome: a randomized, 24-week study. *Int J Obes (Lond)* 2008;32:692–9.
40. Lindholm A, Bixo M, Björn I, Wölner-Hanssen P, Eliasson M, Larsson A, *et al.* Effect of sibutramine on weight reduction in women with polycystic ovary syndrome: a randomized, double-blind, placebo-controlled trial. *Fertil Steril* 2008;89:1221–8.
41. De Santis M, Straface G, Cavaliere AF, Carducci B, Caruso A. Early first-trimester sibutramine exposure : pregnancy outcome and neonatal follow-up. *Drug Saf* 2006;29:255–9.

42. Bray GA. Lifestyle and pharmacological approaches to weight loss: efficacy and safety. *J Clin Endocrinol Metab* 2008;93(11 Suppl 1):S81–8.
43. McGuire MT, Wing RR, Hill JO. The prevalence of weight loss maintenance among American adults. *Int J Obes Relat Metab Disord* 1999;23:1314–19.
44. Wing RR, Hill JO. Successful weight loss maintenance. *Annu Rev Nutr* 2001;21:323–41.
45. Yanovski SZ, Yanovski JA. Obesity. *N Engl J Med* 2002;346:591–602.
46. Cummings DE, Overduin J, Foster-Schubert KE. Gastric bypass for obesity: mechanisms of weight loss and diabetes resolution. *J Clin Endocrinol Metab* 2004;89:2608–15.
47. Maggard MA, Shugarman LR, Suttorp M, Maglione M, Sugerman HJ, Livingston EH, *et al.* Meta-analysis: surgical treatment of obesity. *Ann Intern Med* 2005;142:547–59.
48. Sjöström L, Lindroos AK, Peltonen M, Torgerson J, Bouchard C, Carlsson B, *et al*; Swedish Obese Subjects Study Scientific Group. Lifestyle, diabetes, and cardiovascular risk factors 10 years after bariatric surgery. *N Engl J Med* 2004;351:2683–93.
49. Buchwald H, Varco RL. Ileal bypass in lowering high cholesterol levels. *Surg Forum* 1964;15:289–91.
50. Kremen AJ, Linner JH, Nelson CH. An experimental evaluation of the nutritional importance of proximal and distal small intestine. *Ann Surg* 1954;140:439–48.
51. Pories WJ. Bariatric surgery: risks and rewards. *J Clin Endocrinol Metab* 2008;93(11 Suppl 1):S89–96.
52. Halmi KA, Mason E, Falk JR, Stunkard A. Appetitive behavior after gastric bypass for obesity. *Int J Obes* 1981;5:457–64.
53. Brown EK, Settle EA, Van Rij AM. Food intake patterns of gastric bypass patients. *J Am Diet Assoc* 1982;80:437–43.
54. Kenler HA, Brolin RE, Cody RP. Changes in eating behavior after horizontal gastroplasty and Roux-en-Y gastric bypass. *Am J Clin Nutr* 1990;52:87–92.
55. Sugerman HJ, Starkey JV, Birkenhauer R.A randomized prospective trial of gastric bypass versus vertical banded gastroplasty for morbid obesity and their effects on sweets versus non-sweets eaters. *Ann Surg* 1987;205:613–24.
56. Olbers T, Björkman S, Lindroos A, Maleckas A, Lönn L, Sjöström L, *et al.* Body composition, dietary intake, and energy expenditure after laparoscopic Roux-en-Y gastric bypass and laparoscopic vertical banded gastroplasty: a randomized clinical trial. *Ann Surg* 2006;244:715–22.
57. Morínigo R, Moizé V, Musri M, Lacy AM, Navarro S, Marín JL, *et al.* Glucagon-Like peptide 1, peptide YY, hunger, and satiety after gastric bypass surgery on morbidly obese subjects. *J Clin Endocrinol Metab* 2006;91:1735–40.
58. le Roux CW, Aylwin SJ, Batterham RL, Borg CM, Coyle F, Prasad V, *et al.* Gut hormone profiles following bariatric surgery favor an anorectic state, facilitate weight loss, and improve metabolic parameters. *Ann Surg* 2006;243:108–14.
59. Miras AD, le Roux CW. Bariatric surgery and taste: novel mechanisms of weight loss. *Curr Opin Gastroenterol* 2010;26:140–5.
60. Hey H, Niebuhr-Jørgensen U. Jejuno-ileal bypass surgery in obesity. Gynecological and obstetrical aspects. *Acta Obstet Gynecol Scand* 1981;60:135–40.
61. Deitel M, Stone E, Kassam HA, Wilk EJ, Sutherland DJ. Gynecologic-obstetric changes after loss of massive excess weight following bariatric surgery. *J Am Coll Nutr* 1988;7:147–53.
62. Bastounis EA, Karayiannakis AJ, Syrigos K, Zbar A, Makri GG, Alexiou D. Sex hormone changes in morbidly obese patients after vertical banded gastroplasty. *Eur Surg Res* 1998;30:43–7.
63. Eid GM, Cottam DR, Velcu LM, Mattar SG, Korytkowski MT, Gosman G, *et al.* Effective treatment of polycystic ovarian syndrome with Roux-en-Y gastric bypass. *Surg Obes Relat Dis* 2005;1:77–80.
64. Escobar-Morreale HF, Botella-Carretero JI, Alvarez-Blasco F, Sancho J, San Millán JL. The polycystic ovary syndrome associated with morbid obesity may resolve after weight loss induced by bariatric surgery. *J Clin Endocrinol Metab* 2005;90:6364–9.
65. Teitelman M, Grotegut CA, Williams NN, Lewis JD. The impact of bariatric surgery on menstrual patterns. *Obes Surg* 2006;16:1457–63.
66. Beard JH, Bell RL, Duffy AJ. Reproductive considerations and pregnancy after bariatric surgery: current evidence and recommendations. *Obes Surg* 2008;18:1023–7.
67. Maggard MA, Yermilov I, Li Z, Maglione M, Newberry S, Suttorp M, *et al.* Pregnancy and fertility following bariatric surgery: a systematic review. *JAMA* 2008;300:2286–96.
68. Guelinckx I, Devlieger R, Vansant G. Reproductive outcome after bariatric surgery: a critical review. *Hum Reprod Update* 2009;15:189–201.

10

Chapter 10

Definition of hyperandrogenism

Julian H Barth, Helen P Field, Ephia Yasmin and Adam Balen

The definition of polycystic ovary syndrome (PCOS) has been based on a combination of three characteristics ever since Stein and Leventhal described the first cases in 1935.[1] At that time, no methods for serum androgen measurement were available and the disorder was based on enlarged polycystic ovaries, acne, hirsutism and amenorrhoea. Since then, there have been numerous attempts at defining the syndrome, all of which have attempted to be as inclusive as possible of the myriad of phenotypes that comprise PCOS. There have been three formal definitions over the past two decades that have proposed a combination of clinical, biochemical and imaging criteria[2–4] (see Table 10.1) but these, as we have argued in the past,[5] are still too vague to pin down the syndrome.

Hyperandrogenism in the context of PCOS is a term used loosely to encompass both the clinical features of acne, hirsuties and androgenic alopecia and the laboratory evidence of hyperandrogenaemia. The clinical features are due to androgenic stimulation of the cutaneous pilosebaceous unit but the nature of acne, hirsuties and balding demonstrates that, even within an individual, the response is heterogeneous, so wide variations between women can only be expected and this defies an easy definition. The problem with hyperandrogenaemia is no easier: which androgen(s) should be measured, how often should it/they be measured and when in the menstrual cycle. There also remains the confusion created by the imprecise use of the terms hyperandrogenism and hyperandrogenaemia.

Table 10.1 Criteria for the diagnosis of polycystic ovary syndrome

Organisation	Diagnostic criteria
National Institutes of Health (NIH), 1990	To include all of the following: 1. hyperandrogenism and/or hyperandrogenaemia 2. oligo-ovulation 3. exclusion of related disorders
European Society of Human Reproduction and Embryology (ESHRE)/American Society for Reproductive Medicine (ASRM) Rotterdam consensus meeting, 2003	To include two of the following, including the exclusion of related disorders: 1. oligo-ovulation or anovulation 2. clinical and/or biochemical signs of hyperandrogenism 3. polycystic ovaries
Androgen Excess Society, 2006	To include all of the following: 1. hirsutism and/or hyperandrogenaemia 2. oligo-ovulation/anovulation and/or polycystic ovaries 3. exclusion of androgen excess or related disorders

Clinical hyperandrogenism

Acne, hirsutism and androgenic alopecia are due to androgenic stimulation of the pilosebaceous unit and all occur to a degree in women with PCOS. The exact prevalence of these conditions in the wider population is not precisely known. However, there is considerable evidence suggesting that acne vulgaris is not a disease that solely affects teenagers. Acne does occur in almost all teenagers but a degree of physiological acne occurs in 54% of women over 25 years of age and clinical facial acne in 12%.[6] These figures may underestimate the true incidence as a study of pregnant women reported that 26% complained of acne before pregnancy[7] and a study of PCOS reported that 58% of the women in the control group had acne.[8]

The relationship between acne and biochemical hyperandrogenaemia is well established[9] but the number of women with acne in unselected populations is so great that it makes the link with PCOS unconvincing, particularly since the incidence of acne seems to be greater than that of PCOS. It may therefore be necessary to establish a degree of acne severity that is part of the PCOS spectrum rather than documenting its presence in a similar manner to that for hirsutism. It will be necessary for future studies to be sufficiently powered for this and they will need to include appropriate acne grading to resolve this issue.

The use of hirsutism as a diagnostic criterion is also problematic as its measurement is entirely subjective. There are several grading schemes and the most frequently reported scale, designed by Ferriman and Gallwey[10] in London, was based on neither symptomatic nor pathological criteria. They used an unselected series of hospital patients and defined excess hair growth in mathematical terms: that is, more that two standard deviations above the mean (about 1.2% of the population). This score has become the standard to define hirsutism. DeUgarte *et al.*[11] also studied an unselected group of women and confirmed the findings of Ferriman and Gallwey but noted that many women with lesser hair scores were using hair removal therapies, indicating a mismatch between patient and physician scores. The British Institute & Association of Electrolysis supports the latter as they report that 80% of women have some unwanted hair.[12]

The diagnosis of hirsutism can be very subjective so should it be defined by the woman or by her physician?[13] Is a woman with facial hair but no body or limb hair more or less hirsute than a woman with a hairless face but hairy trunk and limbs? A detailed and sophisticated study of hair growth in Scandinavian women showed that there was an 18% overlap in hair-growth scores between women complaining of hirsutism and a similar-sized control group.[14] And, of course, the same situation occurs with acne, and women who are obese are more likely to find their hair and acne subjectively more troublesome.[13,15]

There are several scoring systems for hirsutism but the vast majority of investigators now use the Ferriman–Gallwey system in which the body is divided into 11 zones, each of which is scored 0–4 on a subjective basis. Nine of the zones are used to compute a hirsutism score. There is no flexibility within this system to allow for non-standard patterns of hair growth. This is a serious deficiency, as women exhibit several different patterns of facial and body hair growth and are more likely to present with hirsutism if they have hair growth on the face, chest and upper back than on other sites.[16] The score is likely to be inflated by hairy thighs, which occur in 45% of premenopausal Scandinavian women,[16] and hair on this site does not appear to respond to antiandrogen therapy.[17]

A greater problem lies in the standardisation of hair-growth scores. We have previously described the differences in mean (and variance) of hair-growth scores between studies.[18] The severity of hirsutism should be fairly similar between studies as the women recruited need to be sufficiently hirsute for adequate hair scores to be made before and after treatment. Yet the difference is great, and we believe that this is largely due to variation in observer scores (Figure 10.1); this has been confirmed by Wild *et al.*[19] who reported a within-patient difference in Ferriman–Gallwey scores of 12 points between different members of their research group, and the maximum score is only 36. Furthermore, only a tiny minority of studies report the investigator variability in this key clinical measurement in comparison with the extensive quality data for laboratory measurements.

The situation with regard to androgenic alopecia is even less clear. While it is undoubtedly an androgen-mediated process, there has been difficulty relating this type of hair loss to increased circulating androgens,[20,21] although an epidemiological link with polycystic ovaries has been demonstrated.[22] Indeed, it may be related more closely to iron deficiency than to androgens.[21] Despite this, there are two well-recognised patterns of androgen-mediated hair loss.[23,24] Proving the link between androgenic alopecia and PCOS is challenging, as outlined above for acne, because the incidence of balding in premenopausal women in the UK is 13%.[25]

Biochemical hyperandrogenism

None of the PCOS guidelines gives any real indication of the definition of the term biochemical hyperandrogenaemia, although some of the issues were raised in the 2003 Rotterdam consensus paper.[3] There is a lack of clarity as to which androgen(s) should be measured, how often it/they should be measured to exclude normal values, what are normal levels of androgens and which analytical techniques should be employed. The latter aspect has been addressed by the Endocrine Society in a 2007 position paper but its strength is in highlighting the problems rather than solutions.[26]

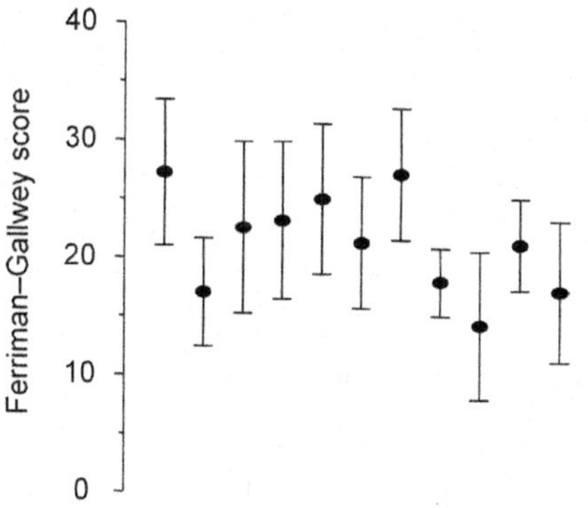

Figure 10.1 Comparison of the hirsutism scores of 11 studies, all of which used the Ferriman–Gallwey hirsutism scoring system (the mean and standard deviation of each study is drawn). This indicates that multicentre comparisons of therapies for hirsuties cannot rely on subjective grading and must be supplemented with criteria that can be objectively compared. If it is assumed that the population of hirsute women presenting to any physician is similar, the wide scatter of values obtained in these studies would indicate marked inter-observer variation. An alternative interpretation might be that there was selection bias in choosing hirsute women but this, too, would argue against the validity of multicentre studies or comparisons between studies. Reproduced with permission from Barth[13]

However, even this paper fails to mention that one of the better-performing direct testosterone immunoassays has a positive bias owing to significant cross-reactivity with dehydroepiandrosterone sulfate (DHEAS).[27]

Firstly, which androgen(s) should be measured? There is an implication that multiple androgens, including testosterone (total [TT] and/or free), DHEAS and possibly androstenedione, should be measured. There are significant issues raised over the analytical performance of free testosterone assays and therefore an alternative is the free androgen index, calculated as (TT/SHBG) × 100 (where SHBG is sex hormone-binding globulin), but this is dependent on the measurement of SHBG, which is itself influenced by the degree of hyperinsulinaemia. There appears to be an underlying philosophy in the guidelines that the aim should be to identify a state of biochemical hyperandrogenism and this is the reason for including free testosterone as it is more frequently elevated. However, this is a circular argument as an elevated androgen is a diagnostic criterion.

The definition of a raised serum androgen will be based on the reference limit prepared by the laboratory. Most laboratories define their reference limits as 95% confidence intervals and therefore 2.5% of the normal population will be above the upper limit of normal. If the four androgens above are measured, there will be a 10% chance that one will be abnormal and this will be increased if calculated variables are included. It should be obvious that if women are investigated on multiple occasions, then the chance of an abnormal result will increase by multiples on each occasion.

Secondly, when should blood be sampled? The variation in hormones throughout the menstrual cycle is well recognised. In particular, testosterone rises towards a peak around ovulation and falls during the luteal phase.[28] This rise and fall is quite reproducible over periods of several months in women with regular cycles.[29] This means that, for a woman with an early-follicular phase testosterone concentration near the upper reference value, a sample taken mid-cycle has the potential to misclassify her as being hyperandrogenaemic (see Figure 10.2).

Thirdly, what is a normal value? The Endocrine Society position statement suggests that each laboratory should collaborate with its endocrinologists to determine its

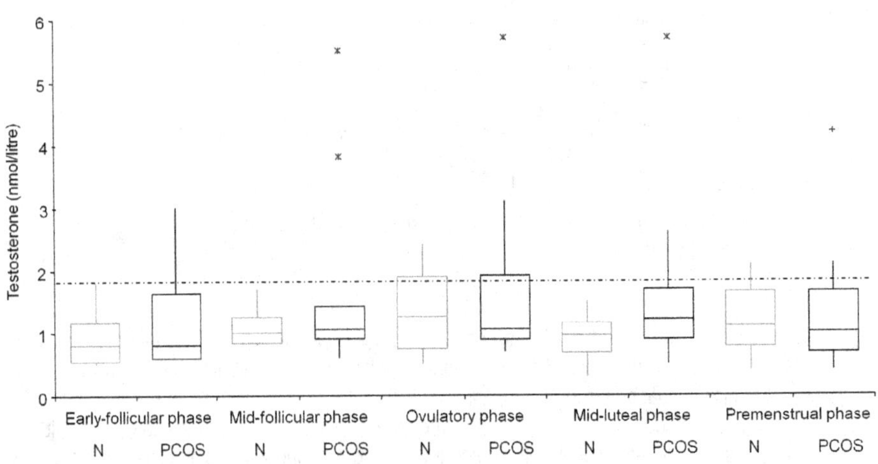

Figure 10.2 Variation in serum testosterone concentrations throughout the menstrual cycle comparing women with PCOS (black columns) and without PCOS (grey columns); box and whisker plots showing 5, 25, 50, 75 and 95 centile values; it can be seen that a number of women would change their status if their blood samples were taken at different points in their cycle

own reference limits for testosterone. This is good practice but reference limits require a minimum population of 120 people and when one considers the range of pre-analytical factors that influence serum testosterone (see Box 10.1), it is clear that this is not practical for any laboratory other than a research unit. The sum of the factors relating to day-to-day variation of total testosterone measurement have been considered by the assessment of its biological variation in both women with and without PCOS: samples taken in the morning throughout the cycle showed an individual index of variation of 0.43% and 0.69%, respectively.[30]

The data in Box 10.1 are based on immunoassays, some of which will have been direct, and will potentially need to be validated with mass spectrometry techniques as these become routinely available.[31]

Finally, it has been proposed that even women with normal circulating androgens on repeated testing can exhibit an occult form of hyperandrogenaemia that is uncovered by human chorionic gonadotrophin (hCG) stimulation testing.[32]

The Rotterdam consensus discarded the use of the luteinising hormone (LH) to follicle-stimulating hormone (FSH) ratio as a diagnostic criterion, which is a good decision. Fauser *et al.*[33] showed that only 50% of women with PCOS had an elevated LH and 43% of those with high LH had PCOS. Given the population of 99 women of whom 35 had ultrasound-proven PCOS, a single LH measurement has a positive predictive value (PPV) of only 18%; if we reduce the prevalence to 7% as in the populations described by Escobar-Morreale *et al.*[34] and Knockenhauer *et al.*[35], the PPV falls further to 3.6%. Gonadotrophins vary hugely throughout the menstrual cycle and their lack of value may be related to poor standardisation of sample timing.

Assessment of anovulation

Anovulation is assessed by measuring the serum progesterone during the mid-luteal phase. The peak value for progesterone only remains for a short time. Indeed, the most common reason for a low value is that the sample was not taken at the appropriate time. The most widely used value in the UK to indicate ovulation is 30 nmol/litre on day 21. It is of note that there is significant bias between methods currently available and this is not reflected by the interpretation given on laboratory report forms.[36] This bias currently ranges from +12% to −14% between the lowest and highest different method means and this clearly introduces further diagnostic confusion regarding the ovulatory status of an individual.

Proposal for new criteria

Diagnostic tests are used to predict whether someone has a disorder. Their accuracy will depend on the incidence of false-positive and false-negative results and the

Box 10.1 Physiological variation in serum testosterone in women
Pulsatile release during the day
Diurnal rhythm: higher in the morning than in the afternoon
Menstrual cycle: mid-cycle peak
Season: no variation in total testosterone but free testosterone shows a 30% difference, being higher in summer than in winter
Age (women with and without PCOS): higher in women in their 20s than in their 40s

prevalence of the disease in the group examined.[37] This requires a robust definition so that the prevalence can be determined. Moreover, the incidence of false tests will vary depending on the case mix of the group under investigation. For example, although it appears that the prevalence of PCOS in randomly selected women is now understood using either the NIH or the Rotterdam criteria, most physicians see women who are selected on the basis of symptoms. Under these circumstances, and contrary to received wisdom, LH has been shown to predict PCOS accurately in 93% of cases.[38] Indeed, this is the main principle behind the development of evidence-based medicine. In an ideal world, consecutive series of women with either a single symptom or various combinations of symptoms would be subjected to formal receiver operating characteristic (ROC) analysis to determine the optimal diagnostic characteristics.

Clinical hyperandrogenism

We would propose that all studies use and cite well-validated scoring systems for acne, balding and hirsutism and include the within- and between-investigator variability. There are well-validated measurement techniques for scoring acne and for training investigators that should be employed.[39] There has been no such proposal for hirsutism, however, but the effect of between-investigator variability on hirsutism can be clearly seen in Figure 1 in the report by Wild *et al.*[19]

Laboratory hyperandrogenism

We would propose that a single sample is taken for serum testosterone in the morning during the early-follicular phase of the cycle. Since the measurement of testosterone is method dependent, each laboratory should ensure that a reference range for women without PCOS has been established for the assay in use. Moreover, the range should be established for the phase of the cycle, as individual women can have a testosterone measurement that rises and falls below the decision limit at different times of the cycle (see Figure 10.2).

Laboratory diagnosis of anovulation

The progesterone method and precision used to confirm anovulation should be cited and the analytical bias relative to an international reference preparation should be stated, such as the Institute for Reference Materials and Measurements.[40]

Summary

The diagnosis of hyperandrogenism is dependent on the accuracy and precision of measurement of the clinical features and the laboratory androgen assays. The heterogeneity of the disease will remain until formal definitions are agreed.

References

1. Stein IF, Leventhal MC. Amenorrhoea associated with bilateral polycystic ovaries. *Am J Obstet Gynaecol* 1935;29:181–91.
2. Zawadzki JK, Dunaif A. Diagnostic criteria for polycystic ovary syndrome: towards a rational approach. In: Dunaif A, Givens JR, Haseltine FP, Merriam GR, editors. *Polycystic Ovary Syndrome.* Boston: Blackwell Scientific; 1992. p. 377–84.

3. The Rotterdam ESHRE/ASRM-Sponsored PCOS Consensus Workshop Group. Revised 2003 consensus on diagnostic criteria and long-term health risks related to polycystic ovary syndrome (PCOS). *Hum Reprod* 2004;19:41–7.
4. Azziz R, Carmina E, Dewailly D, Diamanti-Kandarakis E, Escobar-Morreale HF, Futterweit W, *et al.* Position statement: criteria for defining polycystic ovary syndrome as a predominantly hyperandrogenic syndrome: an Androgen Excess Society guideline. *J Clin Endocrinol Metab* 2006;91:4237–45.
5. Barth JH, Yasmin E, Balen AH. The diagnosis of polycystic ovary syndrome: the criteria are insufficiently robust for clinical research. *Clin Endocrinol* 2007;67:811–15.
6. Goulden V, Stables GI, Cunliffe WJ. Prevalence of facial acne in adults. *J Am Acad Dermatol* 1999;41:577–80.
7. Rushton H, Lyons GM, Firth PS, Abrahams R, James KC. Scalp hair, facial skin and pregnancy. *J Obstet Gynaecol* 1986;7:51–2.
8. Welt CK, Gudmundsson JA, Arason G, Adams J, Palsdottir H, Gudlaugsdottir G, *et al.* Characterising discrete subsets of polycystic ovary syndrome as defined by the Rotterdam criteria: the impact of weight on phenotype and metabolic features. *J Clin Endocrinol Metab* 2006;91:4842–8.
9. Marynick SP, Chakmakjian ZH, McCaffree DL, Herndon JH Jr. Androgen excess in cystic acne. *N Engl J Med* 1983;308:981–6.
10. Ferriman D, Gallwey JD. Clinical assessment of body hair growth in women. *J Clin Endocrinol* 1961;21:1440–7.
11. DeUgarte CM, Woods KS, Bartolucci AA, Azziz R. Degree of facial and body terminal hair growth in unselected black and white women: toward a population definition of hirsutism. *J Clin Endocrinol Metab* 2006;91:1345–50.
12. British Institute & Association of Electrolysis [www.electrolysis.co.uk].
13. Barth JH. How hairy are hirsute women? *Clin Endocrinol* 1997;47:255–60.
14. Lunde O, Grottum P. Body hair growth in women: normal or hirsute. *Am J Phys Anthrop* 1984;64:307–13.
15. Barth JH, Catalan J, Cherry CA, Day AE. Psychological morbidity in women referred for treatment of hirsutism. *J Psychosom Res* 1993;37:615–19.
16. Shah PN. Human body hair – a quantitative study. *Am J Obstet Gynecol* 1957;73:1255–65.
17. Barth JH, Cherry CA, Wojnarowska F, Dawber RP. Cyproterone acetate for severe hirsutism: results of a double-blind dose-ranging study. *Clin Endocrinol* 1991;35:5–10.
18. Barth JH. How robust is the methodology for trials of therapy in hirsute women? *Clin Endocrinol* 1996;45:379–80.
19. Wild RA, Vesely S, Beebe L, Whitsett T, Owen W. Ferriman Gallwey self-scoring I: performance assessment in women with polycystic ovary syndrome. *J Clin Endocrinol Metab* 2005;90:4112–14.
20. De Villez RL, Dunn J. Female androgenic alopecia. The 3 alpha,17 beta-androstanediol glucuronide/sex hormone binding globulin ratio as a possible marker for female pattern baldness. *Arch Dermatol* 1986;122:1011–15.
21. Rushton DH, Ramsay ID, James KC, Norris MJ, Gilkes JJ. Biochemical and trichological characterization of diffuse alopecia in women. *Br J Dermatol* 1990;123:187–97.
22. Cela E, Robertson C, Rush K, Kousta E, White DM, Wilson H, *et al.* Prevalence of polycystic ovaries in women with androgenic alopecia. *Eur J Endocrinol* 2003;149:439–42.
23. Norwood OT. Male pattern baldness: classification and incidence. *South Med J* 1975;68:1359–65.
24. Ludwig E. Classification of the types of androgenic alopecia (common baldness) arising in the female sex. *Br J Dermatol* 1977;97:247–54.
25. Venning VA, Dawber RPR. Patterned androgenic alopecia. *J Am Acad Dermatol* 1988;18:1073–8.
26. Rosner W, Auchus RJ, Azziz R, Sluss PM, Raff H. Utility, limitations, and pitfalls in measuring testosterone: an Endocrine Society position statement. *J Clin Endocrinol Metab* 2007;92:405–13.
27. Warner MH, Kane JW, Atkin SL, Kilpatrick ES. Dehydroepiandrosterone sulphate interferes with the Abbott Architect direct immunoassay for testosterone. *Ann Clin Biochem* 2006;43:196–9.
28. Epstein MT, McNeilly AS, Murray MAF, Hockaday TDR. Plasma testosterone and prolactin in the menstrual cyle. *Clin Endocrinol* 1975;4:531–5.

29. Shultz SJ, Levine BJ, Wideman L, Montgomery MM. Some sex hormone profiles are consistent over time in normal menstruating females: implications for sports injury epidemiology. *Br J Sports Med* 2009 Oct 23. [Epub ahead of print]
30. Jayagopal V, Kilpatrick ES, Jennings PE, Hepburn DA, Atkin SL. The biological variation of testosterone and sex hormone binding globulin (SHBG) in polycystic vary syndrome: implications for SHBG as a surrogate marker of insulin resistance. *J Clin Endocrinol Metab* 2003;88:1528–33.
31. Cawood ML, Field HP, Ford CG, Gillingwater S, Kicman A, Cowan D, *et al.* Testosterone measurement by isotope-dilution liquid chromatography-tandem mass spectrometry: validation of a method for routine clinical practise. *Clin Chem* 2005;51:1472–9.
32. Gilling-Smith C, Story H, Rogers V, Franks S. Evidence for a primary abnormality of thecal cell steroidogenesis in the polycystic ovary syndrome. *Clin Endocrinol* 1997;47:93–9.
33. Fauser BC, Pache TD, Hop WC, de Jong FH, Dahl KD. The significance of a single serum LH measurement in women with cycle disturbances: discrepancies between immunoreactive and bioactive hormone estimates. *Clin Endocrinol* 1992;37:445–52.
34. Escobar-Morreale HF, Asuncion M, Calvo RM, Sancho J, San Millan JL. Receiver operating characteristic analysis of the performance of basal serum hormone profiles for the diagnosis of polycystic ovary syndrome in epidemiological studies. *Eur J Endocrinol* 2001;145:619–24.
35. Knochenhauer ES, Key TJ, Kahsar-Miller M, Waggoner W, Boots LR, Azziz R. Prevalence of the polycystic ovary syndrome in unselected black and white women of the southeastern United States: a prospective study. *J Clin Endocrinol Metab* 1988;83:3078–82.
36. Middle JG. *UK NEQAS for Steroid Hormones Annual Review for Progesterone.* 2006. Available from the author at UK NEQAS, PO Box 3909, Birmingham B15 2UE.
37. Galen RS, Gambino SR. *Beyond Normality: the Predictive Value and Efficiency of Medical Diagnoses.* London: John Wiley & Sons; 1975.
38. Hendriks ML, Brouwer J, Hompes PG, Homburg R, Lambalk CB. LH as a diagnostic criterion for polycystic ovary syndrome in patients with WHO II oligo/amenorrhoea. *Reprod Biomed Online* 2008;16:765–71.
39. Cunliffe WJ. *Acne.* London: Martin Dunitz; 1989. p. 122.
40. Institute for Reference Materials and Measurements [irmm.jrc.ec.europa.eu/html/homepage.htm].

Chapter 11

Treatment of hyperandrogenism in polycystic ovary syndrome

Alison M Layton

Introduction

Hyperandrogenism is the most common endocrinopathy seen in women and may result from ovarian or adrenal overproduction of androgens, altered peripheral metabolism and/or end-organ hypersensitivity. Androgen excess can have profound effects on human skin, especially the skin appendages, sebaceous glands and hair follicles, which are strongly dependent on biologically active androgens.

The development of sudden-onset acne and/or hirsutism, female-pattern hair loss, irregular menses, increased libido, acanthosis nigricans, deepening voice, clitoromegaly or other signs of hyperandrogenism such as cushingoid features requires further investigation. It is important to recognise that women with hyperandrogenism may also have insulin resistance that puts them at increased risk of developing diabetes and cardiovascular disease. The treatment of these women should be managed by an endocrinologist and a gynaecologist to ensure that a comprehensive approach is adopted. The most common cause of hyperandrogenism in women is polycystic ovary syndrome (PCOS) but congenital adrenal hyperplasia as well as ovarian and adrenal tumours may need to be considered.

In the sebaceous gland, androgens stimulate sebocyte proliferation. This is most pronounced in facial sebocytes[1] and leads to increased sebum production. Within the intrafollicular duct of the pilosebaceous unit, androgens increase the rate of mitosis and epithelial proliferation, leading to hyperkeratosis.[2] These events contribute to the pathogenesis and subsequent development of clinical acne.

In the hair follicle, androgens have strong effects on hair growth and act through the androgen receptor on dermal papilla cells.[3] Malfunctions of the androgen receptor are associated with hirsutism and androgenic alopecia in women, reflecting the importance of the androgen receptor in these conditions.[4] Androgens can result in opposite effects on hair follicles in the scalp compared with those in the face and body. In the latter, they may prolong the growth phase and transform vellus hairs to terminal hairs, which contrasts with their ability to shorten the anagen phase in the scalp. Large individual variations in response to normal and elevated androgen levels occur, suggesting significant differences in local androgen metabolism and androgen receptor-mediated activities. It is likely that genetic predisposition also has an important influence on the resultant clinical effects of hyperandrogensim.[5,6]

The dermatological manifestations of abnormal androgen dynamics in PCOS vary within the patient population as a result of the complex interplay between genetics, end-organ susceptibility and hormonal variations. Hyperandrogenism most commonly manifests itself as hirsutism in this population but acne, seborrhoea and/or female-pattern hair loss may also be evident. There is a spectrum of clinical severity in women with these distressing conditions and, however subtle, it is important to recognise and treat these signs as psychological sequelae are very common.

The three main naturally occurring steroids responsible for androgen activity are testosterone and the weak androgens dehydroepiandrosterone (DHEA) and androstenedione. The production, peripheral conversion and binding to sex hormone-binding globulin (SHBG) are important in determining the hormonal activity. Testosterone is converted to the more potent biologically active dihydrotestosterone by 5α-reductase in some peripheral tissues.

Managing the dermatological signs of hyperandrogenism, which generally present as acne, seborrhoea, hirsutism and female-pattern hair loss in PCOS, is achieved by reducing the circulating levels and effects of androgens. Potential mechanisms by which this may occur include:

- direct suppression of androgen production
- change in androgen binding to SHBG
- impairing the peripheral conversion of free testosterone to dihydrotestosterone by inhibiting 5α-reductase type I
- Inhibiting androgens acting at the site of target tissue (see Figure 11.1).

Acne

Acne is a multifactorial inflammatory disease of the pilosebaceous follicle, predominantly involving the skin of the face and trunk. The pathophysiology of acne is slowly

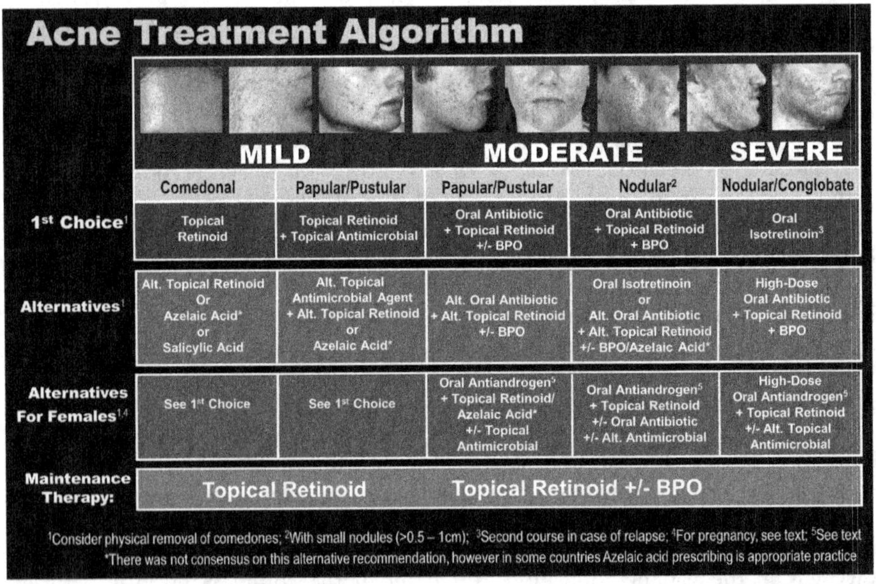
Acne Treatment Algorithm
MILD
MODERATE
SEVERE
Comedonal
Papular/Pustular
Papular/Pustular
Nodular2
Nodular/Conglobate
1st Choice1
Topical Retinoid
Topical Retinoid + Topical Antimicrobial
Oral Antibiotic + Topical Retinoid +/- BPO
Oral Antibiotic + Topical Retinoid + BPO
Oral Isotretinoin3
Alternatives1
Alt. Topical Retinoid Or Azelaic Acid* or Salicylic Acid
Alt. Topical Antimicrobial Agent + Alt. Topical Retinoid or Azelaic Acid*
Alt. Oral Antibiotic + Alt. Topical Retinoid +/- BPO
Oral Isotretinoin or Alt. Oral Antibiotic + Alt. Topical Retinoid +/- BPO/Azelaic Acid*
High-Dose Oral Antibiotic + Topical Retinoid + BPO
Alternatives For Females1,4
See 1st Choice
See 1st Choice
Oral Antiandrogen5 + Topical Retinoid/ Azelaic Acid* +/- Topical Antimicrobial
Oral Antiandrogen5 + Topical Retinoid +/- Oral Antibiotic +/- Alt. Antimicrobial
High-Dose Oral Antiandrogen5 + Topical Retinoid +/- Alt. Topical Antimicrobial
Maintenance Therapy:
Topical Retinoid
Topical Retinoid +/- BPO
1Consider physical removal of comedones; 2With small nodules (>0.5 – 1cm); 3Second course in case of relapse; 4For pregnancy, see text; 5See text
*There was not consensus on this alternative recommendation, however in some countries Azelaic acid prescribing is appropriate practice

Figure 11.1 Acne treatment algorithm; adapted with permission from Gollnick *et al.*[12] (Global Alliance to Improve Outcomes in Acne)

unravelling and, although many factors remain undetermined, better understanding of the mechanisms involved has led to an improvement in acne management over the past decade. Four key factors have been identified in the aetiology of acne:

- increased sebum production
- follicular hyperkeratinisation
- colonisation of the pilosebaceous unit with *Propionibacterium acnes*
- production of inflammation.

Hormonal influences have an important role in the pathogenesis of acne. Increased sebum production due to androgens acting at the sebaceous follicle is a prerequisite for acne in all people.[7–9] Before puberty, the adrenal glands produce increasing amounts of dehydroepiandrosterone sulfate (DHEAS), which can be metabolised into more potent androgens in the skin, driving enlargement of the sebaceous gland and increased sebum production.[10] Subsequent acne relates to increased sensitivity of the sebaceous gland to androgens.[11] In women, aberrant excess production of androgens from the ovary may also cause acne and an endocrinopathy should be excluded in women with persistent late-onset acne or acne associated with hirsutism.[11] Whatever the underlying cause, acne needs to be managed aggressively from the outset using a combination of treatments directed against each of the relevant factors.

The treatment of acne in women with PCOS should embrace a number of aspects, including:

- general advice
- selection of therapy according to clinical lesions/sub-type and appreciation of the pathophysiological events that result from hyperandrogenism
- consideration of therapies according to the woman's lifestyle to aid concordance
- consideration of alternative procedures where medical therapies may not be helpful
- advice on skincare regimens.

General advice

It is important that women have realistic expectations of treatment efficacy and are aware of the potential adverse effects from therapy. The aims of any acne treatment are to:

- prevent comedogenesis
- lower sebum production
- reduce colonisation with and numbers of *Propionibacterium acnes*
- act as a comedolytic, thus reducing established comedones.

Response to therapy may be slow in women with PCOS, hence selecting therapy that will achieve good concordance is vital. Women with PCOS frequently have marked androgen-mediated seborrhoea and, as a result, treatment response to conventional topical therapies combined with antimicrobials is generally less effective in this patient group. Many women will require maintenance therapy as acne pursues a chronic course in PCOS owing to the androgen drive. It is important to recognise triggers for the acne, which may include stress and hormonal influences.

Managing according to clinical sub-type

A number of clinical sub-types may be seen in women with PCOS, including hyperseborrhoea with retentional lesions. The closed comedones are frequently subtle and adequate lighting is required to ensure they do not go unseen when examining these women.

Larger and more extensive macrocomedones may be evident in some women and these often present a cosmetic problem. Inflammatory sub-types include persistent mild to moderate inflammatory acne and/or premenstrual flares of acne. Inflammatory lesions can be deep-seated, long-lasting and present as nodules and cysts predominantly around the chin. Post-inflammatory pigmentation can be a problem, particularly in type 3 and type 4 skin types. Deep-seated inflammatory lesions subsequently result in scarring in many of these women.

Treatment of non-inflammatory lesions

Topical retinoids should be employed as first-line therapy for non-inflammatory lesions in an attempt to prevent comedogenesis and to treat established comedones. Topical retinoids can be irritant and thus they should be applied sparingly for short durations in the first instance and the period of application gradually increased according to tolerance. Adapalene is less irritant than other retinoids and is therefore frequently selected as the first-line topical agent in these patients.[12] Many women with PCOS are unresponsive to topical therapy.

Treatment of mild to moderate inflammatory lesions

For treatment of mild to moderate inflammatory lesions, a combination of topical antimicrobial and retinoid combination therapies should be employed, as outlined in the algorithm in Figure 11.1.

Deep-seated nodular lesions should be treated aggressively in an attempt to avoid scarring and post-inflammatory pigmentation. As topical antimicrobials/retinoid combinations frequently work slowly, short-term topical type IV corticosteroids can be used to achieve a rapid reduction in inflammation.

Topical therapies for post-inflammatory hyperpigmentation

The aims of treatment for post-inflammatory hyperpigmentation are to bleach excess pigment, to avoid new pigment formation and to use exfoliative preparations to help shed pigment. The following agents are used to bleach excess pigment and avoid new pigment forming:

- retinoids
- azelaic acid
- hydroxyquinone
- steroids.

The following medications can aid exfoliation to help shed pigment:

- alpha hydroxy-acids
- chemical peels with glycolic acid, trichloroacetic acid and salicylic acid.

Alternative therapies and procedures

Nodular lesions

For nodular lesions, topical and/or intralesional corticosteroids and/or cryotherapy may be beneficial.

Non-inflammatory lesions

For non-inflammatory lesions, hyfrecation/cautery with or without topical retinoids has been used successfully to reduce closed comedones.[13] Comedo extraction may also be helpful for open comedones. Topical retinoids should be considered as maintenance therapy alongside some form of systemic therapy to avoid further relapse and to manage associated seborrhoea.[12]

Skincare and use of cosmetics

For oily and sensitive skin, it is important to avoid comedogenic products such as isopropyl myristate, cocoa butter, lanolin, butyl stearate and oleic acid. Acnegenic products should also be avoided and, if bleaching agents are used, they should be non-steroid based.

Systemic therapies

Systemic therapies available for acne in women include antibiotics, hormonal therapies, corticosteroids and isotretinoin. Response to systemic therapies is often very slow in women with PCOS. Poor response may in part be due to the relatively higher sebum excretion rate as it has been noted that high sebum excretion rates correlate to poor response to antibiotics,[14] and the acne is frequently recalcitrant such that standard treatments including isotretinoin may have failed or relapsed after initially successful therapy has occurred.[15]

Standard combinations of topical and systemic antibiotic therapies should be tried in women with PCOS but hormonal manipulation usually provides the most effective means of managing acne in these women whether serum androgens are normal or abnormal.[16] Although some women with PCOS may have higher serum androgens compared with women without acne, these levels are often within the normal range. Hormonal therapies are also desirable when menstrual control and/or contraception are required alongside acne therapy in women with PCOS.

All available hormonal treatments have the common goal of opposing the effects of androgens on the sebaceous gland and, to a lesser extent, the follicular keratinocytes.[12] This can be accomplished with the use of estrogens, androgen receptor blockers (cyproterone acetate, chlormadinone acetate, spironalactone, drospirenone, desogestrel or flutamide) or agents designed to inhibit the endogenous production of androgens by the ovary (oral contraceptives, cyproterone acetate or gonadotrophin-releasing hormone [GnRH] agonists) or adrenal gland (low-dose glucocorticoids).

Inhibitors of adrenal androgen production

Glucocorticoids at low doses can suppress the adrenal production of androgens. They are indicated for patients, both male and female, who have elevated DHEAS associated with late-onset congenital adrenal hyperplasia caused by an inherent deficiency of 11-hydroxylase or 21-hydroxylase enzymes. Deficiency of 21-hydroxylase is present in approximately 3% of hirsute women and mutations in the gene encoding this enzyme are found more frequently in women with acne than in those without. Low-dose prednisolone (2.5–5 mg) or dexamethasone (0.25–0.75 mg) given at night (or alternate nights) can be sufficient to suppress adrenal androgen production and subsequently reduce sebum production by up to 50%, with a concomitant improvement in acne.[8,17,18]

Several studies have shown that glucocorticoids given alongside cyclical estrogen can successfully moderate sebum production in recalcitrant acne, with a greater reduction in plasma androgen levels achieved than with either agent alone.[8,19,20] However, the doses of estrogen used in these studies were much higher than the dose in most oral contraceptives (80–100 micrograms), which in practice would need to be balanced against the greater potential for adverse effects such as venous thromboembolism.

Inhibitors of ovarian androgen production

Oral contraceptives. Oral contraceptive pills are the mainstay of therapy for young women with PCOS. Combined oral contraceptives (COCs) all improve acne by reducing androgen secretion in the ovaries and adrenal glands through their estrogenic effects. Estrogen increases the hepatic production of SHBG, which binds testosterone and thus reduces levels of free circulating testosterone. In addition, estrogens suppress the ovarian production of androgens by suppressing gonadotrophin release from the pituitary, resulting in lower serum androgen levels and less seborrhoea. They may also reduce 5α-reductase activity.[21] Most oral contraceptives will achieve 40–50% improvement in acne. Very few good comparative studies are available comparing one systemic agent with another and/or with standard retinoid/antimicrobial combination therapy. COCs can be prescribed safely with other treatment modalities. When using a COC as part of an acne regimen, advice on possible drug interaction leading to reduced contraceptive efficacy is currently advisable. However, there is a paucity of evidence for antibiotic interactions and the COCs, with the exception of rifampicin.[22,23]

All COCs, provided that estrogen is given at a sufficient dose, will reduce sebum production and have the potential to improve acne[12,15] However, the dose of estrogen required to suppress sebum production is often greater than the dose required to suppress ovulation. In recent years, the dose of estrogen in conventional oral contraceptives has been reduced such that many third-generation preparations contain just 20 micrograms of ethinylestradiol, which on its own is insufficient to control seborrhoea in most women with acne.[15] However, a Cochrane systematic review of the effectiveness of COCs for the treatment of facial acne confirmed that all COCs reduced lesion counts, severity grades and self-assessment scores compared with placebo.[24]

The efficacy of estrogen in managing seborrhoea is enhanced by the addition of a progestin with antiandrogenic activity. Progestins traditionally included in COCs include estranes and gonanes, which are derived from 19-nortestosterone and cyproterone acetate. Many progestins have the inherent ability to interact with androgen receptors, thus aggravating acne, hirsutism and androgenic alopecia. There is currently little evidence from randomised controlled trials to support one progestin over another, although it is suggested that third-generation progestins such as gestodene, desogestrel and norgestimate are less selective for the androgen and more selective for the progesterone receptor, making them less problematic in androgen-mediated problems.[25] COCs recommended for the treatment of acne in PCOS are therefore a combined preparation containing estrogen (most commonly ethinylestradiol) and a progestin with low androgenic activity or preferably a progestin with proven antiandrogenic activity. This is supported by limited study data that confirm that cyproterone acetate-containing COCs achieve better efficacy than preparations containing desogestrel or levonorgestrel.[24]

Cyproterone acetate is a progestational antiandrogen that directly inhibits androgen action via its receptor. While not available in the USA, it is widely prescribed as an oral contraceptive formulation in Europe (although not licensed for this in the UK) and for the treatment of severe acne as co-cyprindiol,[26–28] for which it does have a product licence. Co-cyprindiol is able to reduce sebum up to 70% over the 6–9 month course and, in one uncontrolled study of 1161 patients with facial acne investigated over 36 months, 72% improvement was noted over six cycles and 91% improvement in disease was reported at 12 months.[29]

Co-cyprindiol combines 2 mg of cyproterone acetate with 35 micrograms of ethinylestradiol and is currently not licensed as an oral contraceptive in the UK. It has been suggested that the higher amount of estrogen in this agent carries a greater potential for venous thromboembolism when compared with other third-generation COCs.[30] One review of the evidence for efficacy and adverse effects concluded that co-cyprindiol has clear benefits and that the risks of venous thromboembolism are similar to those of other third-generation COCs.[31] A study published in 2009 examined thrombotic risk associated with COCs by type of progestogen and suggested that the highest risk of venous thromboembolism in users of COCs was found with those containing desogestrel and gestodene but confirmed that those containing cyproterone acetate and drospirenone do have a higher risk compared with levonorgestrel. The authors also suggested that venous thromboembolism is less likely after prolonged use of second- and third-generation COCs and most likely in the first 3 months.[32] This fact would support continued use of co-cyprindiol even though androgen-related symptoms and signs might have improved, particularly in light of the fact that relapse on withdrawal of the drug is very high. Women should be clearly informed about the risks.

Co-cyprindiol reduces sebum production by 30% but its success in acne is enhanced by direct effects on androgen-mediated comedogenesis: reductions in inflammatory lesions range from 50% to 75%.[33] It is as effective as oral tetracycline (1 g per day) given over a 6-month period, although it is slower in action.[34] It is therefore of potential benefit to women with acne that is resistant to other therapies. An overall improvement in acne has been reported in up to 90% of women treated with higher doses of cyproterone acetate (50–100 mg per day) with or without ethinylestradiol.[35,36] The clinical effectiveness of co-cyprindiol can therefore be enhanced by prescribing an extra 50–100 mg cyproterone acetate from day 5 to day 14 of the menstrual cycle, but prescribers should be mindful of a possible increase in adverse effects.

General adverse effects of cyproterone acetate, although uncommon, include fatigue, headache, nausea, weight fluctuation, liver dysfunction and blood-clotting abnormalities.[15]

In a comparative study comparing dienogest plus ethinylestradiol with cyproterone acetate plus ethinylestradiol and with placebo, the results showed that both agents were superior to placebo and equivalent in mild to moderate acne over six cycles.[37]

Drospirenone is a novel progestin derived from 17α-spironalactone and thus has both antimineralocorticoid and antiandrogenic activity. It thus increases sodium and water excretion and can lead to potassium retention.[38] Drospirenone combined with ethinylestradiol as Yasmin® (Bayer) is an effective COC. One small company-sponsored randomised comparative double-blind trial examined drospirenone against 2 mg of cyproterone acetate both combined with 35 micrograms of ethinylestradiol over nine cycles and found the efficacy to be similar in improving mild to moderate facial acne.[39] Drospirenone is also available in some countries within a hormonal replacement therapy and it has been shown to increase bone density, thus potentially protecting against osteoporosis in women who are at high risk. In both COCs and hormone replacement therapy, drospirenone represents a unique antimineralocorticoid activity and may produce favourable effects on cardiovascular risk factors in pre- and postmenopausal women. The safety of Yasmin has been compared with that of other oral contraceptives in a large multinational observational study: no increased risks were found of adverse cardiovascular or other serious adverse events in users of drospirenone-containing COCs versus those using other COCs.[40]

The newest COC is YAZ® (Bayer), which contains 20 micrograms of ethinylestradiol and 3 mg of drospirenone in a 24/4 active/inert regimen. It was approved for the treatment of mild to moderate acne in January 2007 based on two multicentre double-blind randomised placebo-controlled trials following 889 women over six cycles. Both trials showed similar results, with a reduction in total lesion counts amounting to 42–46%.[41]

Gonadotrophin-releasing hormone agonists. GnRH agonists, such as nafarelin, leuprorelin and buserelin, have demonstrated efficacy in the treatment of acne and hirsutism in women both with and without endocrine abnormalities.[42] Administered as either a nasal spray or an injection, GnRH agonists inhibit ovarian androgen production by interrupting the cyclical release of luteinising hormone and follicle-stimulating hormone from the pituitary. However, their use is limited somewhat by the potential for adverse effects, including reduced bone mass, headaches and menopausal symptoms caused by the suppression of ovarian estrogen production.

Androgen receptor blockers

Sebum production can be suppressed by antiandrogen agents including cyproterone acetate (as above), spironolactone, drospirenone (as before) and flutamide. The degree of reduction in seborrhoea is drug and dose dependent.[27,28,43]

Spironolactone. Although spironolactone is not approved for the treatment of acne or hitsutism, it has been used for over 20 years. It has inhibitory actions on both the androgen receptor and 5α-reductase and is also known to inhibit androgen biosynthesis by decreasing type II 17β-hydroxysteroid dehydrogenase, thus preventing the conversion of androstenedione to testosterone. It is an effective treatment for acne and can reduce sebum production by 30–75% in a dose-dependent manner.[44–47] It is usually prescribed at a dose of 50–100 mg daily with meals but many women with sporadic outbreaks can be successfully treated with as little as 25 mg daily.[48] Despite a consensus on the clinical benefit observed with spironolactone, there is a surprising paucity of data to confirm its efficacy in acne.[48] In one study of 85 women with acne, 93% showed at least partial improvement in their acne, with 66% showing a marked improvement or complete clearance.[49] As with other hormonal therapies, response is slow and it may take up to 3 months of continuous treatment before any benefit is observed.[50] Enhanced efficacy has been demonstrated in acne when spironolactone is combined with a COC.[51]

Spironolactone has a number of dose-dependent adverse effects. Menstrual irregularities, hyperkalaemia, breast tenderness, fatigue, headache, fluid retention and, rarely, melasma have been observed. Animal studies have reported an association with breast carcinoma in rodents but this has not been replicated in human studies.[52] Owing to potential feminisation effects in a male fetus, spironolactone should be avoided in pregnancy.

Flutamide. Flutamide is most routinely used in the treatment of prostate cancer and is a potent nonsteroidal androgen receptor blocker. It has shown to be efficacious in treating androgen-mediated acne and hirsutism when administered at a dose of 250 mg daily. In a study investigating the effects of flutamide versus placebo on hirsutism in 119 women with PCOS or idiopathic hirsutism,[53] a reduction in baseline hirsutism was seen in both the placebo group (mean baseline reduction 28%) and flutamide group (mean baseline reduction 50%) at 6 months. The improvement was significantly better with flutamide than placebo and no further decrease was noted in the placebo group at 12 months. The doses of flutamide used, 125 mg, 250 mg and 375 mg daily, did not achieve significant differences in benefit, supporting the use of lower doses of flutamide if precribed for hirsutism. In a comparative trial of flutamide and spironalactone, Cusan *et al.*[54] reported superior efficacy with flutamide at reducing total acne count and seborrhoea at 3 months. However, given that spironalactone takes this period to clinically improve acne, few conclusions can be drawn about the overall superiority of flutamide and higher dosages of flutamide are required to achieve the same efficacy as it has less affinity than spironolactone for the androgen receptor. This is of concern as fatal hepatotoxicity has been reported with flutamide at doses greater than 500 mg daily and therefore its use in acne is not advocated.[55]

Finasteride. Finasteride inhibits peripheral androgen metabolism by inhibiting 5α-reductase (mainly type II), the enzyme responsible for converting free testosterone to dihydrotestosterone. 5α-reductase type II is found predominantly in the hair follicle, in contrast to 5α-reductase type I, which is found predominantly in the sebaceous gland. There is little evidence to date to suggest that finasteride is a useful modality in the treatment of acne and certainly no clear advantage over spironolactone has been demonstrated.

Insulin-sensitising drugs

Other possible systemic treatments for acne in adult women include biguanides, such as metformin, which reduce hepatic glucose production and insulin. Metformin 500 mg three times daily has been used and possibly improves hirsutism with prolonged use but there is little impact on acne.[56] To date there is no evidence to support metformin over the COCs for acne or hirsutism.

Conclusion on acne management in PCOS

Persistent and refractory acne may be a problem in women with PCOS and hormonal therapies represent a useful way of treating the associated hyperandrogenism. A focus on early aggressive intervention is paramount to reduce the physical and psychological scarring that can result from acne of any severity.

Clear guidelines now exist to guide clinicians in their prescribing, such as those published by the Global Alliance to Improve Outcomes in Acne (Figure 11.1).[12,57] Topical retinoids are advocated as first-line treatment for any patient with mild to moderate acne, especially with comedonal lesions, and should be employed in combination with benzoyl peroxide, antibiotics and/or hormonal treatments for more severe or treatment-resistant disease. Systemic retinoids provide extremely efficacious therapy for severe disease, including for those people with high sebum production who have not responded to combination therapy. However, the importance of comprehensive counselling for all women of childbearing potential must not be overlooked as the risks of teratogenicity are significant. Maintenance therapy is an important consideration as acne is a chronic disease and frequently recurs without a continuing treatment regimen in women with PCOS. Topical retinoids are recommended for maintenance therapy as they target the microcomedo, the precursor of all acne lesions.

Hirsutism

Hirsutism is the most frequent dermatological problem in women with PCOS and is found in up to 70–80% of cases.[58] It manifests itself as excessive terminal hair growth in women in a typical male-pattern distribution and is a disfiguring cosmetic problem that frequently results in significant psychological distress. Treatment aims to rectify any hormonal imbalance and improve the cosmetic appearance. Options include cosmetic, physical and medical approaches. Medical options work slowly and may take 6–9 months to produce significant effects so combining medications with cosmetic and physical methods is advisable.

Cosmetic and physical approaches include bleaching and/or removal of hair with shaving, waxing/sugaring, tweezing or the use of depilatory creams. Photoepilation with laser and light therapies or electrolysis are also available. Weight loss also has an important part to play in management as obesity has a negative impact on treatments for hirsutism[59] and weight reduction in obese women with PCOS reduces hirsutism in part owing to a reduction in bioavailable (nonprotein-bound) testosterone.[60]

Electrolysis has the potential to achieve permanent hair removal although regrowth commonly occurs and repeated sessions are required at considerable cost and time to patients. In inexperienced hands, electrolysis can result in post-inflammatory changes, pigmentation and scarring, so it is important that only registered electrologists are employed to deliver the treatment.

A number of intense pulse and laser light therapies have been introduced in recent years. These approaches aim to treat hair follicles in the anagen (growing) phase and, as pigment acts as the chromophore, they work more effectively on dark hairs. The ideal patient is one with dark hair and light skin. Repeated treatments are required owing to the varying length of the hair cycle: 3–6 months on the face (contrasting with 5 years or longer on the scalp). Permanent hair removal is still not guaranteed. A number of systems are available but are mainly accessed in the private sector, so proving expensive to the patient. There is a paucity of good-quality randomised controlled studies with adequate follow-up to support one system over another. In the few studies available, there appears to be a short-term effect of approximately 50% hair reduction with the alexandrite and diode lasers up to 6 months post-therapy. Pain, erythema, swelling, thermal damage to hairs and pigmentation are all rare but are reported as possible adverse effects.[61] As with electrolysis, an experienced laser technician should be employed as patient selection is important in achieving good results and adverse effects will then be minimised.

Medical treatments available include topical and systemic treatments. They aim to decrease the rate, and prevent further progression, of hair growth.

Topical therapy

Eflornithine hydrochloride

Topical 11.5% eflornithine hydrochloride is now licensed to treat hirsutism and is able to inhibit hair growth. Eflornithine inhibits the enzyme orthinine decarboxylase, which is key to polyamine synthesis responsible for cell proliferation, migration and differentiation. As a result of blocking orthinine decarboxylase, apoptosis of cells in the dermal papilla occurs and reduced hair growth is the result.

Two studies have evaluated the efficacy and safety of eflornithine hydrochloride over 24 weeks with twice-daily applications. Significant reduction in unwanted hair, as assessed by the clinician, was demonstrated and treatment was well tolerated.[62]

Eflornithine can be combined safely with laser treatments and efficacy is enhanced by adopting this approach.[63] A double-blind placebo-controlled study showed that, for patients who received the placebo (vehicle alone) with laser treatment, complete or almost complete hair removal was achieved in 67.9% compared with 96.4% of those treated with laser combined with eflornithine.[64]

Systemic therapy

As in acne, the aim of systemic therapy for hirsutism is to reduce androgens. The options include COC pills, cyproterone acetate, spironolactone, finasteride, flutamide and insulin sensitisers.

COC pills

The overall effect of a COC containing ethinylestradiol and a progestational agent is antiandrogenic. The commonly prescribed agents used to treat hirsutism include a combination of 30 micrograms of ethinylestradiol with 2 mg of cyproterone acetate or 3 mg of drospirenone. Similar efficacy has been reported with each of these combination products.[65] Response to therapy is slow, frequently taking six to nine cycles, but after six cycles it has been observed that further improvement is limited.[66] Addition of antiandrogens to oral contraceptive pills is frequently adopted in clinical practice; however, a meta-analysis published in 2008, which included five comparisons embracing oral contraceptive pills alone versus antiandrogens combined with oral contraceptive pills, concluded that no significant benefit in end-of-study hirsutism scores was achieved by combining preparations.[64]

Cyproterone acetate

A systematic review[67] examining the use of cyproterone acetate alone or in combination with ethinylestradiol for reducing hair growth in women with hirsutism secondary to ovarian hyperandrogenism found no clinical trials comparing cyproterone acetate with placebo and just one small study comparing cyproterone acetate in combination with ethinylestradiol with placebo. This study demonstrated a significant subjective reduction in hair growth with the active therapy. In studies comparing cyproterone acetate with other treatments including ketoconazole, spironolactone, flutamide and GnRH analogues, no difference in clinical outcome was noted, although these studies were small and lacked standardised outcome measures.[67]

Combining additional cyproterone acetate from day 5 to day 14 of the menstrual cycle with oral contraceptive pills containing 2 mg cyproterone acetate has not demonstrated any additional benefit over 6–9 months, and the adverse effect profile with the additional cyproterone acetate was significantly greater.[48]

Spironolactone

A Cochrane systematic review[68] updated in 2009 examined all randomised controlled comparisons of spironolactone versus placebo or steroids (oral contraceptive pill included), spironolactone of varying dosages, or spironolactone and steroids versus steroids alone when used to reduce hair growth and acne in women. Nine trials were included in the review. Major outcome measures included the Ferriman–Gallwey hirsutism score. The review found that studies in this area were small and scarce but that spironolactone at a dose of 100 mg showed subjective improvements in hair growth (although not significant on Ferriman–Gallwey scores) when compared with placebo in two studies.[68] Individual study data indicated a superiority of spironolactone over other drugs including finasteride 5 mg per day, metformin and low-dose cyproterone acetate but the results could not be generalised.

Gonadotrophin-releasing hormone agonists

A number of researchers have reviewed the effects of GnRH agonists on serum androgen levels in hirsute women and suggested that preliminary results appear promising.[69] However, the use of GnRH is associated with all the signs of hypoestrogenism, including osteoporosis, which clearly negates their routine use in many cases.

Finasteride

Finasteride blocks the conversion of testosterone to the more potent dihydrotestosterone at the hair follicle. It is prescribed at a dose of 5 mg daily for the treatment of hirsutism. Finasteride can cause feminisation of the male fetus so it is important to avoid pregnancy.

Finasteride does not appear to be as beneficial as spironolactone,[68] although it has shown equivalent efficacy to cyproterone acetate and ethinylestradiol combinations in some small studies.[70,71]

Flutamide

Flutamide is a nonsteroidal androgen receptor blocker and has been used at a dose of 250–500 mg daily to treat hirsutism. Feminisation of the male fetus can occur so pregnancy should be avoided. Although in extreme cases this has been used to treat for hirsutism, the potential for life-threatening hepatotoxicity reported at higher dosages limits the usefulness of this agent.[72,73]

A study published in 2009 that compared finasteride 5 mg per day, flutamide 125 mg per day and a combination of both treatments demonstrated that flutamide alone was more effective in treating hirsutism than finasteride alone and the combination of the two drugs was no better than flutamide alone over a 12-month period.[74]

Insulin-sensitising drugs

Hirsutism as a common feature of PCOS is frequently seen in the context of insulin resistance. Metformin inhibits the production of hepatic glucose and enhances the sensitivity of peripheral tissue to insulin, thereby resulting in a decrease in insulin secretion. In women with PCOS, it has been suggested that metformin ameliorates hyperandrogenism and abnormalities of gonadotrophin secretion. This may be due to the concurrent reduction in body mass index that results from metformin usage.

There are limited data in the literature to suggest that hirsutism may improve by reducing hyperinsulinaemia but a study comparing COCs containing cyproterone acetate with metformin in women with PCOS and hirsutism indicated that the cyproterone acetate caused profound androgen suppression that was not seen with metformin.[75] In addition, a meta-analysis comparing other antiandrogens (flutamide and spironolactone) with metformin showed that the antiandrogen group achieved significantly lower hirsutism scores, and adopting a combined approach with metformin alongside the antiandrogen resulted in improved hirsutism scores compared with those achieved with metformin alone.[64] Further studies are required to substantiate the significance of this.

A Cochrane review examining the effectiveness and safety of insulin-sensitising drugs versus oral contraceptive pills (alone or in combination) in improving clinical, hormonal and metabolic effects of PCOS included six appropriate trials.[76] Four compared metformin with oral contraceptive pills and two compared oral contraceptive pills combined with metformin versus oral contraceptive pills alone. Limited data showed no evidence of a difference in effect between metformin and the oral contraceptive pills on hirsutism and acne. Metformin was less effective at reducing serum androgen levels up to 12 months of therapy.

Acarbose, rosiglitazone and pioglitazone represent newer insulin-sensitising agents and are still under evaluation. However, some early studies have suggested that they might lead directly or indirectly to a reduction in hirsutism in women with PCOS.[77–81]

Female-pattern hair loss

Female-pattern hair loss, also sometimes termed androgenic alopecia, is a progressive non-scarring alopecia of scalp terminal hair and results in miniaturisation of the terminal vellus hair types. Ovarian and adrenal androgens have been implicated.

Investigations usually confirm normal androgen blood levels but the women are likely to have a genetic predisposition to this distressing condition, with increased enzyme activation and metabolism at the target end organ. Some will have an increased density of androgen receptors in the target organ.

Current treatment is aimed at managing the underlying hormone dysregulation using an oral contraceptive pill with antiandrogenic activity plus supportive topical therapy with 2% minoxidil.[82]

Minoxidil

A randomised placebo-controlled trial in women comparing 2% and 5% minoxidil found no difference in hair growth between the two concentrations but there were more adverse effects with the 5% solution.[83]

Antiandrogens

Current options include oral contraceptives with low androgen effects and other specific antiandrogen therapies such as spironolactone and cyproterone acetate.

In a 2005 study of 80 women treated with either spironolactone 200 mg daily or cyproterone acetate 50 or 100 mg daily for the first 10 days of the menstrual cycle, 44% of women taking either medication had hair regrowth, 44% had no change and 12% had continued loss.[84]

Reductase inhibitors

Finasteride and dutasteride have been used successfully for males with androgenic hair loss but, unlike minoxidil, there are no studies to show that they are effective in treating female-pattern hair loss.[85] However, in limited cases, finasteride has been shown to benefit some forms of hair loss in women with hyperandrogenism.[86]

Conclusion

The clinical manifestions of hyperandrogenism in PCOS are frequently very visible and, as a result, produce significant psychological morbidity. Greater appreciation of the pathophysiological mechanisms has led to the implementation and development of novel therapies such that many cases can be treated and achieve an acceptable outcome. There is no doubt that further good randomised controlled trials are required to draw firm conclusions on treatment effectiveness for hyperandrogenism in PCOS. Many studies reported to date have examined therapeutic options in women without PCOS but it is likely that the results are generalisable to women suffering from hyperandrogenic states attributable to PCOS.[87]

References

1. Akamatsu H, Zouboulis CC, Orfanos CE. Control of human sebocyte proliferation *in vitro* by testosterone and 5-alpha-dihydrotestosterone is dependent on the localization of the sebaceous glands. *J Invest Dermatol* 1992;99:509–11.
2. Bhamri S, Del Rosso JQ, Bhamri A. Pathogenesis of acne vulgaris: recent advances. *J Drugs Dermatol* 2009;8:615–18.
3. Deplewski D, Rosenfield RL. Role of hormones in pilosebaceous unit development. *Endocr Rev* 2000;21:363–92.
4. Sawaya ME, Shalita AR. Androgen receptor polymorphisms (CAG repeat lengths) in androgenic alopecia, hirsutism and acne. *J Cutan Med Surg* 1998:3:9–15.
5. Flamigni C, Collins WP, Koullapis EN, Craft I, Sommerville IF. Androgen metabolism in human skin. *J Clin Endocrinol Metab* 1971;32:737–43.
6. Rodien P, Mebarki F, Mowszowicz I. Different phenotypes in a family with androgen in sensitivity caused by the same M7801 point mutation in the androgen receptor gene. *J Clin Endocrinol Metab* 1996;81:2994–8.
7. Leyden JJ. New understandings of the pathogenesis of acne. *J Am Acad Dermatol* 1995;32 (Suppl):15–25.
8. Pochi PE. Hormones and acne. *Semin Dermatol* 1982;1:265.
9. Stewart ME, Downing DT, Cook JS, Hansen JR, Strauss JS. Sebaceous gland activity and serum dehydroepiandrosterone sulfate levels in boys and girls. *Arch Dermatol* 1992;128:1345–8.
10. Lucky AW, McGuire J, Rosenfield RL, Lucky PA, Rich BH. Plasma androgens in women with acne vulgaris. *J Invest Dermatol* 1983;81:70–4.
11. Beylot C, Doutre MS, Beylot-Barry M. Oral contraceptives and cyproterone acetate in female acne treatment. *Dermatology* 1998;81:70–4.
12. Gollnick H, Cunliffe W, Berson D. Global Alliance to Improve Outcomes in Acne. Management of acne: a report from a Global Alliance to Improve Outcomes in Acne. *J Am Acad Dermatol* 2003;49(1 Suppl):S1–37.
13. Bottomley WW, Yip J, Knaggs H, Cunliffe WJ. Closed comedones – comparisons of fulguration with topical tretinoin and electrocautery with fulguration. *Dermatology* 1993;186:253–7.
14. Layton AM, Hughes BR, Hull SM, Eady EA, Cunliffe WJ. Seborrhoea – an indicator for poor clinical response in acne patients treated with antibiotics. *Clin Exp Dermatol* 1992;17:173–5.
15. Layton AM. Disorders of the sebaceous glands. In: Burns DA, Breathnach SM, Griffiths S, Cox NH, editors. *Rook's Textbook of Dermatology*. 8th ed. London: Blackwell Publishing; 2010. p. 42.1–42.89.
16. Thiboutot D. Hormones and acne: pathophysiology, clinical evaluation and therapies. *Semin Cutan Med and Surg* 2001;20:144–53.
17. Darley CR, Moore JW, Besser GM, Munro DD, Kirby JD. Low dose prednisolone or oestrogen in the treatment of women with late onset or persistent acne vulgaris. *Br J Dermatol* 1983;108:345–53.
18. Lucky A. Hormonal correlates of acne and hirsutism. *Am J Med* 1995;98:895–945.
19. Saihan E, Burton J. Sebaceous gland suppression in female acne patients by combined glucocorticoid-oestrogen treatment. *Br J Dermatol* 1981;103:139.
20. Pochi P, Strauss J. Sebaceous gland inhibition from combined glucocorticoid-estrogen treatment. *Arch Dermatol* 1976;112:110.
21. Dubé JY, Ngo-Thi NH, Tremblay RR. *In vivo* effects of steroid hormones on the testosterone 5alpha-reductase in skin. *Endocrinology* 1975;97:211–14.

22. Weaver K, Glasier A. Interaction between broad-spectrum antibiotics and the combined oral contraceptive pill. A literature review. *Contraception* 1999;59:71–8.
23. Archer JS, Archer DF. Oral contraceptive efficacy and antibiotic interaction: a myth debunked. *J Am Acad Dermatol* 2002;46:917–23
24. Arowojolu AO, Gallo MF, Lopez LM, Grimes DA, Garner SE. Combined oral contraceptive pills for treatment of acne. *Cochrane Database Syst Rev* 2009;(3):CD004425.
25. Speroff L, De Cherney A. Evaluation of a new generation of oral contraceptives. *Obstet Gynecol* 1993;82:1034–47.
26. Greenwood R, Burke B, Brummitt L, Cunliffe WJ. Cyclic cyproterone/ethinyloestradiol for acne. *Lancet* 1983;ii:796.
27. Hanstead B, Reymann F. Cyproterone acetate in the treatment of acne vulgaris in adult females. *Dermatologica* 1982;164:117–26.
28. Miller JA, Wojnarowska FT, Dowd PM, Ashton RE, O'Brien TJ, Griffiths WA, *et al.* Anti-androgen treatment in women with acne: a controlled trial. *Br J Dermatol* 1986:114:705–16.
29. Aydinik S. Long-term therapy of androgenisation with a low-dose antiandrogen-oestrogen combination. *Clin Trial J* 1990;27:392–402.
30. Vasiakis-Scaramozza C, Jick H. Risk of venous thromboembolism with cyproterone contraceptives. *Lancet* 2001;358:1427–9.
31. Franks S, Layton A, Glasier A. Cyproterone acetate/ethinyl estradiol for acne and hirsutism: time to revise prescribing policy. *Hum Reprod* 2008;23:231–2.
32. van Hylckama Vlieg A, Helmerhorst FM, Vandenbroucke JP, Doggen CJ, Rosendaal FR. The venous thrombotic risk of oral contraceptives, effects of oestrogen dose and progestogen type: results of the MEGA case–control study. *BMJ* 2009;339:b2921.
33. Carlborg L. Cyproterone acetate versus levonorgestrel combined with ethinyl estradiol in the treatment of acne. Results of a multicenter study. *Acta Obstet Gynecol Scand Suppl* 1986;134:29–32.
34. Greenwood R, Brummitt L, Burke B, Cunliffe WJ. Acne: double blind clinical and laboratory trial of tetracycline, oestrogen-cyproterone acetate, and combined treatment. *Br Med J (Clin Res Ed)* 1985;291:1231–5.
35. van Wayjen R, van den Ende A. Experience in the long-term treatment of patient with hirsutism and/or acne with cyproterone acetate containing preparations: efficacy, metabolic and endocrine effects. *Exp Clin Endocrinol Diabetes* 1995;103:241–51.
36. Gollnick H, Albring M, Brill K. The effectiveness of oral CPA in combination with ethinylestradiol in acne tarda facial type. *Ann Endocrinol* 1999;60:157–66.
37. Palombo-Kinne E, Schellschmidt I, Schumacher U, Gräser T. Efficacy of a combined oral contraceptive containing 0.030 mg ethinylestradiol/2 mg dienogest for the treatment of papulopustular acne in comparison with placebo and 0.035 mg ethinylestradiol/2 mg cyproterone acetate. *Contraception* 2009;79:282–9.
38. Krattenmacher R. Drospirenone: pharmacology and pharmacokinetics of a unique progestin. *Contraception* 2000;62:26–38.
39. van Vloten WA, van Haselen CW, van Zuuren EJ, Gerlinger C, Heithecker R. The effect of two combined oral contraceptives containing either drospirenone or cyproterone acetate on acne and seborrhea. *Cutis* 2002;69:1–15.
40. Dinger JC, Heinemann LA, Kühl-Habich D. The safety of a drospirenone-containing oral contraceptive: final results from the European Active Surveillance Study on oral contraceptives based on 142,475 women-years of observation. *Contraception* 2007;75:344–54.
41. Maloney JM, Dietze P Jr, Watson D, Niknian M, Lee-Rugh S, Sampson-Landers C, *et al.* A randomized controlled trial of a low-dose combined oral contraceptive containing 3 mg drospirenone plus 20 microg ethinylestradiol in the treatment of acne vulgaris: lesion counts, investigator ratings and subject self-assessment. *J Drugs Dermatol* 2009;8:837–44.
42. Faloia E, Filipponi S, Mancini V, Morosini P, De Pirro R. Treatment with a gonadotrophin-releasing hormone agonist in acne or idiopathic hirsutism. *J Endocrinol Invest* 1993;16:675–7.
43. George R, Clark S, Thiboutot D. Hormonal therapy for acne. *Semin Cutan Med Surg* 2008;27:188–96.
44. Muhlemann MF, Carter GD, Cream JJ, Wise P. Oral spironalactone: an effective treatment for acne vulgaris in women. *Br J Dermatol* 1986;115:227–32.

45. Goodfellow A, Alaghband-Zadeh J, Carter G, Cream JJ, Holland S, Scully J, *et al.* Oral spironalactone improves acne vulgaris and reduces sebum excretion. *Br J Dermatol* 1984;111:209–14.
46. Lubbos H, Rose LI. Adverse effects of spironalactone therapy in women with acne. *Arch Dermatol* 1998;134:1162–3.
47. Thiboutot D. Acne: hormonal concepts and therapy. *Clin Dermatol* 2004;22:419–28.
48. Farquhar C, Lee O, Toomath R, Jepson R. Spironolactone versus placebo or in combination with steroids for hirsutism and/or acne. *Cochrane Database Syst Rev* 2003;(4):CD000194.
49. Shaw JC. Low dose adjunctive spironalactone in the treatment of acne in a retrospective analysis of 85 patients consecutively treated patients. *J Am Acad Dermatol* 2000;43:498–502.
50. Marcoux D, Thiboutot D. Hormonal therapy for acne. *J Cutan Med Surg* 1996;1(Suppl 1):52–6.
51. Krunic A, Ciurea A, Scheman A. Efficacy and tolerance of acne treatment using both spironolactone and a combined contraceptive containing drospirenone. *J Am Acad Dermatol* 2008;58:60–2.
52. Loube SD, Quirk RA. Breast cancer associated with administration of spironalactone. *Lancet* 1975;i:1428–9.
53. Calaf J, López E, Millet A, Alcañiz J, Fortuny A, Vidal O, *et al*; Spanish Working Group for Hirsutism. Long term efficacy and tolerability of flutamide compared with oral contraception in moderate to severe hirsutism: a 12-month, double-blind, parallel clinical trial. *J Clin Endocrinol Metab* 2007;92:3446–50.
54. Cusan L, Dupont A, Gomez JL, Tremblay RR, Labrie F. Comparison of flutamide and spironolactone in the treatment of hirsutism: a randomized controlled trial. *Fertil Steril* 1995;61:281–7.
55. Wysowski DK, Freiman JP, Tourtelot JB, Horton ML 3rd. Fatal and non-fatal hepatotoxicity associated with flutamide. *Ann Intern Med* 1993;118:860–4.
56. Costello M, Shrestha B, Eden J, Sjoblom P, Johnson N. Insulin-sensitising drugs versus the combined oral contraceptive pill for hirsutism, acne and risk of diabetes, cardiovascular disease, and endometrial cancer in polycystic ovary syndrome. *Cochrane Database Syst Rev* 2007;(1):CD005552.
57. Thiboutot D, Gollnick H, Bettoli V, Dréno B, Kang S, Leyden JJ, *et al*; Global Alliance to Improve Outcomes in Acne. New insights into the management of acne: an update from the Global Alliance to Improve Outcomes in Acne group. *J Am Acad Dermatol* 2009;60(5 Suppl):S1–50.
58. Azziz R, Carmina E, Dewailly D, Diamanti-Kandarakis E, Escobar-Morreale HF, Futterweit W, *et al*; Androgen Excess Society. Position statement: Criteria for defining polycystic ovary syndrome as a predominantly hyperandrogenic syndrome: an Androgen Excess Society Guideline. *J Clin Endocrinol Metab* 2006;91:4237–45.
59. Koulouri O, Conway GS. A systematic review of commonly used medical treatments for hirsutism in women. *Clin Endocrinol (Oxf)* 2008;68:800–5.
60. Pasquali R, Antenucci D, Casimirri F, Venturoli S, Paradisi R, Fabbri R, *et al.* Clinical and hormonal characteristics of obese amenorrhoeic hyperandrogenic women before and after weight loss. *J Clin Endocrinol Metab* 1989;68:173–9.
61. Haedersdal M, Gøtzsche PC. Laser and photoepilation for unwanted hair growth. *Cochrane Database Syst Rev* 2006;(4):CD004684.
62. Wolf JE Jr, Shander D, Huber F, Jackson J, Lin CS, Mathes BM, *et al*; Eflornithine HCl Study Group. Randomized, double-blind clinical evaluation of the efficacy and safety of topical eflornithine HCl 13.9% cream in the treatment of women with facial hair. *Int J Dermatol* 2007;46:94–8.
63. Hamzavi I, Tan E, Shapiro J, Lui H. A randomised bilateral vehicle-controlled study of eflornithine cream combined with laser treatment versus laser treatment alone for facial hirsutism in women. *J Am Acad Dermatol* 2007;57:54–9.
64. Swiglo BA, Cosma M, Flynn DN, Kurtz DM, Labella ML, Mullan RJ, *et al.* Clinical review: Antiandrogens for the treatment of hirsutism: a systematic review and metaanalyses of randomized controlled trials. *J Clin Endocrinol Metab* 2008;93:1153–60.

65. Batukan C, Muderris II, Ozcelik B, Ozturk A. Comparison of two oral contraceptives containing either drospirenone or cyproterone acetate in the treatment of hirsutism. *Gynecol Endocrinol* 2007;23:38–44.
66. Cem B, Ipek M. Efficacy of a new oral contraceptive containing drosperinone and ethinyl oestradiol in long term treatment of hirsutism *Fertil Steril* 2006;85:436–40.
67. van der Spuy ZM, le Roux PA. Cyproterone actetate for hirsutism. *Cochrane Database Syst Rev* 2003;(4):CD000194.
68. Brown J, Farquhar C, Lee O, Toomath R, Jepson RG. Spironolactone versus placebo or in combination with steroids for hirsutism and/or acne. *Cochrane Database Syst Rev* 2009;(2):CD000194.
69. van der Spuy ZM, Tregoning S. Gonadotrophin-releasing hormone analogues for hirsutism (protocol). *Cochrane Database Syst Rev* 2008;(4):CD001126.
70. Beigi A, Sobhi A, Zarrinkoub F. Finasteride versus cyproterone acetate-oestrogen regimens in the treatment of hirsutism. *Int J Gynaecol Obstet* 2004;87:29–33.
71. Sahin Y, Bayram F, Keleştimur F, Müderris I. Comparison of cyproterone acetate plus ethinyl estradiol and finasteride int the treatment of hirsutism. *J Endocrinol Invest* 1998;21:348–52.
72. Falsetti L, Gambera A, Legrenzi L, Iacobello C, Bugari G. Comparison of finasteride versus flutamide in the treatment of hirsutism. *Eur J Endocrinol* 1999;141:361–7.
73. Wallace C, Lalor EA, Crik CL. Hepatotoxicity complicating flutamide treatment of hirsutism. *Ann Int Med* 1993;119:1150.
74. Unluhizarci K, Ozel D, Tanriverdi F, Karaca Z, Kelestimur F. A comparison between finasteride, flutamide, and finasteride plus flutamide combination in the treatment of hirsutism. *J Endocrinol Invest* 2009;32:37–40.
75. Harborne L, Fleming R, Lyall H, Sattar N, Norman J. Metformin or antiandrogen in the treatment of hirsutism in polycystic ovary syndrome. *J Clin Endocrinol Metab* 2003;88:4116–23.
76. Costello MF, Shrestha B, Eden J, Johnson NP, Sjoblom P. Metformin versus oral contraceptive pill in polycystic ovary syndrome: a Cochrane review. *Hum Reprod* 2007;22:1200–9.
77. Pillai A Bang H, Green C. Metformin and glitazones: do they really help PCOS patients? *J Fam Pract* 2007:56:444–53.
78. Penna IA, Canella PR, Reis RM, Silva de Sá MF, Ferriani RA. Acarbose in obese patients with polycystic ovarian syndrome: a double blind placebo controlled study. *Hum Reprod* 2005;20:2396–401.
79. Dereli D, Dereli T, Bayraktar F, Ozgen AG, Yilmaz C. Endocrine and metabolic effects of rosiglitazone in non obese women with PCOS. *Endocr J* 2005:52:299–308.
80. Yilmaz M, Karakoç A, Törüner FB, Cakir N, Tiras B, Ayvaz G, *et al.* The effects of rosglitazone and metformin on menstrual cyclicity and hirsutism in polycystic ovary syndrome. *Gynecol Endocrinol* 2005;21:154–60.
81. Brettenthaler N, De Geyter C, Huber PR, Keller U. Effect of insulin sensitiser pioglitazone on insulin resistance, hyperandrogenism and ovulatory dysfunction in women with polycystic ovary syndrome *J Clin Endocrinol Metab* 2004;89:3835–40.
82. Fraser IS, Kovacs G. Current recommendations for the diagnostic evaluation and follow-up of patients presenting with symptomatic polycystic ovary syndrome. *Best Pract Res Clin Obstet Gynaecol* 2004;18:813–23.
83. Lucky AW, Piacquadio DJ, Ditre CM, Dunlap F, Kantor I, Pandya AG, *et al.* A randomised placebo controlled trial of 5% and 2% topical minoxidil solutions in the treatment of female pattern hair loss. *J Am Acad Dermatol* 2004;50:541–53.
84. Sinclair R, Wewerinke M, Jolley D. Treatment of female pattern hair loss with oral antiandrogens. *Br J Dermatol* 2005;152:466–73.
85. Price VH, Roberts JL, Hordinsky M, Olsen EA, Savin R, Bergfeld W, *et al.* Lack of efficacy of finasteride in postmenopausal women with androgenetic alopecia. *J Am Acad Dermatol* 2000;43(5 Pt 1):768–76.
86. Shum KW, Cullen DR, Messenger AG. Hair loss in women with hyperandrogenism. Four cases responding to finasteride. *J Am Acad Dermatol* 2002;47:733–9.
87. Cahill D. PCOS. *BMJ Clin Evid* 2009;1408:1–19.

12

Chapter 12

Choices in the treatment of anovulatory polycystic ovary syndrome

Roy Homburg

Introduction

Polycystic ovary syndrome (PCOS) is present in approximately 75% of women with infertility due to anovulation[1,2] and it is frequently diagnosed for the first time in the fertility clinic. The majority of women with anovulation or oligo-ovulation due to PCOS have clinical and/or biochemical evidence of hyperandrogenism. Almost all these women will have a typical ultrasonic appearance of the ovaries.[3]

The exact mechanism causing anovulation associated with PCOS is not known and the excess of small antral follicles, hyperandrogenaemia, hyperinsulinaemia and dysfunctional feedback mechanisms have all been implicated. There are, however, a number of strategies to restore ovulation, most of them reliant on increasing follicle-stimulating hormone (FSH) concentrations, either endogenously or exogenously, or reducing insulin levels. These include medical therapies such as clomifene citrate, aromatase inhibitors, metformin and low-dose gonadotrophin therapy and surgical treatment by laparoscopic ovarian diathermy. This chapter describes treatment with clomifene, aromatase inhibitors and gonadotrophins in detail, but metformin only in brief as it is covered in full in Chapter 15. Laparoscopic ovarian diathermy is discussed in Chapter 14.

Weight loss

Whereas obesity expresses and exaggerates the signs and symptoms of insulin resistance, loss of weight can reverse this process by improving ovarian function and the associated hormonal abnormalities[4,5] and may alone induce ovulation and pregnancy. Loss of weight induces a reduction of insulin and androgen concentrations and an increase in sex hormone-binding globulin concentrations. For obese women with PCOS, a loss of just 5–10% of body weight is enough to restore reproductive function in 55–100% within 6 months of weight reduction.[4,6] Weight loss has the undoubted advantages of being effective and cheap with no adverse effects and should be the first line of treatment in obese women with anovulatory infertility associated with PCOS.

Clomifene citrate

Mode of action

Clomifene citrate is a long-established first-line treatment for women with PCOS who have absent or irregular ovulation. Paradoxically, its anti-estrogen action in blocking estradiol receptors in the hypothalamus induces a change in gonadotrophin-releasing hormone pulse frequency, release of FSH from the anterior pituitary and consequent follicular development and estradiol production.

Dose

Clomifene citrate has been given in a dose of 50–250 mg per day for 5 days starting from any of days 2–5 of spontaneous or induced uterine bleeding. The starting dose may be raised in increments of 50 mg per day each cycle until an ovulatory cycle is achieved. However, I have found no advantage in using a dose of more than 150 mg per day, as this seems neither to significantly increase the ovulation rate nor follicular recruitment. The approximately 20% of women who remain resistant to clomifene (that is, remain anovulatory) are thus identified within three cycles.

Results

A compilation of data collected from the literature[7] is presented in Table 12.1. The notable features are an ovulation rate of 73%, a pregnancy rate of 36 % and a live birth rate of 29%.

Clomifene citrate treatment failure

Women who do not respond to clomifene are likely to be more obese, insulin resistant and hyperandrogenic than those who do respond.[8] A course of six ovulatory cycles is usually sufficient to know whether pregnancy will be achieved using clomifene before moving on to more complex treatment, as approximately 75% of the pregnancies achieved with clomifene occur within the first three cycles of treatment[9] and pregnancies are rarely achieved following six ovulatory cycles.

Table 12.1 Published results of treatment with clomifene citrate

Study	Patients	Ovulation	Pregnancy	Termination of pregnancy	Live birth
MacGregor *et al.* (1968)[10]	4098	2869	1393	279	1114
Garcia *et al.* (1977)[47]	159	130	64	16	48
Gysler *et al.* (1982)[9]	428	364	184	24	160
Hammond (1984)[48]	159	137	67	10	57
Kousta *et al.* (1997)[49]	128	113	55	13	42
Messinis *et al.* (1998)[50]	55	51	35	4	31
Imani *et al.* (2002)[11]	259	194	111	11	98
Total	5268 (100%)	3858 (73%)	1909 (36%)	357	1550 (29%)

Although ovulation is restored in approximately 80% of cases, pregnancy is achieved in only about 35–40% of women who are given clomifene.[9–11] There are several possible explanations for this 'gap'. Clomifene induces a discharge of luteinising hormone (LH) as well as FSH, so those with high basal LH levels are less likely to respond and conceive with clomifene treatment.[12] However, the most probable factor involved in this large discrepancy between ovulation and pregnancy rates in women treated with clomifene is its anti-estrogenic effect at the level of the endometrium and cervical mucus. While the depression of the cervical mucus, which occurs in at least 15% of cases, may be overcome by performing intrauterine insemination (IUI), suppression of endometrial proliferation, which is unrelated to dose or duration of treatment but apparently idiosyncratic, indicates a poor prognosis for conception in my experience when endometrial thickness remains less than 8 mm.

Monitoring

Ultrasound evaluation of follicular growth and endometrial thickness on day 11–14 of the cycle is justified by the identification of those who are not responding or have depressed endometrial thickness and is helpful in the timing of natural intercourse or IUI. Although this monitoring means added expense, this is neutralised by the prevention of protracted periods of possibly inappropriate therapy and delay in the inception of more efficient treatment. In our recent study comparing two large groups of ultrasound-monitored and non-monitored clomifene-treated cycles, those that were monitored yielded significantly better pregnancy rates.[13]

Adjuvant treatment

Co-treatment with several proposed adjuvants has been advocated in an attempt to achieve improved results from clomifene treatment. The addition of an ovulation-triggering dose of human chorionic gonadotrophin (hCG) (5000–10 000 IU) is only theoretically warranted when the reason for a non-ovulatory response is that the LH surge is delayed or absent despite the presence of a well-developed follicle. Although the routine addition of hCG at mid-cycle seems to add little to the improvement of conception rates,[14,15] I have found it very useful for the timing of intercourse or IUI, if administered when an ultrasonically demonstrated leading follicle attains a diameter of 18–24 mm.

Dexamethasone 0.5 mg per day at bedtime as an adjunct to clomifene therapy suppresses the adrenal androgen secretion and may induce responsiveness to clomifene in those who did not previously respond (who are mostly hyperandrogenic women with PCOS with elevated concentrations of dehydroepiandrosterone sulfate).[16,17] Although this method meets with some success, medium- to long-term glucocorticoid steroid therapy often induces adverse effects such as increased appetite and weight gain, which is counterproductive for women with PCOS.

The combined treatment of clomifene with metformin is discussed later in this chapter.

Aromatase inhibitors

Aromatase inhibitors are potent nonsteroidal compounds that suppress estrogen biosynthesis by blocking the action of the enzyme aromatase which converts androstendione and testosterone to estrogens. The aromatase inhibitors letrozole

(Femara®, Novartis) and anastrozole (Arimidex®, AstraZeneca) have mainly been employed for the treatment of postmenopausal women with advanced breast cancer. Given orally, they are almost free of adverse effects.

Mode of action

The efficient estrogen-lowering properties of the aromatase inhibitors temporarily release the hypothalamus from the negative feedback effect of estrogen, thus inducing an increased discharge of FSH.[18] Although the end result of an increased discharge of FSH is common to both aromatase inhibitors and clomifene, the differences in their mode of action confer several theoretical advantages to aromatase inhibitors used for ovulation induction:[18,19]

- aromatase inhibitors have no effect on estrogen receptors and therefore no deleterious effect on cervical mucus or endometrium
- aromatase inhibitors do not block hypothalamic estrogen receptors and, therefore, the negative feedback mechanism remains intact; this enables regulation of the FSH discharge when estrogen is produced and should reduce the prevalence of multiple follicle development and, consequently, of multiple pregnancies when compared with clomifene
- the half-life of the aromatase inhibitors is about 2 days, which is much shorter than that of clomifene.

Indications

Indications for the use of aromatase inhibitors in ovulation induction are virtually the same as for clomifene; that is, women with absent or irregular ovulation associated with normal concentrations of endogenous estradiol and FSH (WHO group II, hypothalamic–pituitary dysfunction). A very large majority of these cases are associated with PCOS. In addition to treatment-naïve patients, a trial of treatment with aromatase inhibitors has been suggested for those who are clomifene resistant. Preliminary results have shown that this may be a worthwhile step before proceeding to gonadotrophin therapy.[20]

Dose

Letrozole has been given at a dose of 2.5–5 mg per day for 5 days starting from any of days 2–5 of the cycle, which is similar to clomifene. In the case of failure to ovulate on these doses, as much as 7.5–10 mg per day has been administered,[21] but 5 mg per day would appear to be the optimal dose.[22] Letrozole has virtually no adverse effects. The optimal dose of anastrozole for ovulation induction has yet to be determined.

Evidence

A number of randomised controlled trials have compared the results of ovulation induction for treatment-naïve women with PCOS using clomifene (100 mg per day) with letrozole (2.5–5 mg per day).[23–26] Two meta-analyses of studies comparing pregnancy rates with clomifene or letrozole have demonstrated slight[27] or clear[28] superiority of letrozole, with pregnancy rates ranging from 15% to 33% per patient and around 16% per cycle. In general, both the number of mature follicles and the estradiol levels were lower with the use of letrozole. The multiple pregnancy rate with letrozole, recorded only in an uncontrolled series, was 0.2%.[21]

In a study of women with clomifene-resistant PCOS given letrozole, an ovulation rate of 54.6% and a pregnancy rate of 25% were achieved, suggesting that this treatment should be tried before proceeding to more sophisticated treatments in this group of women.[20]

Although anastrozole (1 mg per day for 5 days) has also been shown to be capable of inducing ovulation and pregnancy, letrozole has been shown to be more successful in those who are clomifene resistant.[29] However, it is very possible that this dose of anastrozole was not optimal for this indication.[30]

Safety

Initial unsubstantiated fears regarding possible teratogenic effects of aromatase inhibitors have largely been quashed by the reporting of a significantly lower incidence of both minor and major congenital anomalies in a very large group of women who conceived using letrozole compared with those who used clomifene.[31] Despite this, the use of aromatase inhibitors for ovulation induction remains off-label in many countries. It is hoped that this limitation will be rescinded in the near future.

As the use of aromatase inhibitors in the treatment of infertility is still in its infancy, many questions still remain to be answered. Trials with aromatase inhibitors for ovulation induction have, reasonably, mimicked treatment with clomifene, being administered on days 3–7 of the cycle and optimal doses have not been fully established. It is a little too early to enthuse about the chances of letrozole and anastrozole becoming standard treatment for ovulation induction. However, now that the initial studies have been completed, there is enough evidence for optimism to encourage further serious trials for this potentially valuable, simple and innocuous treatment.

Metformin

Mode of action

Metformin is an oral biguanide that is well established for the treatment of hyperglycaemia and that does not cause hypoglycaemia in normoglycaemic patients. In women with PCOS, metformin is said to lower fasting insulin concentrations but also probably acts directly on theca cells and attenuates androgen production. The sum total of its actions is often a reduction in insulin and androgen levels and, consequently, a resulting improvement of the clinical sequelae of hyperandrogenism. Although oligomenorrhoea improves in some women with PCOS, significant numbers remain anovulatory.[32] Metformin does not produce consistent significant changes in body mass index or waist to hip ratio but the degree of improvement in ovulation frequency is mainly achieved with weight reduction through lifestyle modification and there is no difference between metformin and placebo in this regard.[33] The improvement has been estimated to represent one extra ovulation every five woman-months.[34]

Dose

Metformin for ovulation induction is given in a dose of 1500–2500 mg per day in two or three divided doses. Gastrointestinal adverse effects are not uncommon.

Evidence

For induction of ovulation, two randomised controlled trials indicate that metformin does not increase live birth rates above those observed with clomifene alone, in either obese or normal-weight women with PCOS.[35,36] In fact, the larger of these two trials[35] demonstrated a selective disadvantage to metformin compared with clomifene and no apparent advantage to adding metformin to clomifene, except perhaps in those with clomifene resistance. Clomifene resulted in higher ovulation, conception, pregnancy and live birth rates compared with metformin, while the combination of both drugs did not result in a significant benefit. Disappointingly, addition of metformin did not reduce the incidence of miscarriage, which was in fact higher in the metformin group. Furthermore, metformin treatment conferred no additional advantage when administered to newly diagnosed women with PCOS.[36] A European Society of Human Reproduction and Embryology (ESHRE)/American Society for Reproductive Medicine (ASRM) consensus meeting therefore concluded that insulin sensitisers should not be used as first-choice agents for induction of ovulation in women with PCOS, while their administration does not appear to reduce the incidence of early pregnancy losses.[37] In addition, data so far do not indicate any advantage to the use of thiazolidinediones over metformin.[38]

Safety

Although data to date suggest that metformin is safe during pregnancy, there is no definitive indication for its use during pregnancy. It does not seem to affect the miscarriage rate and, although there have been suggestions that continuing metformin during pregnancy may be protective against complications,[39] this strategy is currently not widely practised.

Low-dose gonadotrophin therapy

Principle

The aim of the chronic low-dose step-up protocol is to achieve the ovulation of a single follicle. Unlike the conventional protocol, the low-dose protocol employs a dose of gonadotrophin that is not supra-physiological but reaches the threshold for a follicular response without exceeding it and thereby produces monofollicular rather than multifollicular ovulation. This practically eliminates the occurrence of ovarian hyperstimulation syndrome (OHSS) and reduces multiple pregnancies to fewer than 6%.[40]

Regimen

The classic chronic low-dose regimen (Figure 12.1) employs a small starting dose in the first cycle of treatment of 50–75 IU of FSH, which remains unchanged for 14 days.[41] If this does not produce the criteria for hCG administration, a small incremental dose rise of 25–37.5 IU is used every 7 days until follicular development is initiated. Even smaller incremental dose rises of 8.3 IU have been employed with similar results.[42] The dose that initiates follicular development (at least one follicle larger than 10 mm diameter) is continued until the criteria for giving hCG are attained. hCG should not be given if three or more follicles larger than 16 mm diameter are seen, to minimise the chance of a multiple pregnancy. The majority of women on a low-dose protocol develop a single large follicle meeting hCG administration criteria within 14–16 days without any change in the initial dose for 14 days.[40] In the relatively unusual case (typically in very obese women) where a treatment cycle is abandoned after 28–35 days owing to lack of response, a larger starting dose may, of course, be employed in a subsequent attempt.

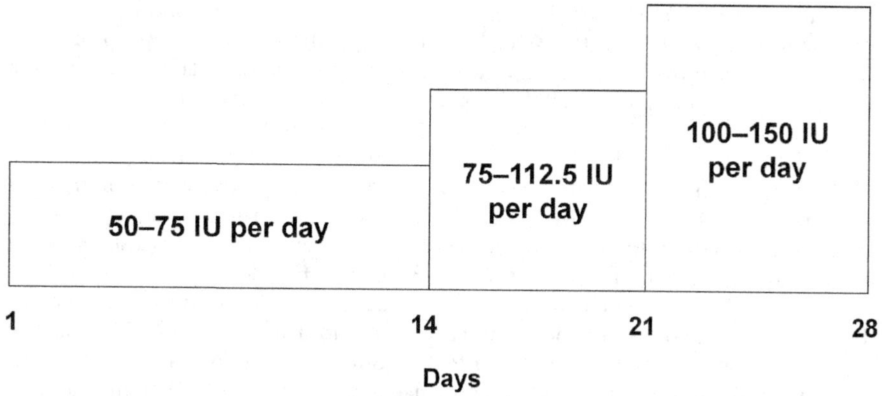

Figure 12.1 A recommended scheme for the first cycle of low-dose step-up follicle-stimulating hormone administration

Evidence

A compilation of reported results from the literature,[40] using a chronic low-dose protocol identical to that described above, is presented in Box 12.1. The prominent features include a remarkably consistent rate of uniovulatory cycles of around 70% in each series. The pregnancy rate of 38% of the patients and 20% per cycle are acceptable compared with past experiences with conventional therapy and taking into account that many of the women in these series received only one cycle of therapy. However, the justification for the adoption of the chronic low-dose protocol may be seen in the extraordinarily low prevalence of OHSS and a multiple pregnancy rate of only 5.7%.

Variations

Some centres reduce the initial no-dose-change time from 14 days to 7 days to shorten the duration of treatment but this may be at the expense of an increased occurrence of multiple follicular ovulations and, consequently, multiple pregnancies.[40] On the basis of physiological principles concerning concentrations of FSH in a natural ovulatory cycle, a step-down protocol has been suggested starting with 150 IU of FSH for 5 days, raising the dose by 37.5 IU every 3 days if necessary until a follicle of 10 mm is obtained. The daily dose is then reduced by 37.5 IU every 3 days until the criteria for giving

Box 12.1 Results of treatment of clomifene-resistant patients with low-dose step-up follicle-stimulating hormone; data from Homburg and Howles[40]

Number of patients	841
Number of cycles	1556
Pregnancies	320 (38 % of patients)
Fecundity per cycle	20 %
Uniovulation	70 %
Ovarian hyperstimulation syndrome	0.14 %
Multiple pregnancies	5.7 %

hCG are reached.[43] However, although pregnancy rates are similar and FSH is given for a shorter duration with this step-down protocol, the low-dose step-up protocol has a lower rate of overstimulation, double the rate of monofollicular ovulation and a higher ovulation rate and is, therefore, preferred by the majority of centres.[44]

From the largest published series of chronic low-dose step-up therapy,[45] the comparison of a starting dose of 75 IU with that of 52.5 IU for an initial 14-day period with an incremental dose rise of 37.5 IU or 22.5 IU, respectively, demonstrated a pregnancy rate per patient, uniovulatory cycle rate and miscarriage rate slightly in favour of the smaller starting dose. In a further series, no difference other than a slight saving in FSH requirements was found between the use of a starting dose of 37.5 IU or 50 IU.[46]

There is now sufficient evidence that low-dose step-up gonadotrophin therapy should be preferred to the now outdated conventional therapy for anovulatory patients and particularly for those with PCOS. Small starting doses in the first cycle for a 14-day initial period without a dose change and then a small incremental dose rise if required seem to give the best results.

References

1. Adams J, Polson DW, Franks S. Prevalence of polycystic ovaries in women with anovulation and idiopathic hirsutism. *Br Med J* 1986;293:355–9.
2. Hull MG. Epidemiology of infertility and polycystic ovarian disease: endocrinological and demographic studies. *Gynaecol Endocrinol* 1987;1:235–45.
3. Adams J, Franks S, Polson DW, Mason HD, Abdulwahid N, Tucker M, *et al.* Multifollocular ovaries: clinical and endocrine features and response to pulsatile gonadotrophin releasing hormone. *Lancet* 1985;ii:1375–8.
4. Kiddy DS, Hamilton-Fairley D, Bush A, Short F, Anyaoku V, Reed MJ, *et al.* Improvement in endocrine and ovarian function during dietary treatment of obese women with polycystic ovary syndrome. *Clin Endocrinol* 1992;36:1105–11.
5. Pasquali R, Antenucci D, Casmirri F, Venturoli S, Paradisi R, Fabbri R, *et al.* Clinical and hormonal characteristics of obese amenorrheic hyperandrogenic women before and after weight loss. *J Clin Endocrinol Metab* 1989;68:173–9.
6. Clark AM, Ledger W, Galletly C, Tomlinson L, Blaney F, Wang X, *et al.* Weight loss results in significant improvement in pregnancy and ovulation rates in anovulatory obese women. *Hum Reprod* 1995;10:2705–12.
7. Homburg R. Clomiphene citrate – end of an era? *Hum Reprod* 2005;20:2043–51.
8. Imani B, Eijkemans MJ, te Velde ER, Habbema JD, Fauser BC. Predictors of patients remaining anovulatory during clomiphene citrate induction of ovulation in normogonadotropic oligomenorrheic infertility. *J Clin Endocrinol Metab* 1998;83:2361–5.
9. Gysler M, March CM, Mishell DR, Bailey EJ. A decade's experience with an individualized clomiphene treatment regimen including its effects on the postcoital test. *Fertil Steril* 1982;37:161–7.
10. MacGregor AH, Johnson JE, Bunde CA. Further clinical experience with clomiphene citrate. *Fertil Steril* 1968;19:616–22.
11. Imani B, Eijkemans MJ, te Velde ER. A nomogram to predict the probability of live birth after clomiphene citrate induction of ovulation in normogonadotropic oligomenorrheic infertility. *Fertil Steril* 2002;77:91–7.
12. Homburg R, Armar NA, Eshel A, Adams J, Jacobs HS. Influence of serum luteinizing hormone concentrations on ovulation, conception and early pregnancy loss in polycystic ovary syndrome. *Br Med J* 1988;297:1024–6.
13. Konig T, Homburg R, Hendriks ML, van Leeuwen A, Hompes PG, Lambalk CB. Do monitoring and hCG administration influence the outcome of clomiphene treatment for anovulatory PCOS? *Annual Meeting of ESHRE, Amsterdam 2009*;Abstract P.335.

14. Agrawal SK, Buyalos RP. Corpus luteum function and pregnancy rates with clomiphene citrate therapy: comparison of human chorionic gonadotrophin-induced versus spontaneous ovulation. *Hum Reprod* 1995;10:328–31.
15. Kosmas IP, Tatsioni A, Fatemi HM, Kolibianakis EM, Tournaye H, Devroey P. Human chorionic gonadotropin administration vs. luteinizing monitoring for intrauterine insemination timing, after administration of clomiphene citrate: a meta-analysis. *Fertil Steril* 2007;87:607–12.
16. Diamant YZ, Evron S. Induction of ovulation by combined clomiphene citrate and dexamethasone treatment in clomiphene citrate non-responders. *Eur J Obstet Gynecol Biol* 1981;11:335–40.
17. Daly DC, Walters CA, Soto-Albors CE, Tohan N, Riddick DH. A randomized study of dexamethasone in ovulation induction with clomiphene citrate. *Fertil Steril* 1984;41:844–8.
18. Mitwally MF, Casper RF Aromatase inhibition: a novel method of ovulation induction in women with polycystic ovary syndrome. *Reprod Technol* 2000;10:244–7.
19. Homburg R. Oral agents for ovulation induction – clomiphene citrate versus aromatase inhibitors. *Hum Fertil* 2008;22:261–4.
20. Elnashar A, Fouad H, Eldosoky M, Saeid N. Letrozole induction of ovulation in women with clomiphene citrate-resistant polycystic ovary syndrome may not depend on the period of infertility, the body mass index, or the luteinizing hormone/follicle stimulating hormone ratio. *Fertil Steril* 2006;85:511–13.
21. Aghassa MM, Asheghan H, Khazali S, Bagheri M. Aromatase inhibitors for ovulation induction in polycystic ovary syndrome. In: Allahbadia G, Agrawal R, editors. *Polycystic Ovary Syndrome.* Tunbridge Wells: Anshan; 2007. p. 341–5.
22. Biljan MM, Tan SL, Tulandi T. Prospective randomized trial comparing the effects of 2.5 and 5.0 mg of letrozole (LE) on follicular development, endometrial thickness and pregnancy rates in patients undergoing superovulation. *Fertil Steril* 2002;76(Suppl 1):S55.
23. Atay V, Cam C, Muhcu M, Cam M, Karateke A. Comparison of letrozole and clomiphene citrate in women with polycystic ovaries undergoing ovarian stimulation. *J Int Med Res* 2006;34:73–6.
24. Badawy A, Abdel Aal I, Abulatta M. Clomiphene or letrozole for ovulation induction in women with polycystic ovary syndrome: a prospective randomized trial. *Fertil Steril* 2009;92:849–52.
25. Bayar U, Basaran M, Kiran S, Coskun A, Gezer S. Use of an aromatase inhibitor in patients with polycystic ovary syndrome: a prospective randomized trial. *Fertil Steril* 2006;86:1447–51.
26. Sohrabvand F, Ansari S, Bagheri M. Efficacy of combined metformin-letrozole in comparison with metformin-clomiphene in clomiphene resistant infertile women with polycystic ovary disease. *Hum Reprod* 2006;21:1432–5.
27. Reqena A, Herrero J, Landeras J, Navarro E, Neyro JL, Salvador C, *et al.* Use of letrozole in assisted reproduction: a systematic review and meta-analysis. *Hum Reprod Update* 2008;14:571–80.
28. Polyzos NP, Tsappi M, Mauri D, Atay V, Cortinovis I, Casazza G. Aromatase inhibtors for infertility in polycystic ovary syndrome. The beginning or the end of a new era? *Fertil Steril* 2008;89:278–80.
29. Al-Omari WR, Sulaiman WR, Al-Hadithi N. Comparison of two aromatase inhibitors in women with clomiphene-resistant polycystic ovary syndrome. *Int J Gynaecol Obstet* 2004;85:289–91.
30. Tredway DR, Buraglio M, Hemsey G, Denton G. A phase I study of the pharmacokinetics, pharmacodynamics, and safety of single- and multiple-dose anastrozole in healthy, premenopausal female volunteers. *Fertil Steril* 2004;82:1587–93.
31. Tulandi T, Martin J, Al-Fadhli R, Kabli N, Forman R, Hitkari J, *et al.* Congenital malformations among 911 newborns conceived after infertility treatment with letrozole or clomiphene citrate. *Fertil Steril* 2006;85:1761–5.
32. Fleming R, Hopkinson ZE, Wallace AM, Greer IA, Sattar N. Ovarian function and metabolic factors in women with oligomenorrhea treated with metformin in a randomized double blind placebo-controlled trial. *J Clin Endocrinol Metab* 2002;87:569–74.
33. Tang T, Glanville J, Hayden CJ, White D, Barth JH, Balen AH. Combined lifestyle modification and metformin in obese patients with polycystic ovary syndrome. A randomized, placebo-controlled, double-blind multicentre study. *Hum Reprod* 2006;21:80–9.
34. Harborne L, Fleming R, Lyall H, Norman J, Sattar N. Descriptive review of the evidence for the use of metformin in polycystic ovary syndrome. *Lancet* 2003;361:1894–901.

35. Legro RS, Barnhart HX, Schlaff WD, Carr BR, Diamond MP, Carson SA, *et al.* Clomiphene, metformin, or both for infertility in the polycystic ovary syndrome. *N Engl J Med* 2007;356;551–66.
36. Moll E, Bossuyt PM, Korevaar JC, Lambalk CB, van der Veen F. Effect of clomifene citrate plus metformin and clomifene citrate plus placebo on induction of ovulation in women with newly diagnosed polycystic ovary syndrome: randomised double blind clinical trial. *BMJ* 2006;332:1485.
37. Thessaloniki ESHRE/ASRM-Sponsored PCOS Consensus Workshop Group. Consensus on infertility treatment related to polycystic ovary syndrome. *Hum Reprod* 2008;23:462–77.
38. Legro RS, Zaino RJ, Demers LM, Kunselman AR, Gnatuk CL, Williams NI, *et al.* The effects of metformin and rosiglitazone, alone and in combination, on the ovary and endometrium in polycystic ovary syndrome. *Am J Obstet Gynecol* 2007;196:402–10.
39. Vanky E, Salvesen KA, Heimstad R, Fougner KJ, Romundstad P, Carlsen SM. Metformin reduces pregnancy complications without affecting androgen levels in pregnant polycystic ovary syndrome women: results of a randomized study. *Hum Reprod* 2004;19:1734–40.
40. Homburg R, Howles CM. Low-dose FSH therapy for anovulatory infertility associated with polycystic ovary syndrome: rationale, results, reflections and refinements. *Hum Reprod Update* 1999;5:493–9.
41. Polson DW, Mason HD, Saldahna MB, Franks S. Ovulation of a single dominant follicle during treatment with low-dose pulsatile follicle stimulating hormone in women with polycystic ovary syndrome. *Clin Endocrinol (Oxf)* 1987;26:205–12.
42. Orvieto R, Homburg R. Chronic ultra-low dose follicle-stimulating hormone regimen for patients with polycystic ovary syndrome: one click, one follicle, one pregnancy. *Fertil Steril* 2009;91(4 Suppl):1533–5.
43. Van Santbrink EJ, Fauser BC. Urinary follicle-stimulating hormone for normogonadotropic clomiphene resistant anovulatory infertility: prospective, randomized comparison between low dose step-up and step-down dose regimens. *J Clin Endocrinol Metab* 1997;82:3597–602.
44. Christin-Maitre S, Hugues JN. A comparative randomized multricentric study comparing the step-up versus the step-down protocol in polycystic ovary syndrome. *Hum Reprod* 2003;18:1621–31.
45. White DM, Polson DW, Kiddy D, Sagle P, Watson H, Gilling-Smith C, *et al.* Induction of ovulation with low-dose gonadotropins in polycystic ovary syndrome: an analysis of 109 pregnancies in 225 women. *J Clin Endocrinol Metab* 1996;81:3821–4.
46. Balasch J, Fábregues F, Creus M, Casamitjana R, Puerto B, Vanrell JA. Recombinant human follicle-stimulating hormone for ovulation induction in polycystic ovary syndrome: a prospective, randomized trial of two starting doses in a chronic low-dose step-up protocol. *J Assist Reprod Genet* 2000;17:561–5.
47. Garcia J, Jones GS, Wentz AC. The use of clomiphene citrate. *Fertil Steril* 1977;28:707–17.
48. Hammond MG. Monitoring techniques for improved pregnancy rates during clomiphene ovulation induction. *Fertil Steril* 1984;42:499–509.
49. Kousta E, White DM, Franks S. Modern use of clomiphene citrate in induction of ovulation. *Hum Reprod Update* 1997;3:359–65.
50. Messinis IE, Milingos SD. Future use of clomiphene in ovarian stimulation. Clomiphene in the 21st century. *Hum Reprod* 1998;13:2362–5.

Chapter 13

Predictors of ovarian response to ovarian stimulation: progress towards individualised treatment in ovulation induction

Bart CJM Fauser

Introduction

Ovarian response can be defined as the endocrine and follicular reaction of the ovaries to a stimulus. The term is used in clinical research and practice both qualitatively (for example, achieving growth of a single dominant follicle and ovulation in anovulatory women undergoing ovulation induction) and quantitatively (for example, the extent of multifollicular development in ovulating women undergoing ovarian stimulation for *in vitro* fertilisation). Achieving a distinct ovarian response usually represents the desired outcome of pharmacological interventions on the hypothalamic–pituitary–ovarian axis in ovulation induction and ovarian stimulation. The considerable individual variability in ovarian response to stimulation, however, necessitates close monitoring and dose adjustment for each woman. The likelihood of pregnancy in a woman undergoing ovulation induction is subject to a large number of factors other than ovarian reserve and ovarian response.[1]

It is of high clinical relevance to identify predictors of ovarian response that will enable clinicians to individualise ovulation induction strategies, thereby minimising complications and the risk of treatment failure while maximising the chances of a continuing pregnancy. The conventional paradigm in many areas of reproductive medicine has been 'one size fits all' or a choice of therapy based on the physician's experience from their own clinical practice, which may have low reproducibility.[2] To improve consistency between clinics, various clinical, endocrine and ovarian ultrasonographic and genetic characteristics have been explored for use as predictors of ovarian response.[3] However, 'the use of observed relationships to make predictions about individuals is an area with many pitfalls; just as it is dangerous to generalise from the particular, we must be very careful about particularising from the general'.[4]

Predictors of ovarian response in ovulation induction

Predicting response to anti-estrogen therapy

Anovulation is a common cause of infertility and is present in at least one-quarter of couples facing conception difficulties.[5] In many women, induction of ovulation with anti-estrogen therapy continues to be first-line therapy. Anti-estrogen is effective in inducing ovulation in 73% of women treated, giving a live birth rate of approximately 29% (pooled results from 5268 women).[6] Using the best evidence to identify those who will remain anovulatory despite anti-estrogen therapy can direct these women towards alternative treatment approaches such as exogenous gonadotrophins, laparoscopic ovarian surgery, insulin-sensitising agents[7] or more complex assisted reproductive technology procedures, especially in women of advanced reproductive age. Furthermore, the process of identifying prognostic factors also provides an insight into ovarian abnormalities and the pathophysiology of anovulation. Three models that have been developed to predict the chances of success with anti-estrogen-induced ovulation in women with World Health Organization (WHO) group II infertility are described below (Table 13.1; Figure 13.1), together with a nomogram that combines predictive factors from two of the models (Figure 13.2).

The predictive value of baseline characteristics was investigated in a prospective study of 201 women with WHO group II anovulatory infertility who underwent 432 cycles of clomifene citrate ovulation induction, with all but 45 achieving ovulation.[8] The most predictive characteristics were the free androgen index (FAI, calculated from the testosterone to sex hormone-binding globulin ratio) and body mass index (BMI), with areas under the receiver operating characteristic curve (AUCs) of 0.76 and 0.70, respectively. Entering FAI, BMI, ovarian volume and cycle history (oligomenorrhoea versus amenorrhoea) into a regression model achieved a fairly accurate prediction, with an overall AUC of 0.82. By scoring each characteristic based on its value at screening (for example, a woman with a BMI over 35 kg/m^2 would gain 15 points for that characteristic whereas one whose BMI is below 20 kg/m^2 would gain no points), a total score can be calculated. A higher score would predict a greater chance

Table 13.1 Prediction models for treatment response in ovulation induction

Treatment	Outcome	Number of women (achieving outcome/total in study)	Predictive factors	AUC *c* statistic
Clomifene citrate[7]	Ovulation	156/201	Amenorrhoea, BMI, FAI	0.82
Clomifene citrate[10]	Pregnancy	73/159	Age, oligomenorrhoea	AUC not calculated
Clomifene citrate[13]	Live birth	625 (different interventions)	FAI, proinsulin, BMI, age, duration of infertility	No AUC
FSH[16]	Continuing pregnancy	57/154	IGF-I, testosterone, age	0.67
FSH[17]	Continuing pregnancy	57/85	Oligomenorrhoea, FAI, duration of infertility	0.72
Clomifene citrate/ FSH[15]	Live birth	134/240	Age, insulin to glucose ratio, duration of infertility	0.61

AUC = area under the receiver operating characteristic curve; BMI = body mass index; FAI = free androgen index; FSH = follicle-stimulating hormone; IGF-I = insulin-like growth factor I

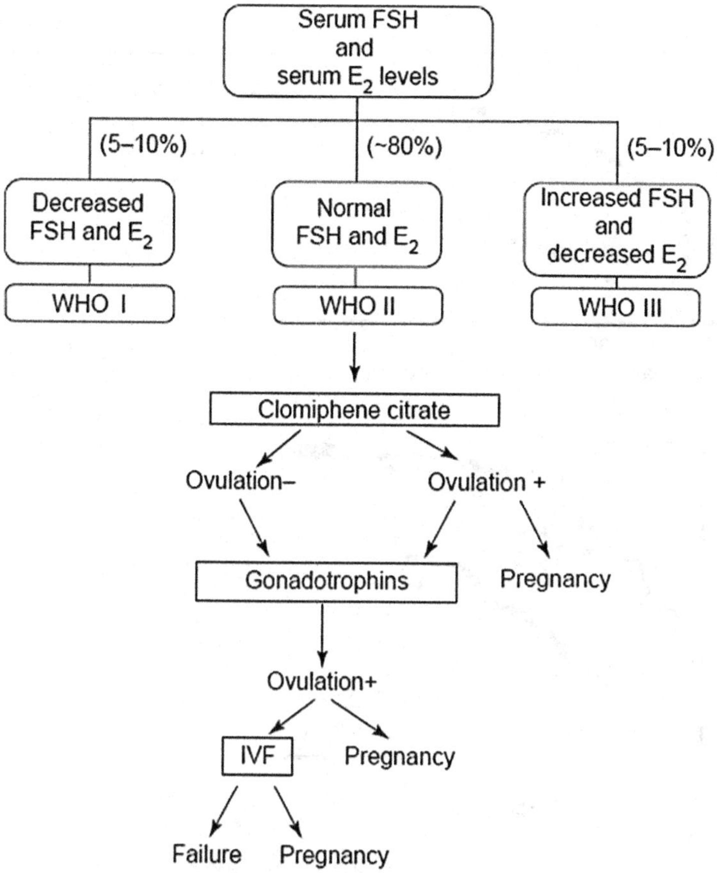

	Cumulative pregnancy rate	**Cumulative singleton live birth rate**
CC	47%	37%
FSH	58%[a]	43%
CC + FSH	78%	71%
IVF	68%	28%
CC + FSH + IVF	83%	77%

Figure 13.1 Ovulation induction treatment algorithm (upper panel) and treatment outcomes (bottom panel) in WHO group II anovulatory infertility; CC = clomifene citrate; FSH = follicle-stimulating hormone; IVF = *in vitro* fertilisation

of that woman remaining anovulatory.[8] Although this model had moderately good predictive power, the requirement to assess FAI has limited its use as this variable is not commonly measured.

To determine whether the discriminatory power of this model could be improved, additional endocrine factors potentially involved in the ovarian abnormalities of woman with WHO group II anovulatory infertility were investigated. As the characteristics identified in the earlier study as being predictive of clomifene citrate resistance, namely obesity, hyperandrogenism and amenorrhoea, are all signs and symptoms of polycystic

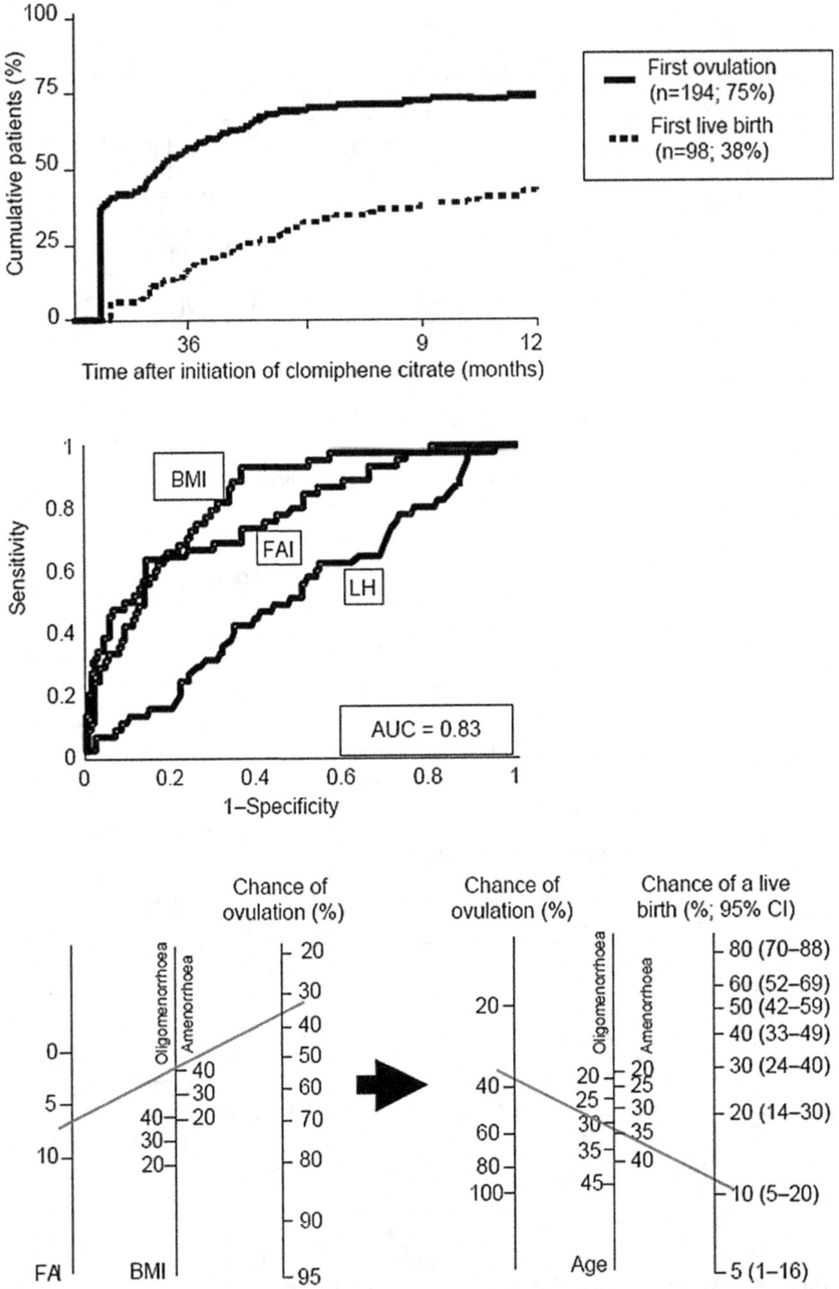

Figure 13.2 First ovulation and live birth (upper panel), area under the receiver operating characteristic curve of predictors for clomifene citrate ovulation induction (middle panel) and a two-step nomogram to predict live birth (bottom panel) following clomifene citrate; AUC = area under the receiver operating characteristic curve; BMI = body mass index; FAI = free androgen index; LH = luteinising hormone; reproduced with permission from Imani *et al.*[12]

ovary syndrome (PCOS),[9] additional endocrine abnormalities associated with PCOS were evaluated. Women who remained anovulatory had significantly higher fasting insulin levels, insulin to glucose ratios and serum leptin levels, and significantly lower insulin-like growth factor-binding protein-1 (IGFBP-1) levels than the women who did ovulate ($P \leq 0.02$).[10] These factors and those previously identified were entered into a forward stepwise logistic regression analysis. The strongest predictive factor to remain in the model was the FAI. The final model had an AUC of 0.85 and included FAI, cycle history, leptin concentration and mean ovarian volume. Although replacing BMI with leptin in the model marginally improved the predictive power, leptin is seldom measured in clinical practice, which would severely limit the use of this version of the model.

The two models described above are designed to predict the chances of a woman failing to ovulate after anti-estrogen treatment. A model that predicts the chances of conception in those in whom ovulation is induced is the next step in predicting outcome for individual women. In a proportional hazards analysis, the woman's age and her cycle history were the only factors identified as predictors of time to conception.[11] The disparity between the characteristics predictive of conception and the characteristics previously shown to be predictive of ovulation (body weight and hyperandrogenaemia) is most probably because ovarian response is only one of many variables associated with pregnancy likelihood. However, this observation also raised an interesting hypothesis. These results suggested that the regulation of endogenous follicle-stimulating hormone (FSH) to stimulate follicle growth and ovulation may differ from the regulation of endogenous FSH needed to ensure oocyte quality. It is the latter threshold that predicts the chances of conception in ovulatory cycles.

Combining prediction models for success in ovulation induction and success in conception would allow prediction of the likelihood of conception before anti-estrogen therapy is initiated, allowing women with a low percentage chance of a live birth to be directed towards another first-line treatment modality. This has been achieved through use of an integrated double nomogram that uses the predictive factors for anovulation[8] in one section and those for pregnancy[11] in another section. Although the nomogram was based on these earlier studies, it was tailored for use in clinical practice by including only characteristics that are routinely measured.[12] The nomogram consists of two steps (Figure 13.2). The goodness of fit of the model was assessed using data from a prospective study of 259 women starting treatment with clomifene citrate. Calibrating the predicted probability of a live birth against the observed live birth rate revealed no significant lack of fit ($P = 0.49$); however, the AUC was not determined.[12] The nomogram was tested in a retrospective study using the case notes of 104 anovulatory women.[13] The investigators found a negative predictive value of 80% (95% CI 60–99%), indicating that the nomogram could identify 80% of non-responders to clomifene citrate; nevertheless, they considered it insufficiently accurate for clinical use. More recently, FAI, proinsulin levels and BMI have been shown to predict live birth following clomifene citrate in an independent data set.[14,15]

Predicting response to gonadotrophins

Gonadotrophins are commonly used as a second-line treatment to restore ovarian function in women with WHO group II anovulation who have not responded to anti-estrogen therapy. Models have been developed to predict the chances of pregnancy in women using clomifene citrate therapy first line and gonadotrophin therapy second line,[16] the chances of ovulation in women in whom clomifene citrate has failed[17] and the chances of ovulation in women with PCOS,[18] and the gonadotrophin dose threshold (Figure 13.3).[19] These models are discussed below (Table 13.1).

Predictor variables were entered into a Cox regression analysis to construct a multivariate prediction model. The final model included three variables that were negatively correlated with pregnancy at 12 months leading to a singleton live birth:

- the age of the woman
- the insulin to glucose ratio
- the duration of infertility.

The *c* statistic for the model was 0.61 (optimism-corrected), indicating only a moderate ability to discriminate between outcomes. To use this model in clinical

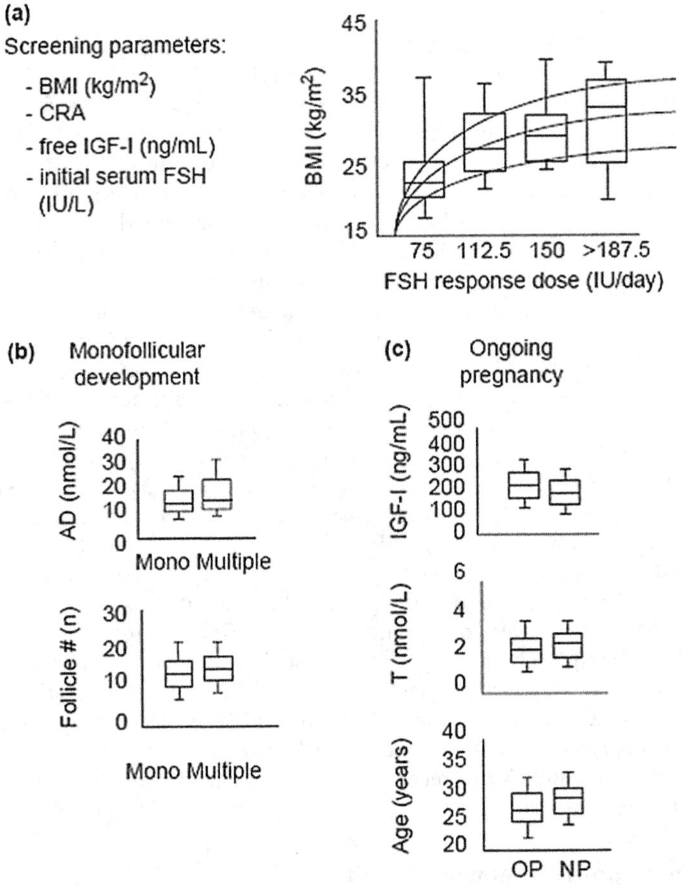

Figure 13.3 Follicle-stimulating hormone (FSH) response dose (upper panel) and follicle development/continuing pregnancy in relation to various clinical and endocrine parameters (bottom panel) using gonadotrophin ovulation induction in women with WHO group II anovulatory infertility; AD = androstenedione; BMI = body mass index; CRA = clomifene citrate-resistant anovulation; IGF-I = insulin-like growth factor I; NP = not pregnant; OP = ongoing pregnancy; T = testosterone; reproduced with permission from (a) Imani *et al*,[36] (b) and (c) Mulders *et al.*[17]

practice, physicians would need to arbitrarily select the most appropriate cut-off for their clinical setting, offering women an alternative first-line treatment for which the chances of success were only 10%, 20% or whatever level they considered acceptable. If a 30% chance of success is taken to represent a poor prognosis, the model predicted that 25 of 240 women (10%) would be below this cut-off.[16]

To predict the individual outcome of ovulation induction with gonadotrophins in women for whom clomifene citrate induction of ovulation was unsuccessful, a model has been developed based on characteristics at screening. Women ($n = 154$) who underwent a total of 544 gonadotrophin cycles in a prospective follow-up study formed the cohort for the model; the first cycle always followed a low-dose step-up protocol, and the second cycle followed a step-down protocol.[17] The factors identified as most strongly predictive of continuing pregnancy were:

- the age of the woman
- testosterone concentration
- insulin-like growth factor I (IGF-I) levels.

For this multivariate model, however, the AUC was only 0.67. Factors most predictive of multifollicular growth were androstenedione concentration and the number of ovarian follicles (AUC = 0.62).

A separate study in women with PCOS found that the following were associated with a higher chance of continuing pregnancy:[18]

- oligomenorrhoea
- shorter duration of infertility
- a lower FAI.

The predictive model had a moderate discriminatory power (AUC = 0.72). This allowed women with a less than 5% probability of attaining a continuing pregnancy to be distinguished from those with a more than 25% chance.

Imani *et al.*[19] have developed a model to predict a woman's FSH dose threshold from characteristics measured at screening and during cycle monitoring. In this prospective cohort study, normogonadotrophic, anovulatory women received daily exogenous FSH in a low-dose step-up regimen (from 75 IU per day with weekly increments of 37.5 IU per day). The FSH dose threshold was defined as the FSH dose on the day that follicle growth exceeded 10 mm in diameter. The multiple regression analysis model of the association between clinical characteristics and FSH dose was: $[4 \times \text{BMI}\ (\text{kg/m}^2)] + [32 \times \text{clomifene citrate resistance (yes} = 1 \text{ or no} = 0)] + [7 \times \text{initial free IGF-I (ng/ml)}] + [6 \times \text{initial serum FSH (IU/litre)}] - 51$. The accuracy of the model was expressed by R^2, with a value of 0.54, and the average error in dose prediction was 31 IU. To make the model easier to use, free IGF-I was substituted for the insulin to glucose ratio, which is more often measured in clinical practice: the R^2 reduced from 0.54 to 0.49, indicating that the modified model explained approximately 49% of the variability in FSH dose.

This model was also validated externally. The cohort of women in the external validation ($n = 85$) had PCOS and none had ovulated with clomifene citrate treatment (some women in the development cohort had ovulated but failed to conceive with clomifene citrate treatment). The clinical characteristics of the two populations were similar, with the exception of more pronounced hyperandrogenism in the PCOS validation population.[20] The model overestimated the FSH threshold dose by 25 IU on average in the validation cohort, with higher discrepancies at higher predicted doses. Prescribing a dose higher than the stimulation threshold may lead to cycle cancellations through overstimulation. The R^2 of the model in the test cohort was 0.11, meaning that it could explain only 11% of the variation in FSH dose threshold between women. This emphasises the necessity to validate a model before routine clinical application and, furthermore, it implies that the external validity of a model will depend on how closely the external validation cohort resembles the original development cohort of patients.

To identify predictive factors that are common to all studies, a systematic review and meta-analysis assembled data from earlier studies of gonadotrophin ovulation induction in women with WHO group II anovulation.[21] The combined results of 13 eligible studies suggested that obesity and insulin resistance are both associated with adverse outcomes, including increased total dose of FSH administered, cancelled cycles and decreased ovulation and pregnancy rates. These predictive factors would need prospective validation before use in clinical practice. Combined results of medical ovulation induction are shown in Figures 13.4 and 13.5.

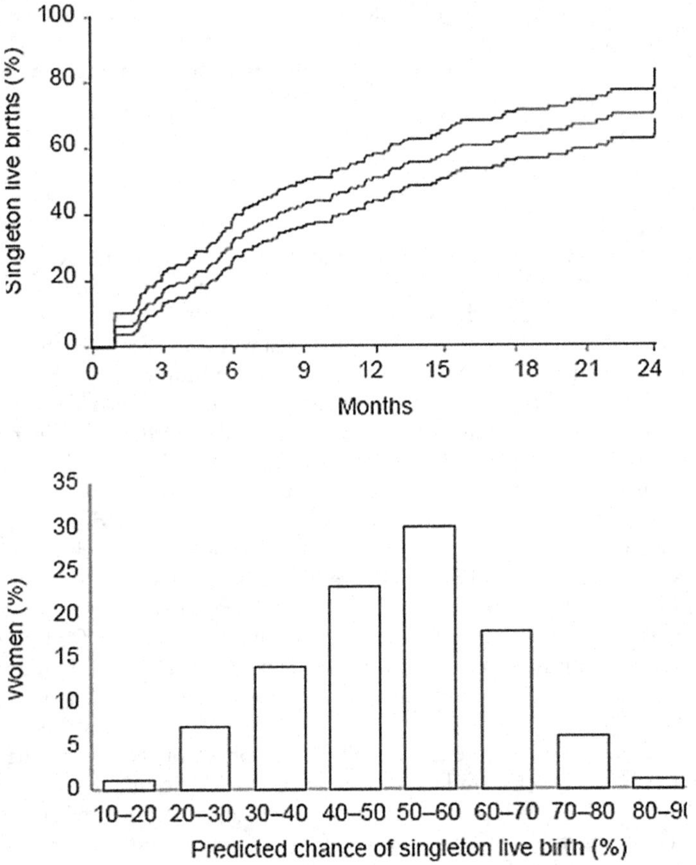

Figure 13.4 Cumulative singleton live birth rate and distribution of predicted chances for singleton live birth following a clomifene citrate/gonadotrophin ovulation induction strategy in women with WHO group II anovulatory infertility; reproduced with permission from Eijkemans *et al.*[16]

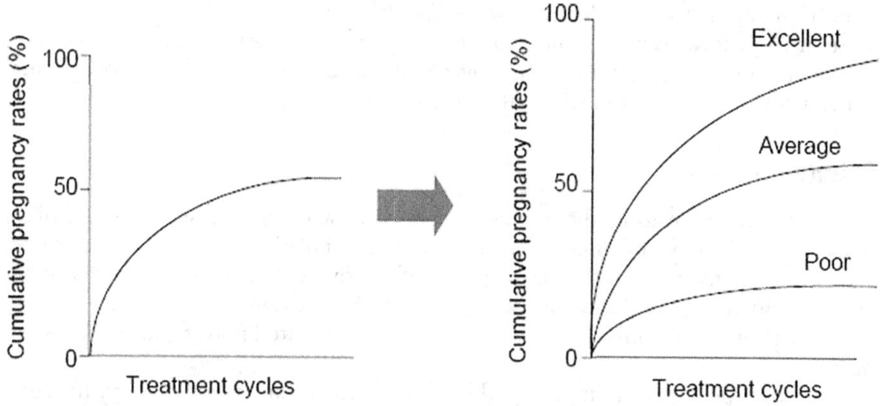

Figure 13.5 Schematic representation of a shift from a 'one size fits all' ovulation induction treatment strategy towards more patient-tailored prediction of outcomes; reproduced with permission from van Santbrink *et al.*[3]

Might genetic predictors be useful?

Since the human genome was mapped, much progress has been made in the search for genes related to ovarian function.[22] Genetic polymorphisms such as single-nucleotide polymorphisms (SNPs) may become the preferred predictive factors of ovarian response. The genetic test closest to reaching the clinic is that for polymorphisms of the FSH receptor gene (*FSHR*), which may help to predict the most appropriate dose of FSH for each woman. Mutations in *FSHR* are associated with primary amenorrhoea,[23,24] and a common SNP in *FSHR* (rs6166, causing a change from an asparagine [A] to a serine [S] residue at codon position 680; p.S680N) is associated with a different sensitivity to both exogenous[25] and endogenous[26] FSH. Moreover, anovulatory women may have a different *FSHR* genotype compared with normo-ovulatory women.[27] As a group, women with the S/S genotype have a higher FSH threshold than those with the A/A genotype[26,28,29] and may benefit from a higher dose of FSH when undergoing multifollicular stimulation.[30] The question of whether this polymorphism is associated with pregnancy rates remains controversial and requires further study in larger populations. Furthermore, recent observations suggest that antiMüllerian hormone (*AMH*) and AMH receptor type II (AMHR2) polymorphism is also associated with FSH sensitivity in the human ovary.[31]

Although progress has been slow, genetic factors may eventually help in predicting ovarian response and the likelihood of ovarian hyperstimulation syndrome. So far, most progress has come from initiatives to identify the contribution of genetic factors to ovarian dysfunction in women with PCOS.[32,33] Distinct SNPs in genes involved in steroid biosynthesis and in the hypothalamic–pituitary–gonadal axis have been identified in women with WHO group II anovulation and PCOS. A common SNP in the aromatase gene (*AR*) may also be of interest. Other PCOS genes of interest include *AMH* and *AMHR2*.[34]

The challenge will be to study whether a certain SNP pattern related to ovarian dysfunction in PCOS is also associated with ovarian response to stimulation. In addition, certain SNP patterns may be identified related to FSH sensitivity in normo-ovulatory women. This, again, may impact on the optimal dosing required for ovarian simulation for *in vitro* fertilisation. It seems likely that, with the novel molecular research tools now available, much attention in clinical research will focus on this crucial area in the near future. This may reveal entirely new possibilities for making individualised ovarian stimulation protocols a reality.

Conclusion

Predicting and managing the variability between women is a significant clinical challenge in mono- or multifollicular ovarian stimulation protocols.[35] Research into predictive factors and the construction of multivariate models are the first steps towards evidence-based individualised treatment. As yet, however, predictive models have a limited use in clinical practice because of their limited power and the need for validation.

Predictive power will improve when more factors are identified, particularly genetic factors. Validation will improve with further studies that apply the prediction model prospectively in a different patient population but with similar characteristics to that in which the model was developed. Only when these criteria have been met can the validation be trusted. So far, the results from validation studies that have met these criteria have been encouraging. Practical considerations also need attention: it is important for a prediction model to be simple enough for physicians to remember and incorporate into daily work, and to include only variables that are routinely measured.

Despite problems in using the current predictive tests in clinical practice, the wide variation in patients' characteristics mean that individualised patient-tailored approaches remain mandatory for safe and effective ovarian stimulation. The current practice of individualised treatment is based only on clinical experience and has poor reproducibility. The challenge is to design studies to identify better response prediction and further test the added value of individualised approaches.

References

1. Fauser BC, Diedrich K, Devroey P. Predictors of ovarian response: progress towards individualized treatment in ovulation induction and ovarian stimulation. *Hum Reprod Update* 2008;14:1–14.
2. Wiegerinck MA, Bongers MY, Mol BW, Heineman MJ. How concordant are the estimated rates of natural conception and *in-vitro* fertilization/embryo transfer success? *Hum Reprod* 1999;14:689–93.
3. van Santbrink EJ, Eijkemans MJ, Laven JS, Fauser BC. Patient-tailored conventional ovulation induction algorithms in anovulatory infertility. *Trends Endocrinol Metab* 2005;16:381–9.
4. Altman DG. Statistics and ethics in medical research. VII – Interpreting results. *Br Med J* 1980;281:1612–14.
5. Smith S, Pfeifer SM, Collins JA. Diagnosis and management of female infertility. *JAMA* 2003;290:1767–70.
6. Homburg R. Clomiphene citrate – end of an era? A mini-review. *Hum Reprod* 2005;20:2043–51.
7. Legro RS, Barnhart HX, Schlaff WD, Carr BR, Diamond MP, Carson SA, *et al.* Clomiphene, metformin, or both for infertility in the polycystic ovary syndrome. *N Engl J Med* 2007;356:551–66.
8. Imani B, Eijkemans MJ, te Velde ER, Habbema JD, Fauser BC. Predictors of patients remaining anovulatory during clomiphene citrate induction of ovulation in normogonadotropic oligoamenorrheic infertility. *J Clin Endocrinol Metab* 1998;83:2361–5.
9. The ESHRE/ASRM-Sponsored PCOS Consensus Workshop Group. Revised 2003 consensus on diagnostic criteria and long-term health risks related to polycystic ovary syndrome. *Fertil Steril* 2004;81:19–25.
10. Imani B, Eijkemans MJ, de Jong FH, Payne NN, Bouchard P, Giudice LC, *et al.* Free androgen index and leptin are the most prominent endocrine predictors of ovarian response during

clomiphene citrate induction of ovulation in normogonadotropic oligoamenorrheic infertility. *J Clin Endocrinol Metab* 2000;85:676–82.

11. Imani B, Eijkemans MJ, te Velde ER, Habbema JD, Fauser BC. Predictors of chances to conceive in ovulatory patients during clomiphene citrate induction of ovulation in normogonadotropic oligoamenorrheic infertility. *J Clin Endocrinol Metab* 1999;84:1617–22.
12. Imani B, Eijkemans MJ, te Velde ER, Habbema JD, Fauser BC. A nomogram to predict the probability of live birth after clomiphene citrate induction of ovulation in normogonadotropic oligoamenorrheic infertility. *Fertil Steril* 2002;77:91–7.
13. Ghobadi C, Nguyen TH, Lennard MS, Amer S, Rostami-Hodjegan A, Ledger WL. Evaluation of an existing nomogram for predicting the response to clomiphene citrate. *Fertil Steril* 2007;87:597–602.
14. Rausch ME, Legro RS, Barnhart HX, Schlaff WD, Carr BR, Diamond MP, *et al.* Predictors of pregnancy in women with polycystic ovary syndrome. *JCEM* 2009;94:3458–66.
15. Fauser BC, Eijkemans MJ. Predicting pregnancy in women with polycystic ovary syndrome. *JCEM* 2009;94:3183–4.
16. Eijkemans MJ, Imani B, Mulders AG, Habbema JD, Fauser BC. High singleton live birth rate following classical ovulation induction in normogonadotrophic anovulatory infertility (WHO 2). *Hum Reprod* 2003;18:2357–62.
17. Mulders AG, Eijkemans MJ, Imani B, Fauser BC. Prediction of chances for success or complications in gonadotrophin ovulation induction in normogonadotrophic anovulatory infertility. *Reprod Biomed Online* 2003;7:170–8.
18. van Wely M, Bayram N, van der Veen F, Bossuyt PM. Predicting ongoing pregnancy following ovulation induction with recombinant FSH in women with polycystic ovary syndrome. *Hum Reprod* 2005;20:1827–32.
19. Imani B, Eijkemans MJ, Faessen GH, Bouchard P, Giudice LC, Fauser BC. Prediction of the individual follicle-stimulating hormone threshold for gonadotropin induction of ovulation in normogonadotropic anovulatory infertility: an approach to increase safety and efficiency. *Fertil Steril* 2002;77:83–90.
20. van Wely M, Fauser BC, Laven JS, Eijkemans MJ, van der Veen F. Validation of a prediction model for the follicle-stimulating hormone response dose in women with polycystic ovary syndrome. *Fertil Steril* 2006;86:1710–15.
21. Mulders AG, Laven JS, Eijkemans MJ, Hughes EG, Fauser BC. Patient predictors for outcome of gonadotrophin ovulation induction in women with normogonadotrophic anovulatory infertility: a meta-analysis. *Hum Reprod Update* 2003;9:429–49.
22. Layman LC. Editorial: *BMP15* – the first true ovarian determinant gene on the X-chromosome? *J Clin Endocrinol Metab* 2006;91:1673–6.
23. Doherty E, Pakarinen P, Tiitinen A, Kiilavuori A, Huhtaniemi I, Forrest S, *et al.* A Novel mutation in the FSH receptor inhibiting signal transduction and causing primary ovarian failure. *J Clin Endocrinol Metab* 2002;87:1151–5.
24. Meduri G, Touraine P, Beau I, Lahuna O, Desroches A, Vacher-Lavenu MC, *et al.* Delayed puberty and primary amenorrhea associated with a novel mutation of the human follicle-stimulating hormone receptor: clinical, histological, and molecular studies. *J Clin Endocrinol Metab* 2003;88:3491–8.
25. Perez Mayorga M, Gromoll J, Behre HM, Gassner C, Nieschlag E, Simoni M. Ovarian response to follicle-stimulating hormone (FSH) stimulation depends on the FSH receptor genotype. *J Clin Endocrinol Metab* 2000;85:3365–9.
26. Greb RR, Grieshaber K, Gromoll J, Sonntag B, Nieschlag E, Kiesel L, *et al.* A common single nucleotide polymorphism in exon 10 of the human follicle stimulating hormone receptor is a major determinant of length and hormonal dynamics of the menstrual cycle. *J Clin Endocrinol Metab* 2005;90:4866–72.
27. Laven JS, Mulders AG, Suryandari DA, Gromoll J, Nieschlag E, Fauser BC, *Simoni M.* FSH receptor polymorphisms in women with normogonadotropic anovulatory infertility. *Fertil Steril* 2003;80:986–92.
28. Sudo S, Kudo M, Wada S, Sato O, Hsueh AJ, Fujimoto S. Genetic and functional analyses of polymorphisms in the human FSH receptor gene. *Mol Hum Reprod* 2002;8:893–9.

29. de Koning CH, Benjamins T, Harms P, Homburg R, van Montfrans JM, Gromol J, *et al.* The distribution of FSH receptor isoforms is related to basal FSH levels in subfertile women with normal menstrual cycles. *Hum Reprod* 2006;21:443–6.
30. Behre HM, Greb RR, Mempel A, Sonntag B, Kiesel L, Kaltwasser P, Seliger E, *et al.* Significance of a common single nucleotide polymorphism in exon 10 of the follicle-stimulating hormone (FSH) receptor gene for the ovarian response to FSH: a pharmacogenetic approach to controlled ovarian hyperstimulation. *Pharmacogenet Genomics* 2005;15:451–6.
31. Kevenaar ME, Themmen AP, Laven JS, Sonntag B, Fong SL, Uitterlinden AG, *et al.* Anti-Mullerian hormone and anti-Mullerian hormone type II receptor polymorphisms are associated with follicular phase estradiol levels in normo-ovulatory women. *Hum Reprod* 2007;22:1547–54.
32. Escobar-Morreale HF, Lugue-Ramirez M, San Millan JL. The molecular-genetic basis of functional hyperandrogenism and the PCOS. *Endocr Rev* 2005;26:251–82.
33. Diamanti-Kandarakis E, Piperi C. Genetics of PCOS: searching for the way out of the labyrinth. *Hum Reprod Upd* 2005;11:631–43.
34. Simoni M, Tempfer CB, Destenaves B, Fauser BC. Functional genetic polymorphisms and female reproductive disorders: Part I: polycystic ovary syndrome and ovarian response. *Hum Reprod Upd* 2008;14:459–84.
35. van Santbrink EJ, Fauser BC. Is there a future for ovulation induction in the current era of assisted reproduction? *Hum Reprod* 2003;18:2499–502.
36. Imani B, Eijkemans MJ, Faessen GH, Bouchard P, Giudice LC, Fauser BC. Prediction of the individual follicle-stimulating hormone threshold for gonadotropin induction of ovulation in normogonadotropic anovulatory infertility: an approach to increase safety and efficiency. *Fertil Steril* 2002;77:83–90.

14

Chapter 14

Surgical management of anovulatory infertility in polycystic ovary syndrome

Adam Balen

Introduction

The management of anovulatory infertility in polycystic ovary syndrome (PCOS) has traditionally involved the use of clomifene citrate and then gonadotrophin therapy or laparoscopic ovarian surgery in those who are clomifene resistant. The principles of therapy are first to optimise health (for example, weight loss for those who are overweight) before commencing therapy and then induce regular unifollicular ovulation, while minimising the risks of ovarian hyperstimulation syndrome and multiple pregnancy. Weight loss improves the endocrine profile and the likelihood of ovulation and a healthy pregnancy.

From the 1930s to the early 1960s, wedge resection of the ovary was the only treatment for PCOS. Wedge resection required a laparotomy and removal of up to 75% of each ovary, and often resulted in extensive pelvic adhesions. The modern-day, minimal access alternative to gonadotrophin therapy for clomifene-resistant PCOS is laparoscopic ovarian surgery, usually employing diathermy or laser. Laparoscopic ovarian surgery has therefore replaced ovarian wedge resection as the surgical treatment for clomifene resistance in women with PCOS. It is free of the risks of multiple pregnancy and ovarian hyperstimulation and does not require intensive ultrasound monitoring. Furthermore, ovarian diathermy is said to be as effective as routine gonadotrophin therapy in the treatment of clomifene-insensitive PCOS, although the evidence for this will be discussed in this chapter. In addition, laparoscopic ovarian surgery is a useful therapy for anovulatory women with PCOS who need a laparoscopic assessment of their pelvis or who live too far away from the hospital to be able to attend for the intensive monitoring required for gonadotrophin therapy. Laparoscopic ovarian surgery, by its effect on reducing serum luteinising hormone (LH) concentrations, is recommended for women who persistently hypersecrete LH, either during natural cycles or in response to clomifene. Surgery does, of course, carry its own risks and should be performed only by properly trained laparoscopic surgeons.

History

Wedge resection of the ovaries was initially described in 1935 by Stein and Leventhal[1] at the time that polycystic ovaries were diagnosed during a laparotomy. It was found that ovarian biopsies taken to make the diagnosis led to subsequent ovulation. The rationale was to 'normalise' ovarian size and hence the endocrinopathy by removing between 50% and 75% of each ovary. A large review in 1963 of 187 reports summarised data on 1079 ovarian wedge resections, with an overall rate of ovulation of 80% and pregnancy of 62.5% (range 13.5–89.5%).[2] Another 30 or so years later, Donesky and Adashi[3] were able to increase the summated experience in the literature to 1766 treatments, with an average pregnancy rate of 58.8%. Because of the realisation that significant postoperative adhesion formation occurred and that initial favourable reports of pregnancy rates were not sustained, wedge resection became less popular in the 1970s, and at the same time medical therapies for ovulation induction appeared to be more successful.

Methods and dose

Commonly employed methods for laparoscopic surgery include monopolar electrocautery (diathermy) and laser. In the first reported series, laparoscopic ovarian diathermy (LOD; also known as laparoscopic ovarian drilling) resulted in ovulation in 90% and conception in 70% of the 62 women treated.[4] The outcome of 62 pregnancies from a later series from the same group was no different from the normal population[5] and the miscarriage rate was 15%. A number of subsequent studies have produced similarly encouraging results, although the techniques used and degree of ovarian damage vary considerably. Gjønnaess[4] cauterised each ovary at five to eight points, for five to six seconds at each point with 300–400 W. Using a similar technique, Dabirashrafi *et al.*[6] reported mild to moderate adhesion formation in 20% of patients. Naether *et al.*[7] treated 5–20 points per ovary with 400 W for approximately one second. They found that the rate of adhesions was 19.3% and that this was reduced to 16.6% by peritoneal lavage with saline.[8] They also reported that the post-diathermy fall in serum testosterone concentration was proportional to the degree of ovarian damage, with up to 40 cauterisation sites being used in some patients.[9]

The greater the amount of damage to the surface of the ovary, the greater the risk of periovarian adhesion formation. This led Armar *et al.*[10] to develop a strategy of minimising the number of diathermy points. This is a logical technique in which the ovary is simply cauterised at four points and the lowest effective dose used. The high pregnancy rate (86% of those with no other pelvic abnormality) indicates that the small number of diathermy points used leads to a low rate of significant adhesion formation.[11] We also currently advocate the use of adhesion barriers to reduce the risk further.

The difficulty when deciding how to perform LOD is in not knowing the 'dose response' for a particular patient. While we demonstrated some years ago in a small study[12] that LOD using 40 W for four seconds in four places on one ovary can lead to bilateral ovarian activity and ovulation (our usual protocol involves the same on each ovary), our ovulation rate was 50% and conception rate 40% (some patients were sensitised to exogenous stimulation). It has been proposed[13] that the degree of ovarian destruction should be determined by the size of the ovary. Naether *et al.*[13] reported their method of laparoscopic electrocautery of the ovarian surface, which causes greater destruction of the ovary than the method we use as they apply 400 W at 5–20 sites on each ovary. Despite such a large amount of ovarian destruction, in their series of 206 patients 45% of those who conceived required additional ovarian stimulation (with an 8% multiple pregnancy rate) and the overall miscarriage rate was 20%. There is also no doubt that different patient populations are being treated, as we only recommend operation for women with irregular, anovulatory cycles who have not responded to anti-estrogen therapy, while in Naether's series approximately 24% of the women operated on had regular cycles and 15% were ovulating before their operation.[13]

Amer and colleagues performed a retrospective assessment of the effect of the amount of energy used on the outcome of LOD[14] and then proceeded to assess this prospectively.[15] They found no difference in their retrospective analyses between the use of three up to ten punctures but suggested that two punctures was too few.[14] There are many variables in the potential for response, including the anthropometric characteristics of the patient and ovarian morphology. In the prospective study,[15] using a modified Monte Carlo protocol and a standardised energy of 150 J per puncture, the rates of ovulation and pregnancy were respectively 67% and 67% with four punctures per ovary ($n = 12$), 44% and 56% with three punctures per ovary ($n = 9$), 33% and 17% with two punctures per ovary ($n = 6$) and 33% and 0% with one puncture per ovary ($n = 12$), indicating a clear dose response, although the study only included a relatively small number of women.

Risks of adhesion formation and ovarian failure

The risk of periovarian adhesion formation can be reduced by abdominal lavage and early second-look laparoscopy, with adhesiolysis if necessary.[16] Others have also used liberal peritoneal lavage to good effect.[10] Greenblatt and Casper[17] found no correlation between the degree of ovarian damage and subsequent adhesion formation, nor did they find benefit from the adhesion barrier Interceed® (Ethicon), as assessed by second-look laparoscopy. In another interesting study,[18] 40 women undergoing laser photocoagulation of the ovaries using a neodymium-doped yttrium aluminium garnet (Nd:YAG) laser set at 50 W at 20–25 points per ovary were randomised to a second-look laparoscopy and adhesiolysis. Of those who underwent a second-look laparoscopy, adhesions that were described as minimal or mild were found in 68%, yet adhesiolysis did not appear to be necessary as the cumulative conception rate after 6 months was 47% compared with 55% in the expectantly managed group, a difference that was not statistically significant.

Laser treatment seems to be as efficacious as diathermy and it has been suggested that it may result in less adhesion formation,[19,20] although the only study to compare the two techniques[20] was non-randomised, reported similar ovulation and pregnancy rates and did not examine adhesion formation. Various types of laser have been used, from the CO_2 laser to the Nd:YAG and potassium-titanyl-phosphate (KTP) lasers. As with the use of lasers in other spheres of laparoscopic surgery, whether laser or diathermy is employed appears to depend on the preference of the surgeon and the availability of the equipment.

An additional concern is the possibility of ovarian destruction leading to ovarian failure, which is obviously a disaster in a woman wishing to conceive. Cases of ovarian failure have been reported after both wedge resection and laparoscopic surgery. An unfortunate vogue has developed whereby women with polycystic ovaries who have over-responded to superovulation for *in vitro* fertilisation are subjected to LOD as way of reducing the likelihood of subsequent ovarian hyperstimulation syndrome.[21] If one accepts that appropriately performed LOD works by sensitising the ovary to follicle-stimulating hormone (FSH), and LOD certainly makes the clomifene-resistant polycystic ovary sensitive to clomifene,[22] then one could extrapolate that LOD before superovulation for *in vitro* fertilisation should make the ovary more and not less likely to overstimulate. The amount of ovarian destruction that is required to reduce the chance of overstimulation is therefore likely to be considerable and one should be very cautious before proceeding with such an approach because of concerns about permanent ovarian atrophy.

Endocrine changes after laparoscopic ovarian surgery

With restoration of ovarian activity after LOD, serum concentrations of LH and testosterone fall. A fall in serum LH concentrations may both increase the chance of conception and reduce the risk of miscarriage.[11,23] Whether patients respond to LOD appears to depend on their pretreatment characteristics, with those with high basal LH concentrations having a better clinical and endocrine response.[12,24] A Cochrane meta-analysis did not, however, find any difference in miscarriage rates compared with the use of gonadotrophins (OR 0.61; 95% CI 0.17–2.16).[25] While hyperinsulinaemia plays a major role in the pathophysiology of anovulatory PCOS, the procedure of LOD does not appear to influence insulin sensitivity.[26] With respect to insulin resistance, there has been much recent interest in insulin-lowering drugs such as metformin for enhancing reproductive function, although the overall benefit is not as high as originally postulated (see Chapter 15). Nonetheless, while a prospective randomised controlled trial (RCT) in 120 women who were clomifene resistant found no significant difference in rates of ovulation (approximately 55% in each group), those treated with metformin had significantly higher pregnancy rates (18.6% versus 13.4%; $P<0.05$) and live birth rates (82.1% versus 64.5%; $P<0.05$).[27]

Pregnancy rates

Most early studies were of an observational nature and have also since been reported in large reviews.[2,3] An unfortunate feature of many of the papers that describe laparoscopic treatment or wedge resection is the poor characterisation of the patients such that many appear to have been ovulating before treatment. Furthermore, as the polycystic ovary becomes more sensitive to either endogenous or exogenous FSH after LOD, many practitioners have taken a pragmatic approach by commencing ovarian stimulation with either clomifene or gonadotrophins if ovulatory activity is not immediately induced.[22,28] The first RCT suggested that LOD was as effective as routine gonadotrophin therapy in the treatment of clomifene-insensitive PCOS.[29] In this study, 88 women were randomised prospectively to receive either human menopausal gonadotrophins (hMG)/FSH or LOD. There were no differences in the rates of ovulation or pregnancy between those stimulated with hMG or FSH compared with LOD, although those treated with LOD had fewer cycles with multiple follicular growth and a lower rate of miscarriage.[29] The largest RCT to date was a multicentre study performed in the Netherlands in which 168 women resistant to clomifene were randomised to either LOD ($n=83$) or ovulation induction with recombinant FSH (rFSH; $n=65$).[30] The initial cumulative pregnancy rate after 6 months was 34% in the LOD arm versus 67% with rFSH. Those who did not ovulate in response to LOD were then given first clomifene and then rFSH, and by 12 months the cumulative pregnancy rate was similar in each group at 67%.[30] It has to be emphasised that those treated with LOD took longer to conceive and 54% required additional medical ovulation induction therapy. Interestingly, in this study it was difficult to predict those who would fail to respond to LOD and, somewhat counter-intuitively, it was those who were younger at menarche, had lower LH : FSH ratios and lower glucose levels.[31] The Dutch researchers also looked at health-related quality of life and found no major significant differences, although those women who did not conceive found the use of rFSH more burdensome.[32] Furthermore, an economic comparison found no major difference, although the cost of caring for multiple pregnancies was not included.[33] In contrast, a smaller study in New Zealand[34] found a significant reduction in both direct and indirect costs, with the cost of a live birth estimated as NZ$19,640 for those who were treated with LOD compared with NZ$29,836 for those who received gonadotrophins.

It has been suggested that to demonstrate a 20% increase in pregnancy rate over 6 months from 50% to 70%, with an 80% power, at least 235 patients would be required in each arm of a study to compare LOD with gonadotrophin therapy. The current meta-analysis in the Cochrane database includes a total of only 303 women.[25] The continuing pregnancy rate following LOD compared with gonadotrophins differed according to the length of follow-up. Overall, the pooled odds ratio for all studies was not statistically significant (OR 1.27; 95% CI 0.77–1.98). Multiple pregnancy rates were reduced in the LOD arms of the four trials where there was a direct comparison with gonadotrophin therapy (OR 0.16; 95% CI 0.03–0.98). There was no difference in miscarriage rates in the LOD group when compared with gonadotrophin in these trials (OR 0.61; 95% CI 0.17–2.16).

The duration of follow-up varied among the studies that were included in the meta-analysis. Furthermore, it is difficult to produce a temporal comparison as not all women receiving gonadotrophin therapy were treated in consecutive months and it is therefore necessary to compare treatment cycles. The meta-analysis found that, when comparing 6 months after LOD with six cycles of gonadotrophin therapy, the cumulative continuing pregnancy rate was higher among women who received gonadotrophins (OR 0.48; 95% CI 0.28–0.81). Thus it was concluded that there is insufficient evidence of a difference in cumulative continuing pregnancy rates between LOD after 6–12 months follow-up and three to six cycles of ovulation induction with gonadotrophins as a primary treatment for subfertile women with anovulatory PCOS. The greatest advantage is that multiple pregnancy rates are considerably reduced.

LOD has traditionally been used as a second-line therapy in clomifene-resistant women with PCOS. A recent RCT of 72 anovulatory women with PCOS showed no difference in pregnancy rates when LOD was compared with clomifene as first-line therapy.[35]

Transvaginal approach

A few groups have been exploring the use of transvaginal hydrolaparoscopy to both assess the pelvis and provide therapy without the need for laparoscopy, although this approach has not been adopted widely. A number of small reports now exist of bipolar ovarian capsular drilling[36] and even transvaginal ultrasound-guided ovarian laser treatment,[37] although there are no large RCTs and, in the author's opinion, it is unlikely that these treatments will gain widespread popularity.

Summary

Laparoscopic ovarian surgery is free of the risks of multiple pregnancy and ovarian hyperstimulation and does not require intensive ultrasound monitoring. It is a useful therapy for anovulatory women with PCOS who fail to respond to clomifene and who persistently hypersecrete LH, who need a laparoscopic assessment of their pelvis, or who live too far away from the hospital to be able to attend for the intensive monitoring required of gonadotrophin therapy. Those who respond best are usually those with an elevated LH and those who respond poorly are those who are obese and have significant hyperandrogenism and more than 3 years' duration of infertility.[38] Surgery does, of course, carry its own risks and must be performed only by fully trained laparoscopic surgeons. Compared with medical ovulation induction, the additional advantage of LOD is that it need only be performed once and intensive monitoring is not required as there is no danger of multiple ovulation or ovarian hyperstimulation. Furthermore, only minimal ovarian damage is required to achieve this effect. There is still uncertainty, however, about the right dose of diathermy to reliably stimulate the resumption of ovulatory cycles. The chance of achieving a continuing pregnancy within 6 months is less than with carefully conducted ovulation induction with gonadotrophins but, if adjuvant ovulation induction agents are used in those who do not initially respond, the 12-month pregnancy rates are similar.

Key points

- Laparoscopic ovarian surgery can achieve unifollicular ovulation with no risk of ovarian hyperstimulation syndrome or of high-order multiples, and detailed monitoring is not required.
- Gonadotrophin preparations can be expensive but do provide a quicker cumulative pregnancy rate.
- LOD may achieve a normalisation of endocrinology, with a fall in LH and testosterone concentrations, but no change in insulin sensitivity.
- LOD is a single treatment using existing equipment.
- The risks of surgery are minimal but include the risks of general anaesthesia, laparoscopy, adhesion formation and destruction of normal ovarian tissue.

Clinical practice points

- Laparoscopic ovarian surgery is an alternative to gonadotrophin therapy for clomifene-resistant anovulatory PCOS.
- Women with an elevated serum LH concentration tend to respond best.
- The treatment is best suited to those for whom frequent ultrasound monitoring is impractical.
- Surgery should be performed by appropriately trained personnel.
- Minimal damage should be caused to the ovaries.
- Irrigation with an adhesion barrier is recommended.

Future avenues for research

Research is required into mechanisms by which LOD works, dose response and predictors for response.

References

1. Stein IF, Leventhal ML. Amenorrhoea associated with bilateral polycystic ovaries. *Am J Obstet Gynaecol* 1935;29:181–91.
2. Goldzieher JW, Axelrod LR. Clinical and biochemical features of polycystic ovarian disease. *Fertil Steril* 1963;14:631–53.

3. Donesky BW, Adashi EY. Surgically induced ovulation in the polycystic ovary syndrome: wedge resection revisited in the age of laparoscopy. *Fertil Steril* 1995;63:439–63.
4. Gjönnaess H. Polycystic ovarian syndrome treated by ovarian electrocautery through the laparoscope. *Fertil Steril* 1984;41:20–5.
5. Gjønnaess H. The course and outcome of pregnancy after ovarian electrocautery with PCOS: the influence of body weight. *Br J Obstet Gynaecol* 1989;96:714–19.
6. Dabirashrafi H, Mohamad K, Behjatnia Y, Moghadami-Tabrizi N. Adhesion formation after ovarian electrocauterization on patients with PCO syndrome. *Fertil Steril* 1991;55:1200–1.
7. Naether OG, Fischer R, Weise HC, Geiger-Kotzler L, Delfs T, Rudolf K. Laparoscopic electrocoagulation of the ovarian surface in infertile patients with polycystic ovarian disease. *Fertil Steril* 1993;60:88–94.
8. Naether OG, Fischer R. Adhesion formation after laparoscopic electrocoagulation of the ovarian surface in polycystic ovary patients. *Fertil Steril* 1993;60:95–9.
9. Naether O, Weise HC, Fischer R. [Results of treatment with surface cauterization of polycystic ovaries in sterility patients]. *Geburtshilfe Frauenheilkd* 1991;51:920–4. Article in German.
10. Armar NA, McGarrigle HH, Honour JW, Holownia P, Jacobs HS, Lachelin GC. Laparoscopic ovarian diathermy in the management of anovulatory infertility in women with polycystic ovaries: endocrine changes and clinical outcome. *Fertil Steril* 1990;53:45–9.
11. Armar NA, Lachelin GC. Laparoscopic ovarian diathermy: an effective treatment for anti-oestrogen resistant anovulatory infertility in women with polycystic ovaries. *Br J Obstet Gynaecol* 1993;100:161–4.
12. Balen AH, Jacobs HS. A prospective study comparing unilateral and bilateral laparoscopic ovarian diathermy in women with the polycystic ovary syndrome. *Fertil Steril* 1994;62:921–5.
13. Naether lG, Baukloh V, Fischer R, Kowalczyk T. Long-term follow-up in 206 infertility patients with polycystic ovarian syndrome after laparoscopic electrocautery of the ovarian surface. *Hum Reprod* 1994;9:2342–9.
14. Amer SA, Li TC, Cooke ID. Laparoscopic ovarian diathermy in women with polycystic ovary syndrome: a retrospective study on the influence of the amount of energy used on the outcome. *Hum Reprod* 2002;17:1046–51.
15. Amer SA, Li TC, Cooke ID. A prospective dose-finding study of the amount of thermal energy required for laparoscopic ovarian diathermy. *Hum Reprod* 2003;18:1693–8.
16. Naether OG. Significant reduction in adnexal adhesions following laparoscopic electrocautery of the ovarian surface by lavage and artificial ascites. *Gynaecol Endoscopy* 1995;4:17–19.
17. Greenblatt E, Casper RF. Adhesion formation after laparoscopic ovarian cautery for PCOS: lack of correlation with pregnancy rate. *Fertil Steril* 1993;60:766–9.
18. Gürgan T, Urman B, Aksu T, Yarali H, Develioglu O, Kisnisci HA. The effect of short-interval laparoscopic lysis of adhesions on pregnancy rates following Nd-YAG laser photocoagulation of polycystic ovaries. *Obstet Gynecol* 1992;80:45–7.
19. Daniell JF, Miller N. Polycystic ovaries treated by laparoscopic laser vaporization. *Fertil Steril* 1989;51:232–6.
20. Heylen SM, Puttemans PJ, Brosens LH. Polycystic ovarian disease treated by laparoscopic argon laser capsule drilling: comparison of vaporization versus perforation technique. *Hum Reprod* 1994;9:1038–42.
21. Rimmington MR, Walker SM, Shaw RW. The use of laparoscopic ovarian electrocautery in preventing cancellation of *in-vitro* fertilization treatment cycles due to risk of ovarian hyperstimulation syndrome in women with polycystic ovaries. *Hum Reprod* 1997;7:1443–7.
22. Farhi J, Soule S, Jacobs H. Effect of laparoscopic ovarian electrocautery on ovarian response and outcome of treatment with gonadotrophins in clomifene citrate resistant patients with PCOS. *Fertil Steril* 1995;64:930–5.
23. Balen AH, Tan SL, Jacobs HS. Hypersecretion of luteinising hormone: a significant cause of infertility and miscarriage. *Br J Obstet Gynaecol* 1993;100:1082–9.
24. Abdel Gadir A, Alnaser HM, Mowafi RS, Shaw RW. The response of patients with polycystic ovarian disease to human menopausal gonadotrophin therapy after ovarian electrocautery or a luteinizing hormone-releasing hormone agonist. *Fertil Steril* 1992;57:309–13.

25. Farquhar C, Vandekerckhove P, Arnot M, Lilford R. Laparoscopic "drilling" by diathermy or laser for ovulation induction in anovulatory polycystic ovary syndrome. *Cochrane Database Syst Rev* 2000;(2):CD001122.
26. Tulandi T, Saleh A, Morris D, Jacobs HS, Payne NN, Tan SL. Effects of laparoscopic ovarian drilling on serum vascular endothelial growth factor and on insulin responses to the oral glucose tolerance test in women with polycystic ovary syndrome. *Fertil Steril* 2000;74:585–8.
27. Palomba S, Orio F, Nardo LG, Falbo A, Russo T, Corea D, *et al.* Metformin administration versus laparoscopic ovarian diathermy in clomifene citrate-resistant women with polycystic ovary syndrome: A prospective parallel randomized double-blind placebo-controlled trial. *JCEM* 2004;89:4801–9.
28. Ostrzenski A. Endoscopic carbon dioxide laser ovarian wedge resection in resistant polycystic ovarian disease. *Int J Fertil* 1992;37:295–9.
29. Abdel Gadir A, Mowafi RS, Alnaser HM, Alrashid AH, Alonezi OM, Shaw RW. Ovarian electrocautery versus human menopausal gonadotrophins and pure follicle stimulating hormone therapy in the treatment of patients with polycystic ovarian disease. *Clin Endocrinol (Oxf)* 1990;33:585–92.
30. Bayram N, van Wely M, Kaaijk EM, Bossuyt PM, van der Veen F. Using an electrocautery strategy or recombinant FSH to induce ovulation in polycystic ovary syndrome: a randomised controlled trial. *BMJ* 2004;328:192–5.
31. van Wely M, Bayram N, van der Veen, Bossuyt PM. Predictors for treatment failure after laparoscopic electrocautery of the ovaries in women with clomiphene citrate resistant polycystic ovary syndrome. *Hum Reprod* 2005;20:900–5.
32. van Wely M, Bayram N, Bossuyt PM, van der Veen F. Laparoscopic electrocautery of the ovaries versus recombinant FSH in clomiphene citrate-resistant polycystic ovary syndrome. Impact on women's health-related quality of life. *Hum Reprod* 2004;19:2244–50.
33. van Wely M, Bayram N, van der Veen F, Bossuyt PM. An economic comparison of a laparoscopic electrocautery strategy and ovulation induction with recombinant FSH in women with clomiphene citrate-resistant polycystic ovary syndrome. *Hum Reprod* 2004;19:1741–5.
34. Farquhar CM, Williamson K, Brown PM, Garland J. An economic evaluation of laparoscopic ovarian diathermy versus gonadotrophin therapy for women with clomiphene citrate resistant polycystic ovary syndrome. *Hum Reprod* 2004;19:1110–15.
35. Amer SA, Li TC, Metwally M, Emarh M, Ledger WL. Randomized controlled trial comparing laparoscopic ovarian diathermy with clomiphene citrate as a first-line method of ovulation induction in women with polycystic ovary syndrome. *Hum Reprod* 2009;24:219–25.
36. Gordts S, Gordts S, Puttemans P, Valkenburg M, Campo R, Brosens I. Transvaginal hydrolaparoscopy in the treatment of polycystic ovary syndrome. *Fertil Steril* 2009;91:2520–6.
37. Zhu WJ, Li XM, Chen XM, Lin Z, Zhang L. Transvaginal, ultrasound-guided ovarian interstitial laser treatment in anovulatory women with clomifene-citrate-resistant polycystic ovary syndrome. *BJOG* 2006;113:810–16.
38. Amer SA, Li TC, Ledger WL. Ovulation induction using laparoscopic ovarian drilling in women with polycystic ovary syndrome: predictors of success. *Hum Reprod* 2004;19:1719–24.

15

Chapter 15

The role of insulin-sensitising drugs in the treatment of polycystic ovary syndrome

Richard S Legro

Introduction

Insulin-sensitising agents are frequently used in the treatment of women with polycystic ovary syndrome (PCOS) but, to date, the results have fallen short of expectations. Despite their limited benefits, these drugs are widely used in PCOS, and they are probably overprescribed. Insulin-sensitising agents are a class of drugs that work primarily or in part by improving peripheral insulin sensitivity to lower insulin levels and, ultimately, to lower circulating glucose levels. The classic example is the thiazolidinediones (pioglitazone and rosiglitazone). Given the intense endocrine interaction of tissues involved in glucose homeostasis, drugs that target one organ or function often have cross-over benefit on other aspects of glucose homeostasis. For instance, the biguanides primarily suppress hepatic gluconeogenesis but also exert some peripheral insulin-sensitising action, and it is this action that has led to the use of metformin in women with PCOS.

While insulin-sensitising agents improve many symptoms and presenting complaints of women with PCOS, they do not represent a cure. They exert varying effects depending on the condition being treated. In many situations, there is no or only minimal benefit. The risk/benefit ratio for their use must thus be examined for each indication. This chapter explores the use of insulin sensitisers, primarily metformin, for varying indications related to PCOS and discusses the evidence to develop a risk/benefit ratio for their use. These drugs were developed to treat type 2 diabetes and have been adapted as treatments for the symptoms of PCOS. One drug, D-chiro-inositol, which initially showed promise to induce ovulation,[1] disappointed in phase II studies and its development was eventually halted. An update of the meta-analyis of insulin-sensitising agents in PCOS was published in 2009[2] and its results are discussed in this chapter.

Metformin

Metformin remains the most widely studied insulin sensitiser in PCOS. It circulates unbound to proteins and is excreted unmetabolised in the urine. Gastrointestinal symptoms (diarrhoea, nausea, vomiting, abdominal bloating, flatulence and anorexia) are the most common reactions to metformin and are approximately 30% more frequent in women treated with metformin than in those receiving a placebo. For this reason, the dose is often escalated in a stepwise fashion to increase tolerance. An extended-release version with equal efficacy is available with a gastrointestinal adverse effect profile identical to that of placebo.[3]

There is a small risk of lactic acidosis among women taking this medication that may be triggered by exposure to intravenous iodinated radiocontrast agents in susceptible individuals. This most commonly occurs in women with poorly controlled diabetes and impaired renal function. The dose for reproductive medicine indications tends to be empirical as no adequately powered and designed dose-ranging studies have been performed for these indications. The dose tends to range from 1500 to 2550 mg per day. None of the indications for metformin discussed in this chapter has received US Food and Drug Administration (FDA) approval.

Premature pubarche

Premature pubarche is the premature onset of puberty in children and, like PCOS, may be more common with increasing obesity in the population. In females, premature pubarche has been associated with a relative adrenal hyperandrogenism and hyperinsulinaemia.[4] Further long-term follow-up of these girls suggests that they are at increased risk of developing ovarian hyperandrogenism, polycystic ovaries and oligomenorrhoea; that is, full-blown PCOS after menarche.[5] The driving force in this disorder is unknown but, similarly to PCOS, there may be a vicious circle between hyperinsulinaemia and hyperandrogenism, first with the adrenal gland and then with the ovary. Thus many researchers have tried to slow both the progression of puberty and the development of a PCOS phenotype through the use of metformin.

Randomised trials, primarily from one group in Spain, have shown that metformin improves many aspects of premature pubarche, including slowing the onset of puberty, reducing total and visceral fat, improving circulating lipid levels and lowering testosterone levels.[6–8] They have also combined treatment with flutamide in treating this population.[9] Larger trials and replication in other populations would solidify the use of this drug. Metformin has been approved for the treatment of diabetes in children and is generally safe in this population. The major adverse effects remain primarily gastrointestinal, with heartburn, diarrhoea and flatulence. However, the drug has not been studied as extensively in children under the age of 10 years; that is, in the age group that girls with premature pubarche present. Certain insulin-sensitising drugs may not be suitable in this population, such as thiazolidinediones, because of concerns about weight gain, the inducement of a larger fat mass or more serious adverse effects such as hepatotoxicity or cardiotoxicity.

Infertility

No other indication for insulin sensitisers has been studied as extensively as the treatment of infertility in PCOS with metformin. The rationale for the use of metformin in infertility is that it lowers both circulating insulin levels and testosterone levels and leads to increased ovulation. With increased ovulation, women with PCOS have an improved chance of pregnancy. The five trials summarised in Table 15.1 are all randomised double-blind multicentre trials that used metformin and clomifene citrate alone or in combination for the treatment of infertility in women with PCOS.

Table 15.1 Summary of large randomised blinded trials of metformin and clomifene citrate for infertility that have reported pregnancy and/or live birth results

Study	*n*	Treatment	Results	Conclusion
Palomba *et al.* (2005)[37]	100	Metformin + placebo vs clomifene + placebo	Live birth rate: metformin 52%; clomifene 18%	Metformin superior to clomifene
Moll *et al.* (2006)[13]	225	Clomifene + placebo vs clomifene + metformin	Continuing pregnancy: clomifene 46%; clomifene + metformin 40%	No benefit of combined therapy with clomifene + metformin
Legro *et al.* (2007)[10]	626	Clomifene + placebo vs metformin + placebo vs clomifene + metformin	Live birth rate: clomifene 23%; metformin 7%; clomifene + metformin 27%	Clomifene superior to metformin; no benefit of combined therapy with clomifene + metformin
Palomba *et al.* (2007)[38]	80	Metformin vs clomifene	Cumulative pregnancy rate: metformin 63%; clomifene 49%	No benefit of metformin over clomifene
Zain *et al.* (2009)[11]	115	Clomifene vs metformin vs clomifene + metformin	Live birth rate: clomifene 15%; metformin 8%; clomifene + metformin 18%	No benefit of metformin over clomifene; no benefit of combined therapy with clomifene + metformin

All trials studied participants for up to at least six cycles, there were no adjuvant medications such as human chorionic gonadotrophin to trigger ovulation, and conception was by timed intercourse without inseminations. Two of the trials were conducted by the same group in Italy and their results are disparate from the multicentre Dutch, Malaysian and US trials. Each trial had a unique design and endpoint. However, as a solo agent, metformin has been markedly inferior as a first-line treatment to clomifene, which in the largest trial to date (the PPCOS study)[10] was found to be three times more successful at achieving live birth than metformin and twice as successful in the Malaysian trial.[11] This has been supported by most larger multicentre trials that have looked at the two drugs head to head. Furthermore, there was no change over time in the pregnancy rate with metformin, suggesting that there is not a critical pretreatment period necessary after which the benefit of metformin kicks in (Figure 15.1). It is equally relatively ineffective over time. More importantly, these trials revealed that, given an ovulation, an ovulation on clomifene is twice as fecund as an ovulation on metformin, implying that all ovulations are not alike. The European Society of Human Reproduction and Embryology (ESHRE)/American Society for Reproductive Medicine (ASRM) consensus conference in 2008 recommended against the use of metformin alone as the first-line agent for the treatment of infertility in PCOS.[12]

Metformin may have more of a use as an adjuvant agent for infertility in PCOS. While several individual trials did not show a benefit of metformin added to clomifene compared with clomifene alone,[10,11,13] a meta-analysis has found cumulative evidence of a benefit. Metformin plus clomifene increased the likelihood of pregnancy (OR 2.67; 95% CI 1.45–4.94; number needed to treat 4.6) when compared with clomifene alone.[14] Furthermore, there may be some benefit in treating obese women with PCOS with the combination of metformin and clomifene. A systematic review of metformin noted that, in women resistant to clomifene, metformin plus clomifene

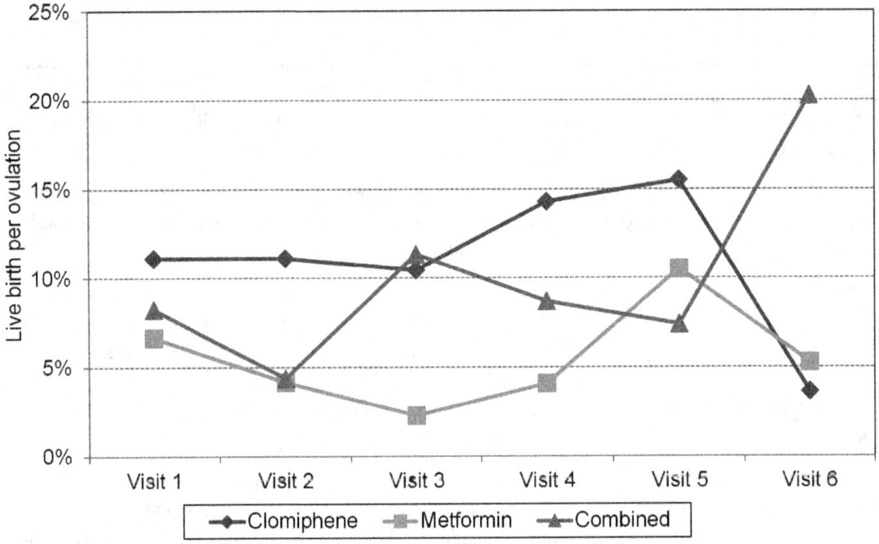

Figure 15.1 Live birth per ovulation by monthly visit in women with polycystic ovary syndrome being treated with clomifene citrate, metformin or a combination of both; there was a significant time trend (towards improvement) in the combined arm ($P<0.05$), with no statistically significant changes in fecundity rates over time with clomifene or metformin alone; data from Legro *et al.*[10]

led to higher live birth rates than clomifene alone (RR 6.4; 95% CI 1.2–35); metformin also led to higher live birth rates than laparoscopic ovarian diathermy (RR 1.6; 95% CI 1.1–2.5).[15] Another interesting adjuvant use of metformin in infertile women with PCOS is to prevent the development of ovarian hyperstimulation syndrome (OHSS) in those receiving gonadotrophin therapy as part of an *in vitro* fertilisation cycle. A large trial noted a marked reduction in the incidence of OHSS[16] and a meta-analysis has also supported this use.[17] This review found no evidence that metformin treatment before or during assisted reproductive technology cycles improved live birth or clinical pregnancy rates. The risk of OHSS in women with PCOS undergoing *in vitro* fertilisation or intracytoplasmic sperm injection cycles was reduced with metformin (pooled OR 0.27; 95% CI 0.16–0.47).[17] This indication, that is, to slow follicular recruitment and/or development during gonadotrophin stimulation, would support the relative anti-fecundity of metformin observed with ovulation induction.

Metformin has been recommended for use in fertility treatment partly because it is thought to be associated with monofollicular ovulation and lower multiple pregnancy rates. None of the trials was adequately powered to detect differences in multiple pregnancy rates. In the PPCOS study,[10] the multiple pregnancy rate in the clomifene-only group was 6.0% ($n=3$; one triplet), 0% in the metformin-only group and 3.1% in the combination therapy group ($n=2$). This number (around 5%) is at or below what has been reported from large series of women conceiving on clomifene[18] and well below the expectations of many of an enhanced multiple pregnancy rate in response to clomifene in women with PCOS.[19] However, given the low number of multiple pregnancies overall, there was no statistically significant difference in multiple pregnancy rates between treatment groups. The Dutch study reported one triplet (none survived) and one twin pregnancy in women on clomifene therapy.[13] Further research is needed, although given the relatively small multiple pregnancy rate, a very large number of pregnancies will be required to detect a significant reduction from a 5–6% multiple pregnancy rate with clomifene. The benefit of multiple pregnancy reduction must be balanced against the substantially lower pregnancy rates with metformin alone.

The risk/benefit ratio of metformin use for infertility is very favourable. These are adult women and serious adverse reactions such as ketoacidosis are rare in this healthy population. There are no major interactions with the commonly used adjuvant infertility medications. Metformin is not protein bound, is not metabolised and is excreted primarily in urine. There is no known fetal toxicity or teratogenecity (see below). However most of these studies have stopped the drug at the time of a positive pregnancy test.

There have been fewer studies of thiazolidinediones for infertility. These have been small and they have rarely looked at pregnancy. The published studies have been underpowered to address the benefit on pregnancy and live birth. The risk/benefit ratio is also less favourable for this indication as thiazolidinediones may be associated with fetal loss, based on animal studies, and exposure in early pregnancy would best be avoided. The recent increase in cardiovascular events and mortality seen with rosiglitazone in type 2 diabetes is concerning and should lead to caution in their use for infertility.[20]

Miscarriage and pregnancy complications

Metformin has been proposed to prevent early first-trimester miscarriage. There are some data to suggest that both hyperinsulinaemia and hyperandrogenism are more common among women with recurrent miscarriage. Similarly, there has been concern that women with PCOS are more likely to experience first-trimester miscarriage than other women.[21] Metformin is theorised to improve pregnancy continuation by lowering insulin and androgen levels, analogously to their use for inducing ovulation. The quality of the data for these studies tends to be low: they are usually case series of improved outcomes after giving metformin compared with the prior outcomes when it was not given.

The trials discussed in Table 15.1 offer some insight into early pregnancy loss but all of them stopped study medication in women upon determination of pregnancy. These trials thus cannot address the potential risk/benefit ratio of continuing medication through the first trimester or throughout pregnancy, as some groups have advocated.[22] It is concerning that there was a non-significant and unexpected trend towards an increased first-trimester miscarriage rate in the metformin group versus the clomifene group (40% in the metformin group versus 23% in the clomifene and 25% in the combined group) in the PPCOS trial. No similar trend in miscarriage rates was noted in the other trials but they were significantly smaller. The Italian group in another small trial did report a significant reduction in miscarriage rates in clomifene-resistant women who conceived after metformin use compared with laparoscopic ovarian diathermy.[23] A 2009 review of the published studies found that metformin had no effect on first-trimester miscarriage rates.[24]

Women with PCOS are suspected to be at increased risk of pregnancy complications. A meta-analysis found that women with PCOS demonstrated a significantly higher risk of gestational diabetes (OR 2.94; 95% CI 1.70–5.08), pregnancy-induced hypertension (OR 3.67; 95% CI 1.98–6.81), pre-eclampsia (OR 3.47; 95% CI 1.95–6.17) and preterm birth (OR 1.75; 95% CI 1.16–2.62). Their babies had a significantly higher risk of admission to a neonatal intensive care unit (OR 2.31; 95% CI 1.25–4.26) and higher perinatal mortality (OR 3.07; 95% CI 1.03–9.21), unrelated to multiple births.[25] These same maternal complications were noted in the same decreasing frequency in the PPCOS study, where pregnancies were followed until completion.[10]

This has led some to recommend that metformin be continued throughout pregnancy in women with PCOS. The justification is that insulin resistance plays a role in the aetiology of both pre-eclampsia and gestational diabetes, and these can be improved with an insulin sensitiser. As will be discussed and advocated below, metformin is effective in preventing diabetes in an adult population, so it remains within the same paradigm to give it to prevent gestational diabetes. A small single-centre randomised trial from Norway has shown a remarkable reduction in maternal morbidity in women with PCOS with the use of metformin continually throughout pregnancy[26] and this has led to the conducting of a larger multicentre trial whose results are unfortunately not yet available.

A 2006 meta-analysis looked at the major malformation rate after first-trimester metformin exposure (Figure 15.2).[27] Eight studies were included in the meta-analysis, with an odds ratio of 0.50 (95% CI 0.15–1.60). After adjustment for publication bias, metformin treatment in the first trimester was associated with a statistically significant 57% protective effect. After pooling the studies, the malformation rate in the disease-matched control group was approximately 7.2%, statistically significantly higher than the rate found in the metformin group (1.7%). However, this meta-analysis was limited by the small number of women in the metformin exposure group ($n = 172$) and in the control group ($n = 235$).

Without further documentation of the efficacy and the fetal risks of continuous use, it is premature to recommend the use of metformin as a preventive agent for any indication in pregnant women with PCOS.

Hirsutism

There are not enough data to conclude whether insulin-sensitising agents improve hirsutism, at least to the patient's satisfaction. Many trials have not reported the effects on hirsutism or were too short to determine a benefit. A meta-analysis tried to address the comparative effectiveness of metformin versus the oral contraceptive pill. Limited data from only six trials and 174 participants demonstrated no evidence of difference in effect between metformin and the oral contraceptive pill on hirsutism and acne.[28] The initial meta-analysis found no benefit. The largest trial to date in women with

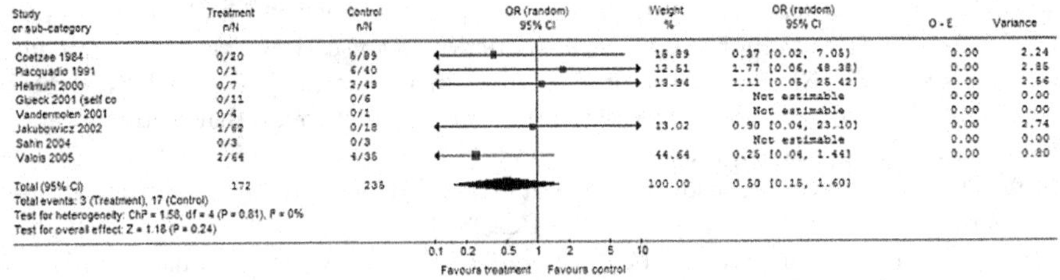
Meta-Analysis: All groups
Review: Metformin
Comparison: 01 Malformations (all groups)
Outcome: 01 Malformations (all groups)
Study or sub-category
Treatment n/N
Control n/N
OR (random) 95% CI
Weight %
OR (random) 95% CI
O - E
Variance
Coetzee 1984 0/20 5/89 15.89 0.37 [0.02, 7.05] 0.00 2.24
Piacquadio 1991 0/1 6/40 12.51 1.77 [0.06, 48.38] 0.00 2.85
Hellmuth 2000 0/7 2/43 13.94 1.11 [0.05, 25.42] 0.00 2.56
Glueck 2001 (self co 0/11 0/6 Not estimable 0.00 0.00
Vandermolen 2001 0/4 0/1 Not estimable 0.00 0.00
Jakubowicz 2002 1/62 0/18 13.02 0.90 [0.04, 23.10] 0.00 2.74
Sahin 2004 0/3 0/3 Not estimable 0.00 0.00
Valois 2005 2/64 4/35 44.64 0.25 [0.04, 1.44] 0.00 0.80
Total (95% CI) 172 235 100.00 0.50 [0.15, 1.60]
Total events: 3 (Treatment), 17 (Control)
Test for heterogeneity: Chi² = 1.58, df = 4 (P = 0.81), I² = 0%
Test for overall effect: Z = 1.18 (P = 0.24)
0.1 0.2 0.5 1 2 5 10
Favours treatment
Favours control

Figure 15.2 Meta-analysis of fetal major malformations after first-trimester exposure to metformin; reproduced with permission from Gilbert *et al.*[27]

PCOS that tracked hirsutism involved the use of troglitazone, a thiazolidinedione that has since been removed from the market owing to hepatotoxicity.[29] This study, which lasted 44 weeks, was also longer than most studies. It was a phase II dose-ranging study and involved four treatment arms – one placebo arm and three active drug arms. There was a significant decrease in the Ferriman–Gallwey score only with the highest dose of troglitazone compared with placebo (-2.21 ± 0.49 versus 0.22 ± 0.53; $P<0.05$) (Figure 15.3). This small decrease, while statistically significant, is of uncertain cosmetic benefit.

Diabetes prevention

The strongest evidence for the use of metformin in women with PCOS is with regard to diabetes prevention in high-risk individuals. The evidence for this is largely based on studies conducted in similar populations. For instance, the Diabetes Prevention Program showed a 31% (95% CI 17–43%) reduction in the conversion to type 2 diabetes with metformin compared with placebo in individuals with impaired glucose tolerance.[30] Impaired glucose tolerance is common in women with PCOS and may approach 30–40% in obese populations.[31,32]

Thiazolidinediones appear to be similarly if not more effective than metformin at delaying the development of diabetes. For example, although the troglitazone arm was stopped prematurely during the Diabetes Prevention Program owing to hepatotoxicity, it was more effective than metformin during the time period that it was studied.[33] Similarly, it was very effective in preventing the conversion to type 2 diabetes in women with gestational diabetes when it was used post-pregnancy, halving the conversion rate to diabetes compared with placebo.[34] Rosiglitazone has also been effective at preventing diabetes in an at-risk population. The risk/benefit ratio of the thiazolidinediones may be more favourable when the goal is prevention of diabetes in a pre-diabetic population.

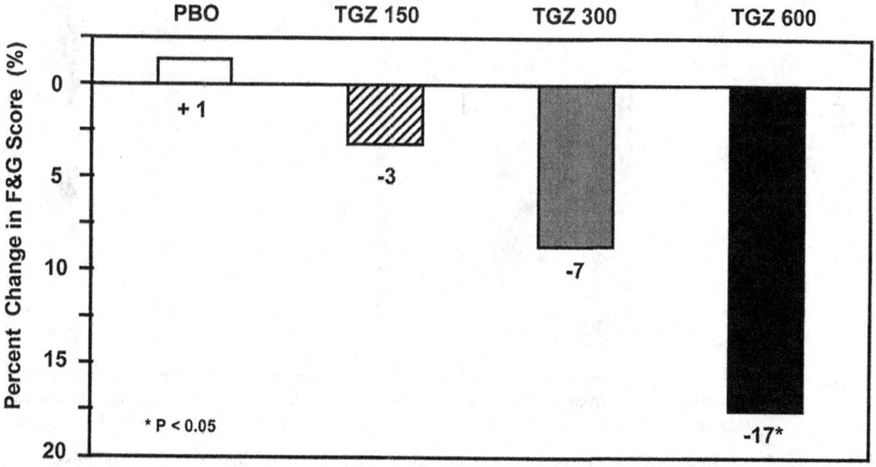

Figure 15.3 Decrease in mean Ferriman–Gallwey hirsutism score relative to baseline with treatment with the insulin-sensitiser troglitazone (TGZ) compared with placebo (PBO) in women with PCOS; reproduced with permission from Azziz *et al.*[29] © 2001, The Endocrine Society

Weight loss and a reduction of centripetal fat was shown in the Diabetes Prevention Program with metformin. This has not universally been shown with the drug but weight loss is often noticed in women with PCOS on metformin. The PPCOS trial noted a significant reduction in weight of almost 1 body mass index (BMI) unit (Figure 15.4).[10] A 2009 meta-analysis of treatment with metformin in women with PCOS showed a statistically significant decrease in BMI compared with placebo (weighted mean difference −0.68; 95% CI −1.13 to −0.24).[35] There was some indication of greater effect with high-dose metformin (> 1500 mg per day) and longer duration of therapy (> 8 weeks).

Endometrial cancer prevention

The effects of insulin-sensitising agents on the endometrium have not been well studied. Theoretically, any treatment that improves ovulation and decreases the exposure of the endometrium to chronic unopposed estrogen will be beneficial. One study[36] performed endometrial biopsies before and after treatment with metformin or rosiglitazone alone or in combination and found that abnormal histology (simple hyperplasia) tended to normalise (two cases of simple hyperplasia reverted to normal histology). There were no discernible effects on the histology of the women who had normal morphology at baseline. However, this study was too small ($n = 16$)to assess the long-term endometrial effects of these drugs.

Conclusion

In 2009, the *Cochrane Database of Systematic Reviews* updated their analysis of insulin-sensitising agents in women with PCOS.[2] The main conclusion was: 'Metformin is

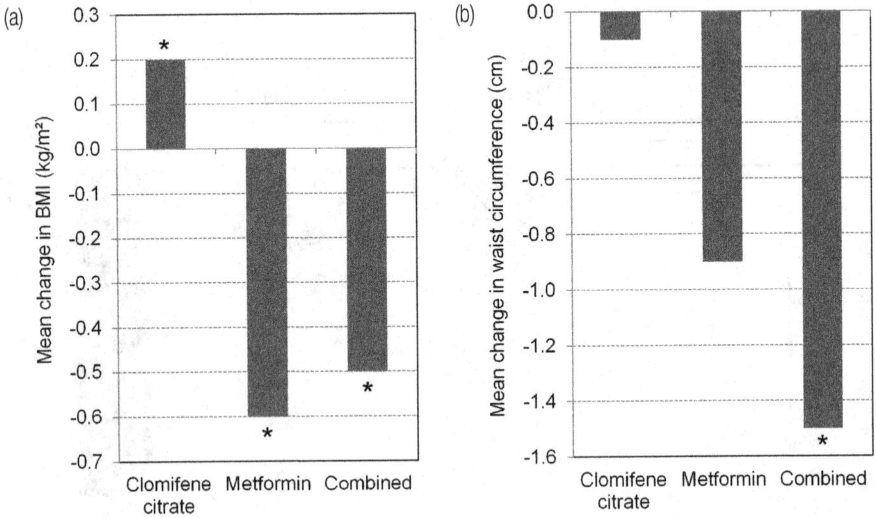

Figure 15.4 Change in parameters of women on metformin, clomifene citrate or a combination of both in the PPCOS study[10] from baseline to study completion or study dropout (owing to pregnancy or other cause): (a) mean change in body mass index; (b) mean change in waist circumference; * $P < 0.05$, relative to baseline

still of benefit in improving clinical pregnancy and ovulation rates. However, there is no evidence that metformin improves live birth rates whether it is used alone or in combination with clomiphene, or when compared with clomiphene. Therefore, the use of metformin in improving reproductive outcomes in women with PCOS appears to be limited.' The conclusions from this chapter largely agree with the Cochrane analysis and are as follows:

- Metformin has many potential uses in reproductive medicine but its impact in properly designed trials has been modest to date.
- Metformin may delay pubertal progression and development of a PCOS phenotype in girls with premature pubarche.
- Metformin is relatively ineffective as a solo agent to treat infertility and furthermore has a relative anti-fecundity compared with clomifene alone. Clomifene remains the first choice for infertility therapy and the gold standard treatment for women with PCOS.
- There may be benefits of combined therapy with clomifene and metformin on live birth rates in select subpopulations, for example in a very obese population.
- Metformin may be useful to prevent OHSS in women with PCOS when used in conjunction with gonadotrophins.
- The use of metformin to prevent pregnancy loss or to prevent pregnancy complications is still experimental and better trials are needed to guide therapy.
- Limited data do not support that metformin has any increased teratogenic effects.
- Metformin does result in modest improvements in the PCOS phenotype, with reductions in circulating insulin and testosterone levels, weight loss and improved menstrual/ovulatory frequency.
- Metformin delays diabetes development in women at high risk but its effects at preventing cardiovascular disease are unclear; further studies in women with PCOS are needed.

Acknowledgements

This work was supported by PHS K24 HD01476, U54 HD034449, a GCRC grant MO1 RR 10732, and construction grant C06 RR016499 to Pennsylvania State University.

References

1. Nestler JE, Jakubowicz DJ, Reamer P, Gunn RD, Allan G. Ovulatory and metabolic effects of D-chiro-inositol in the polycystic ovary syndrome. *New Engl J Med* 1999;340:1314–20.
2. Tang T, Lord JM, Norman RJ, Yasmin E, Balen AH. Insulin-sensitising drugs (metformin, rosiglitazone, pioglitazone, D-chiro-inositol) for women with polycystic ovary syndrome, oligo amenorrhoea and subfertility. *Cochrane Database Syst Rev* 2009;(4):CD003053.
3. Fujioka K, Brazg RL, Raz I, Bruce S, Joyal S, Swanink R, *et al.* Efficacy, dose-response relationship and safety of once-daily extended-release metformin (Glucophage XR) in type 2 diabetic patients with inadequate glycaemic control despite prior treatment with diet and exercise: results from two double-blind, placebo-controlled studies. *Diabetes Obes Metab* 2005;7:28–39.
4. Ibañez L, Potau N, Zampolli M, Prat N, Virdis R, Vicenscalvet E. Hyperinsulinemia in postpubertal girls with a history of premature pubarche and functional ovarian hyperandrogenism. *J Clin Endocrinol Metab* 1996;81:1237–43.

5. Ibañez L, de Zegher F, Potau N. Anovulation after precocious pubarche: early markers and time course in adolescence. *J Clin Endocrinol Metab* 1999;84:2691–5.
6. Ibañez L, Ferrer A, Ong K, Amin R, Dunger D, de Zegher F. Insulin sensitization early after menarche prevents progression from precocious pubarche to polycystic ovary syndrome. *J Pediatr* 2004;144:23–9.
7. Ibañez L, Ong K, Valls C, Marcos MV, Dunger DB, de Zegher F. Metformin treatment to prevent early puberty in girls with precocious pubarche. *J Clin Endocrinol Metab* 2006;91:2888–91.
8. Ibañez L, Lopez-Bermejo A, Diaz M, Marcos MV, de Zegher F. Metformin treatment for four years to reduce total and visceral fat in low birth weight girls with precocious pubarche. *J Clin Endocrinol Metab* 2008;93:1841–5.
9. Ibañez L, Valls C, Ferrer A, Ong K, Dunger DB, De Zegher F. Additive effects of insulin-sensitizing and anti-androgen treatment in young, nonobese women with hyperinsulinism, hyperandrogenism, dyslipidemia, and anovulation. *J Clin Endocrinol Metab* 2002;87:2870–4.
10. Legro RS, Barnhart HX, Schlaff WD, Carr BR, Diamond MP, Carson SA, *et al*; Cooperative Multicenter Reproductive Medicine Network. Clomiphene, metformin, or both for infertility in the polycystic ovary syndrome. *N Engl J Med* 2007;356:551–66.
11. Zain MM, Jamaluddin R, Ibrahim A, Norman RJ. Comparison of clomiphene citrate, metformin, or the combination of both for first-line ovulation induction, achievement of pregnancy, and live birth in Asian women with polycystic ovary syndrome: a randomized controlled trial. *Fertil Steril* 2009;91:514–21.
12. Thessaloniki ESHRE/ASRM-Sponsored PCOS Consensus Workshop Group. Consensus on infertility treatment related to polycystic ovary syndrome. *Fertil Steril* 2008;89:505–22.
13. Moll E, Bossuyt PM, Korevaar JC, Lambalk CB, van der Veen F. Effect of clomifene citrate plus metformin and clomifene citrate plus placebo on induction of ovulation in women with newly diagnosed polycystic ovary syndrome: randomised double blind clinical trial. *BMJ* 2006;332:1485.
14. Creanga AA, Bradley HM, McCormick C, Witkop CT. Use of metformin in polycystic ovary syndrome: a meta-analysis. *Obstet Gynecol* 2008;111:959–68.
15. Moll E, van der Veen F, van Wely M. The role of metformin in polycystic ovary syndrome: a systematic review. *Hum Reprod Update* 2007;13:527–37.
16. Tang T, Glanville J, Orsi N, Barth JH, Balen AH. The use of metformin for women with PCOS undergoing IVF treatment. *Hum Reprod* 2006;21:1416–25.
17. Costello MF, Chapman M, Conway U. A systematic review and meta-analysis of randomized controlled trials on metformin co-administration during gonadotrophin ovulation induction or IVF in women with polycystic ovary syndrome. *Hum Reprod* 2006;21:1387–99.
18. Asch RH, Greenblatt RB. Update on the safety and efficacy of clomiphene citrate as a therapeutic agent. *J Reprod Med* 1976;17:175–80.
19. Casper RF, Mitwally MF. Review: aromatase inhibitors for ovulation induction. *J Clin Endocrinol Metab* 2006;91:760–71.
20. Nissen SE, Wolski K. Rosiglitazone revisited: an updated meta-analysis of risk for myocardial infarction and cardiovascular mortality. *Arch Intern Med* 2010 Jun 28. [Epub ahead of print]
21. Homburg R, Armar NA, Eshel A, Adams J, Jacobs HS. Influence of serum luteinising hormone concentrations on ovulation, conception, and early pregnancy loss in polycystic ovary syndrome. *BMJ* 1988;297:1024–6.
22. Jakubowicz DJ, Iuorno MJ, Jakubowicz S, Roberts KA, Nestler JE. Effects of metformin on early pregnancy loss in the polycystic ovary syndrome. *J Clin Endocrinol Metab* 2002;87:524–9.
23. Palomba S, Orio F Jr, Nardo LG, Falbo A, Russo T, Corea D, *et al*. Metformin administration versus laparoscopic ovarian diathermy in clomiphene citrate-resistant women with polycystic ovary syndrome: a prospective parallel randomized double-blind placebo-controlled trial. *J Clin Endocrinol Metab* 2004;89:4801–9.
24. Palomba S, Falbo A, Orio F Jr, Zullo F. Effect of preconceptional metformin on abortion risk in polycystic ovary syndrome: a systematic review and meta-analysis of randomized controlled trials. *Fertil Steril* 2009;92:1646–58.
25. Boomsma CM, Eijkemans MJ, Hughes EG, Visser GH, Fauser BC, Macklon NS. A meta-analysis of pregnancy outcomes in women with polycystic ovary syndrome. *Hum Reprod Update* 2006;12:673–83.

26. Vanky E, Salvesen KA, Heimstad R, Fougner KJ, Romundstad P, Carlsen SM. Metformin reduces pregnancy complications without affecting androgen levels in pregnant polycystic ovary syndrome women: results of a randomized study. *Hum Reprod* 2004;19:1734–40.
27. Gilbert C, Valois M, Koren G. Pregnancy outcome after first trimester exposure to metformin: a meta-analysis. *Fertil Steril* 2006;86:658–63.
28. Costello M, Shrestha B, Eden J, Sjoblom P, Johnson N. Insulin-sensitising drugs versus the combined oral contraceptive pill for hirsutism, acne and risk of diabetes, cardiovascular disease, and endometrial cancer in polycystic ovary syndrome. *Cochrane Database Syst Rev* 2007;(1):CD005552.
29. Azziz R, Ehrmann D, Legro RS, Whitcomb RW, Hanley R, Fereshetian AG, *et al*; PCOS/Troglitazone Study Group. Troglitazone improves ovulation and hirsutism in the polycystic ovary syndrome: a multicenter, double blind, placebo-controlled trial. *J Clin Endocrinol Metab* 2001;86:1626–32.
30. Knowler WC, Barrett-Connor E, Fowler SE, Hamman RF, Lachin JM, Walker EA, *et al*; Diabetes Prevention Program Research Group. Reduction in the incidence of type 2 diabetes with lifestyle intervention or metformin. *New Engl J Med* 2002;346:393–403.
31. Legro RS, Kunselman AR, Dodson WC, Dunaif A. Prevalence and predictors of risk for type 2 diabetes mellitus and impaired glucose tolerance in polycystic ovary syndrome: a prospective, controlled study in 254 affected women. *J Clin Endocrinol Metab* 1999;84:165–9.
32. Gambineri A, Pelusi C, Manicardi E, Vicennati V, Cacciari M, Morselli-Labate AM, *et al.* Glucose intolerance in a large cohort of mediterranean women with polycystic ovary syndrome: phenotype and associated factors. *Diabetes* 2004;53:2353–8.
33. Knowler WC, Hamman RF, Edelstein SL, Barrett-Connor E, Ehrmann DA, Walker EA, *et al*; Diabetes Prevention Program Research Group. Prevention of type 2 diabetes with troglitazone in the Diabetes Prevention Program. Diabetes 2005;54:1150–6.
34. Buchanan TA, Xiang AH, Peters RK, Kjos SL, Marroquin A, Goico J, *et al.* Preservation of pancreatic beta-cell function and prevention of type 2 diabetes by pharmacological treatment of insulin resistance in high-risk hispanic women. *Diabetes* 2002;51:2796–803.
35. Nieuwenhuis-Ruifrok AE, Kuchenbecker WK, Hoek A, Middleton P, Norman RJ. Insulin sensitizing drugs for weight loss in women of reproductive age who are overweight or obese: systematic review and meta-analysis. *Hum Reprod Update* 2009;15:57–68.
36. Legro RS, Zaino RJ, Demers LM, Kunselman AR, Gnatuk CL, Williams NI, *et al.* The effects of metformin and rosiglitazone, alone and in combination, on the ovary and endometrium in polycystic ovary syndrome. *Am J Obstet Gynecol* 2007;196:402.e1–10; discussion 402.e10–1.
37. Palomba S, Orio F Jr, Falbo A, Manguso F, Russo T, Cascella T, *et al.* Prospective parallel randomized, double-blind, double-dummy controlled clinical trial comparing clomiphene citrate and metformin as the first-line treatment for ovulation induction in nonobese anovulatory women with polycystic ovary syndrome. *J Clin Endocrinol Metab* 2005;90:4068–74.
38. Palomba S, Orio F Jr, Falbo A, Russo T, Tolino A, Zullo F. Clomiphene citrate versus metformin as first-line approach for the treatment of anovulation in infertile patients with polycystic ovary syndrome. *J Clin Endocrinol Metab* 2007;92:3498–503.

16

Chapter 16

The role of *in vitro* maturation of oocytes for anovulatory polycystic ovary syndrome

Tim Child

In vitro fertilisation (IVF) and embryo transfer is an established and successful form of treatment for infertility. Recent data from the Human Fertilisation and Embryology Authority (HFEA) show consistently improving IVF success rates.[1] The live birth rate per IVF cycle is mainly dependent on female age: during 2007, the average live birth rate per cycle started for women younger than 35 years in the UK was 32.3%, although many clinics are achieving rates of over 40%. During standard IVF treatment, *in vivo* matured metaphase II (MII) stage oocytes are aspirated from follicles measuring 14–20 mm in diameter. To achieve this, gonadotrophin ovarian stimulation is used, most commonly after achieving pituitary suppression using a gonadotrophin-releasing hormone (GnRH) agonist (long-protocol IVF).

However, these high rates of success are achieved at the expense of two major complications, namely multiple pregnancy and ovarian hyperstimulation syndrome (OHSS). Over 25% of the IVF live births described above were multiple. This results from the fairly routine transfer of multiple embryos to the uterine cavity in an attempt to overcome low implantation rates, particularly in older women. Moreover, in order to have multiple embryos available for transfer, ovarian stimulation is required, which places the woman at risk of developing OHSS. There has been much recent focus on reducing both the rate of multiple pregnancy and also the rate of OHSS.[2] Prolonged embryo culture to day 5 or 6 (blastocyst stage) with replacement of a single embryo maintains pregnancy rates while significantly reducing the multiple pregnancy rate. However, the rate of embryo attrition means that multiple oocytes need to be retrieved and successfully fertilised to allow sufficient good-quality day 3 embryos to continue culture to day 5.

OHSS is a recognised complication of ovarian stimulation. Known risk factors include younger female age (less than 35 years), gonadotrophin stimulation, previous OHSS, and ovaries of polycystic morphology. A number of studies have shown that the presence of ovaries of polycystic morphology, regardless of whether there are additional features of the full polycystic ovary syndrome (PCOS), significantly increase the risk of developing moderate to severe OHSS.[3] In its most severe form, OHSS is characterised by ascites, pleural effusions, ovarian enlargement and electrolyte and haemostatic disturbances.

A number of strategies have been suggested for the prevention of OHSS but unfortunately none is entirely satisfactory. These include reduced daily gonadotrophin dose ('mild IVF'), the use of gonadotrophin antagonists rather than agonists during IVF, gonadotrophin withdrawal for a period before human chorionic gonadotrophin (hCG) injection ('coasting'), cryopreservation ('freeze-all') and replacement of frozen–thawed embryos in a subsequent cycle, and intravenous albumin transfusion at the time of oocyte retrieval.[4] The only way to avoid the risk of developing OHSS entirely is to avoid stimulating the ovaries. Natural-cycle IVF, with the retrieval of a single mature oocyte from the dominant follicle, is of limited success, with live birth rates per cycle in single figures. Clearly, women with anovulatory PCOS do not produce dominant follicles so natural-cycle treatment is not an option anyway. Stimulated ovaries are not necessary for *in vitro* maturation (IVM) of immature oocytes retrieved from the resting antral follicles. IVM is therefore an approach with the potential to increase both the simplicity and safety of assisted reproductive technology (ART) treatment through the absence of the need for ovarian stimulation. IVM may be particularly applicable for women with anovulatory PCOS, which is the focus of this chapter.

In vitro maturation of immature oocytes

The basis of clinical IVM is the maturation *in vitro* of oocytes from the germinal vesicle stage of development to the MII stage. What follows is the protocol used in the Oxford Fertility Unit (as of January 2010, the only UK clinic offering IVM). The protocol is heavily based on the McGill University (Montreal) protocol where the author spent 2 years researching IVM. Variations on this protocol will then be discussed.

IVM is offered in Oxford to women with ovaries of polycystic morphology (regardless of whether they also have other features of the full syndrome) who are aged less than 38 years. A pretreatment scan confirms that the ovaries contain sufficient antral follicles and are accessible transvaginally. While ovaries stuck high in the pelvis due to endometriosis or adhesions may be accessed transvaginally during standard IVF when enlarged following gonadotrophin stimulation, the same is not true for small, unstimulated ovaries. Women have the process of the IVM cycle explained, including the lower chance of success compared with IVF. We also explain that the treatment is less well established than IVF, with limited numbers of children born and follow-up studies performed. On the positive side, we explain that, to date, IVM babies appear to be as normal as those from IVF and that, with IVM, the woman will not develop OHSS.

Women call on day 1 of their menstrual cycle (either spontaneous or induced) and undergo a transvaginal ultrasound scan between day 2 and day 5 to confirm the ovarian antral follicle count and accessibility and the absence of pathology such as corpus luteum cysts. Anovulatory women are given a date for immature oocyte retrieval between day 7 and day 14 of the cycle. For ovulatory women, we aim to perform the retrieval before there is a dominant follicle greater than 14 mm in diameter, so a second ultrasound scan may be performed to assist with timing.

The only drug used before immature oocyte retrieval is hCG 10 000 IU subcutaneously 40 hours before collection. Women undergoing IVF in Oxford receive hCG 35 hours before oocyte retrieval.

During IVM, immature oocytes are aspirated from resting antral follicles measuring 2–8 mm in diameter. The first successful use of IVM was reported by Cha *et al.*[5] in 1991 and, in their case, the oocytes were retrieved at laparotomy. The successful aspiration of immature oocytes using transvaginal ultrasound was reported by Trounson *et al.*[6] in 1994 and this has been the standard retrieval technique since then. The small antral follicle size means that narrow-gauge single-channel needles are used (such as K-OPS-7035-RWH-ET; Cook, Australia) with a reduced aspiration pressure of 7.5 kPa. Flushing of the tiny follicles is not generally possible (so double-channel needles are not required) and the needle, passing through the dense ovarian stroma, tends to block. Consequently, a multiple-puncture technique is used, with the needle being passed into a number of antral follicles and then withdrawn from the vagina before aspirating heparinised culture medium from a test tube to keep the needle clear and to flush the immature oocytes from the collecting system. The oocyte collection takes around 20 minutes to perform and standard IVF 'conscious sedation' is used together with a local anaesthetic paracervical block.

Test tubes containing the aspirate are passed to the embryologist, who pours the contents through a 70 micrometre mesh cell strainer. Oocytes are identified and their maturity assessed, without stripping of the granulosa cells, using the sliding method.[7] Any mature oocytes collected are prepared for intracytoplasmic sperm injection (ICSI), while immature oocytes are cultured in specially designed IVM culture medium, now available commercially in the UK (Sage/Cooper Surgical, Rochford Medical UK), supplemented with 75 mIU/ml follicle-stimulating hormone (FSH) and luteinising hormone (LH). The majority of oocytes, over 60%, mature by 24 hours of culture. Once mature, ICSI is used for insemination (see below) and from then on standard IVF embryo culture techniques are used. In the UK, one or at most two embryos are transferred to the endometrial cavity 2–5 days after ICSI. Since oocytes from one collection may be fertilised on three different days (mature on day of oocyte retrieval or by 24 or 48 hours after), it is not unusual that, at the time of transfer, there are embryos at differing developmental stages.[8]

Endometrial priming using estradiol valerate 6 mg daily by mouth begins from the day of oocyte retrieval. Progesterone luteal support is given in the form of 200 mg vaginal pessaries twice daily starting the following day. Ideally, estrogen priming would be commenced from the start of the cycle (as it is during frozen embryo replacement treatments) since this would be a more physiological approach. However, data suggest that exogenous estrogen before immature oocyte retrieval reduces oocyte potential.[9] This truncated endometrial priming regimen, lasting only a few days between oocyte retrieval and embryo transfer, is likely to be a limitation of the IVM technique and may partly explain the lower success rates. If pregnant, the woman continues with estrogen and progesterone supplementation until 10–12 weeks of gestation.

Variations

There are a number of variations to this basic IVM protocol that will now be discussed.

Patient selection

The pregnancy rate with unstimulated IVM is related to the number of immature oocytes retrieved[10] and embryos produced. This can be predicted by the baseline antral follicle count (AFC) measured using transvaginal ultrasonography.[10] Immature oocytes are retrieved from around 50% of the antral follicles present on scan.[10] Consequently, it is expected that women with ovaries of polycystic morphology, with many antral follicles, should have a higher pregnancy rate than those with normal ovaries. This has been confirmed in a number of observational studies. One of the largest compared 56 cycles in women with normal ovaries with 68 cycles in women with anovulatory PCOS and 53 in those with ovulatory PCO (ovaries of polycystic morphology but regular ovulatory cycles).[11] The numbers of immature oocytes collected in the PCOS and the ovulatory PCO groups were very similar (mean 11.3 and 10.0, respectively), as were the live birth rates (14.9% and 17.3% per cycle, respectively). However, women with normal ovaries had a low number of oocytes collected (mean 5.1) and a correspondingly poor live birth rate of 2%.

The majority of published reports of IVM cycles and successes have focused on women with ovaries of polycystic morphology (ovulatory or anovulatory) (see below). More recently, improved IVM success rates have been reported in women with normal ovaries.[12] There is particular interest in IVM in women with normal ovaries in Italy following the change in law that now only allows a maximum of three oocytes to be inseminated per ART cycle. Under these restrictions, the IVF success rates are limited and there may be less of a reason for a woman with normal ovaries to undergo gonadotrophin stimulation with the retrieval of numerous oocytes never destined to be inseminated. However, in countries where no restriction exists, the pregnancy rate with IVF for women with normal ovaries is expected to be far superior to IVM. Consequently, in Oxford we do not offer IVM to such women, as those aged less than 35 years are achieving pregnancy rates with IVF of around 50% per cycle.

hCG priming

During standard IVF, hCG (or LH) is administered 35–38 hours before oocyte recovery to promote nuclear maturation. A randomised controlled trial (RCT) involving 24 unstimulated IVM cycles for women with PCOS was undertaken at McGill University.[13] Women were randomised to receive either no hCG priming or 10 000 IU hCG 36 hours before immature oocyte recovery. Priming with hCG significantly increased both the speed of nuclear maturation following oocyte retrieval and the final number of mature oocytes. Seventy-eight percent of oocytes in the hCG group matured by 24 hours after oocyte retrieval compared with 4.9% in the non-primed group ($P<0.05$). By 48 hours after oocyte retrieval, 84% of hCG-primed oocytes had reached MII compared with 69% of unprimed oocytes ($P<0.05$). The majority of clinics performing IVM use hCG priming. A further RCT from Montreal comparing two different hCG priming doses, 10 000 versus 20 000 IU, reported no difference in outcome.[14]

More recently it has been suggested that extending the interval between hCG priming and immature oocyte recovery from 35 to 38 hours increases the rates of oocyte maturation and embryo implantation,[15] although this was a retrospective study.

Gonadotrophin ovarian stimulation

Studies examining gonadotrophin stimulation during the early part of an IVM cycle have had conflicting results. Although FSH priming may increase the numbers of oocytes collected, it is not apparent that this translates into higher pregnancy rates. Mikkelsen and Lindenberg[16] used FSH 150 IU on cycle days 3–5 in women with PCOS, but without hCG priming, and reported an increase in clinical pregnancies. However, when hCG priming was used in all IVM cycles, the addition of FSH stimulation did not improve the outcome.[17] Son *et al.*[18] also found that hCG priming resulted in faster rates of oocyte maturation and significantly higher blastocyst development rates compared with either no priming or the use of low-dose human menopausal gonadotrophin (hMG).

ICSI

Hardening of the zona pellucida during *in vitro* culture results in a significantly lower fertilisation rate following standard oocyte insemination compared with when ICSI is used. Consequently, nearly all reported IVM cycles have included ICSI in the protocol as standard. However, a retrospective cohort study suggested that, for men with normal semen parameters (who would normally use standard insemination as opposed to ICSI during IVF), the lower fertilisation rate achieved after insemination was compensated for by a significantly higher implantation rate.[19] When ICSI was used during IVM (for the couples where male factor was also an issue), the fertilisation rate was 69% compared with 38% following standard insemination during IVM (for couples with no male factor). The implantation rate per embryo was 14.8% following ICSI and 24.2% after standard insemination ($P < 0.05$). In the subgroup of women with PCOS, the results were even more striking, with implantation rates of 12.5% (ICSI) and 34.5% (standard insemination), although smaller cycle numbers led to a lack of statistical significance. An RCT is required to assess whether these promising results can be substantiated. Avoiding ICSI would greatly simplify IVM cycle management and reduce the costs of IVM.

Endometrial priming

Estradiol valerate is started following immature oocyte recovery. If started before oocyte retrieval, the implantation potential of immature oocytes appears to be reduced.[9] This truncated regimen of endometrial priming is a limitation of the current protocol as embryo transfer may occur after only 3 days of estrogen and 2 days of progesterone treatment. An alternative regimen of freezing all fertilised IVM oocytes for subsequent transfer in a pituitary-suppressed hormone replacement therapy cycle did not appear particularly advantageous.[20] Endometrial thickness on the day of embryo transfer is related to the rates of implantation and clinical pregnancy although subjective assessment of 'endometrial quality' (heterogenous, homogeneous or triple line) was not.[21]

Metformin co-treatment

An RCT involving 56 women with clomifene citrate-resistant PCOS undergoing 70 IVM cycles reported that treatment with metformin 1 g per day for 12 weeks before IVM resulted in significantly higher implantation (15.3% versus 6.2%) and clinical pregnancy rates (38.2% versus 16.7%).[22]

Timing of immature oocyte retrieval in relation to follicular diameter

There are conflicting data on the effect of the presence of a dominant follicle at the time of oocyte retrieval on IVM outcome, although most women with anovulatory PCOS will only infrequently, if ever, produce one. An RCT suggested in 1999 that the blastocyst rate was significantly reduced if a dominant follicle of over 10 mm in diameter was present at immature oocyte retrieval.[23]

More recently, retrospective studies have suggested a significantly higher success rate if dominant follicles are present. Certainly the pregnancy rate is increased in unstimulated IVM cycles where one or more mature oocytes are present at oocyte retrieval.[9] This has led to the idea of 'natural-cycle' IVM and IVF, where the aim is to collect both *in vivo* matured oocytes and immature oocytes for IVM during the same retrieval procedure.[24] It appears that if the retrieval is performed too late, with the dominant follicle greater than 14 mm in diameter, then the potential of the sibling immature oocytes retrieved is reduced.[9] Thus, if this approach is taken, the optimal maximum diameter at retrieval may be around 12–14 mm.

Results

Data consistently confirm a lower success rate of clinical IVM compared with standard IVF in women with PCO. To date, no RCTs have compared the two techniques. Our group performed a case–control study with 107 cycles of IVM and 107 cycles of IVF for women with anovulatory PCOS or ovulatory PCO.[25] The cycles were matched for female age, ovulatory status and other fertility diagnoses such as male factor, tubal damage and endometriosis. Following oocyte maturation in the IVM group, the mean number of mature oocytes available was significantly higher in the IVF group (7.8 versus 12.0). Fertilisation rates were similar so the number of embryos produced was also significantly higher in the IVF group (6.1 versus 9.3). The implantation rate was significantly greater in the IVF group at 17.1% compared with 9.5% for IVM cycles, with corresponding live birth rates per cycle of 26.2% (IVF) and 15.9% (IVM), although the difference was not statistically significant. As expected, there were no cycles complicated by moderate or severe OHSS in the IVM group, whereas the rate was 11.2% in IVF cycles.

Miscarriage rates appear to be higher in IVM cycles compared with IVF.[26] However, when IVM or IVF cycles only in women with PCOS are considered, the miscarriage rates are similar, suggesting that the IVM technique does not itself increase the loss rate; it is the patient population who are at greater risk.

Suikkari reviewed the published data on IVM success rates in 2008.[27] In women with ovaries of polycystic morphology (PCOS or ovulatory PCO) (nine studies), 108 live births occurred after a total of 671 IVM cycles, which is a live birth rate of 16.1%.

In Oxford, we began undertaking IVM in February 2007. Since that time, we have performed 124 unstimulated IVM cycles for women with PCOS and ovulatory PCO. The pregnancy and clinical pregnancy rates per oocyte collection procedure are 28% and 21%, respectively. The mean (and standard deviation) patient age was 32.9 years (3.7 years), with the oldest woman being 39 years of age. The mean numbers of oocytes collected were 17.4 (9.0), matured *in vitro* 11.2 (7.0) and normally fertilised 7.4 (4.9). Live birth data are more limited (as the programme has only been running for 3 years) but, based on the first 68 cycles, the live birth rate was 21% (14 deliveries; 12 singletons and two twins).

Safety

For women requiring ART who have PCOS, IVM is safer than IVF because of the avoidance of OHSS. PCOS is one of the major risk factors for development of OHSS.

The immature oocyte retrieval procedure involves a multiple-puncture technique and greater pain levels. Initially, spinal anaesthesia was used by some groups during IVM retrievals, but we have found good effect combining standard IVF 'conscious sedation' with a paracervical local anaesthetic block. Following 124 IVM retrievals in Oxford, one woman required overnight hospital admission owing to pain, which was thought most likely to be due to a small intraperitoneal bleed from the ovarian punctures.

Over 1000 IVM babies have been born worldwide, with retrospective data on neonatal outcomes being collected by the Montreal group led by RC Chian. The combined data were presented at the 2008 meeting of the European Society of Human Reproduction and Embryology (ESHRE) and suggest no obvious concerns. However, formal prospective paediatric follow-up studies are limited. Buckett *et al.*[28] reported similar obstetric outcomes and congenital abnormality rates between babies born following IVM, IVF and ICSI. Neurological development of IVM children at

2 years of age appears to be normal.[29,30] The lack of good follow-up data means that couples considering IVM need to be aware of the lack of long-term safety knowledge and should be invited to participate in longitudinal paediatric studies.

Data suggest the possibility of higher rates of abnormal meiotic spindle and chromosome configurations in oocytes matured *in vitro*.[31] A small study reported a non-significant higher rate of aneuploid embryos (12 out of 20; 60%) compared with 33% in an IVF control group including 200 embryos following day 3 blastomere biopsy and fluorescence *in situ* hybridisation analysis.[32] Of the eight euploid IVM embryos, five (63%) went on to reach blastocyst stage compared with only three of 12 (25%) aneuploid IVM embryos. This might explain the observation of lower blastocyst, implantation and success rates of IVM compared with IVF, although the study data were obviously very limited. The authors suggested that a higher rate of chromosome abnormalities, together with other possible cytoplasm alterations due to altered maturation of organelles, may account for early cleavage arrest and a low implantation rate. However, in view of the data suggesting similar miscarriage rates and incidence of congenital disorders in newborn infants after IVM and conventional IVF protocols, they considered it possible that, once an IVM embryo has implanted, subsequent embryo development would not differ from standard IVF.

There is increasing interest and concern regarding the possibility of an association between ART treatments and imprinting disorders such as Angelman syndrome and Beckwith–Wiedemann syndrome.[33,34] Any increased incidence may in part be due to hormonal stimulation and/or *in vitro* culture. IVM avoids hormonal ovarian stimulation although it does involve prolonged *in vitro* culture. A 2008 study[33] involving immature oocytes retrieved from unstimulated and stimulated (IVF) cycles, followed by their *in vitro* maturation and analysis, suggested greater disruption to normal DNA methylation patterns in the IVF oocytes, probably owing to the gonadotrophin stimulation. Clearly, more work is required in all areas of ART.

Summary

IVM is a promising technique for women with anovulatory PCOS. The success rates are currently lower than those achieved with IVF but IVM is safer and easier to undertake for the woman and it avoids gonadotrophin stimulation and the attendant risk of OHSS. IVM is also likely to be cheaper, although this might only happen if ICSI can be shown to be redundant for couples with normal sperm function. While IVM is apparently safer for the woman, long-term paediatric studies are required before IVM can be fully assessed, which is also the case for other ART treatments.

References

1. Human Fertilisation and Embryology Authority [www.hfea.gov.uk].
2. Bensdorp AJ, Slappendel E, Koks C, Oosterhuis J, Hoek A, Hompes P, *et al.* The INeS study: prevention of multiple pregnancies: a randomised controlled trial comparing IUI COH versus IVF e SET versus MNC IVF in couples with unexplained or mild male subfertility. *BMC Womens Health* 2009;9:35.
3. Swanton A, Storey L, McVeigh E, Child T. IVF outcome in women with PCOS, PCO and normal ovarian morphology. *Eur J Obstet Gynecol Reprod Biol* 2010;149:68–71.
4. Practice Committee of American Society for Reproductive Medicine. Ovarian hyperstimulation syndrome. *Fertil Steril* 2008;90(5 Suppl):S188–93.
5. Cha KY, Koo JJ, Ko JJ, Choi DH, Han SY, Yoon TK. Pregnancy after *in vitro* fertilization of human follicular oocytes collected from nonstimulated cycles, their culture *in vitro* and their transfer in a donor oocyte program. *Fertil Steril* 1991;55:109–13.

6. Trounson A, Wood C, Kausche A. *In vitro* maturation and the fertilization and developmental competence of oocytes recovered from untreated polycystic ovarian patients. *Fertil Steril* 1994;62:353–62.
7. Russell JB, Knezevich KM, Fabian KF, Dickson JA. Unstimulated immature oocyte retrieval: early versus midfollicular endometrial priming. *Fertil Steril* 1997;67:616–20.
8. Child TJ, Abdul-Jalil AK, Tan SL. Embryo morphology, cumulative embryo score,and outcome in an oocyte *in vitro* maturation program. *Fertil Steril* 2002;77:424–5.
9. Son WY, Chung JT, Herrero B, Dean N, Demirtas E, Holzer H, *et al.* Selection of the optimal day for oocyte retrieval based on the diameter of the dominant follicle in hCG-primed *in vitro* maturation cycles. *Hum Reprod* 2008;23:2680–5.
10. Tan SL, Child TJ, Gulekli B. *In vitro* maturation and fertilization of oocytes from unstimulated ovaries: predicting the number of immature oocytes retrieved by early follicular phase ultrasonography. *Am J Obstet Gynecol* 2002;186:684–9.
11. Child TJ, Abdul-Jalil AK, Gulekli B, Tan SL. *In vitro* maturation and fertilization of oocytes from unstimulated normal ovaries, polycystic ovaries, and women with polycystic ovary syndrome. *Fertil Steril* 2001;76:936–42.
12. Fadini R, Dal Canto MB, Renzini MM, Brambillasca F, Comi R, Fumagalli D, *et al.* Predictive factors in *in-vitro* maturation in unstimulated women with normal ovaries. *Reprod Biomed Online* 2009;18:251–61.
13. Chian RC, Gülekli B, Buckett WM, Tan SL. Priming with human chorionic gonadotropin before retrieval of immature oocytes in women with infertility due to the polycystic ovary syndrome. *N Engl J Med* 1999;341:1624–6. Erratum in: *N Engl J Med* 2000;342:224.
14. Gulekli B, Buckett WM, Chian RC, Child TJ, Abdul-Jalil AK, Tan SL. Randomized, controlled trial of priming with 10,000 IU versus 20,000 IU of human chorionic gonadotropin in women with polycystic ovary syndrome who are undergoing *in vitro* maturation. *Fertil Steril* 2004;82:1458–9.
15. Son WY, Chung JT, Chian RC, Herrero B, Demirtas E, Elizur S, *et al.* A 38 h interval between hCG priming and oocyte retrieval increases *in vivo* and *in vitro* oocyte maturation rate in programmed IVM cycles. *Hum Reprod* 2008;23:2010–16.
16. Mikkelsen AL, Lindenberg S. Benefit of FSH priming of women with PCOS to the *in vitro* maturation procedure and the outcome: a randomized prospective study. *Reproduction* 2001;122:587–92.
17. Lin YH, Hwang JL, Huang LW, Mu SC, Seow KM, Chung J, *et al.* Combination of FSH priming and hCG priming for *in-vitro* maturation of human oocytes. *Hum Reprod* 2003;18:1632–6.
18. Son WY, Yoon SH, Lim JH. Effect of gonadotrophin priming on *in-vitro* maturation of oocytes collected from women at risk of OHSS. *Reprod Biomed Online* 2006;13:340–8.
19. Söderström-Anttila V, Mäkinen S, Tuuri T, Suikkari AM. Favourable pregnancy results with insemination of *in vitro* matured oocytes from unstimulated patients. *Hum Reprod* 2005;20:1534–40.
20. Suikkari AM, Tulppala M, Tuuri T, Hovatta O, Barnes F. Luteal phase start of low-dose FSH priming of follicles results in an efficient recovery, maturation and fertilization of immature human oocytes. *Hum Reprod* 2000;15:747–51.
21. Child TJ, Gulekli B, Sylvestre C, Tan SL. Ultrasonographic assessment of endometrial receptivity at embryo transfer in an *in vitro* maturation of oocyte program. *Fertil Steril* 2003;79:656–8.
22. Wei Z, Cao Y, Cong L, Zhou P, Zhang Z, Li J. Effect of metformin pretreatment on pregnancy outcome of *in vitro* matured oocytes retrieved from women with polycystic ovary syndrome. *Fertil Steril* 2008;90:1149–54.
23. Cobo AC, Requena A, Neuspiller F, Aragonés M, Mercader A, Navarro J, *et al.* Maturation *in vitro* of human oocytes from unstimulated cycles: selection of the optimal day for ovum retrieval based on follicular size. *Hum Reprod* 1999;14:1864–8.
24. Lim JH, Yang SH, Xu Y, Yoon SH, Chian RC. Selection of patients for natural cycle *in vitro* fertilization combined with *in vitro* maturation of immature oocytes. *Fertil Steril* 2009;91:1050–5.
25. Child TJ, Phillips SJ, Abdul-Jalil AK, Gulekli B, Tan SL. A comparison of *in vitro* maturation and *in vitro* fertilization for women with polycystic ovaries. *Obstet Gynecol* 2002;100:665–70.

26. Buckett WM, Chian RC, Dean NL, Sylvestre C, Holzer HE, Tan SL. Pregnancy loss in pregnancies conceived after *in vitro* oocyte maturation, conventional *in vitro* fertilization, and intracytoplasmic sperm injection. *Fertil Steril* 2008;90:546–50.
27. Suikkari AM. *In-vitro* maturation: its role in fertility treatment. *Curr Opin Obstet Gynecol* 2008;20:242–8.
28. Buckett WM, Chian RC, Holzer H, Dean N, Usher R, Tan SL. Obstetric outcomes and congenital abnormalities after *in vitro* maturation, *in vitro* fertilization, and intracytoplasmic sperm injection. *Obstet Gynecol* 2007;110:885–91.
29. Söderström-Anttila V, Salokorpi T, Pihlaja M, Serenius-Sirve S, Suikkari AM. Obstetric and perinatal outcome and preliminary results of development of children born after *in vitro* maturation of oocytes. *Hum Reprod* 2006;21:1508–13.
30. Shu-Chi M, Jiann-Loung H, Yu-Hung L, Tseng-Chen S, Ming-I L, Tsu-Fuh Y. Growth and development of children conceived by *in-vitro* maturation of human oocytes. *Early Hum Dev* 2006;82:677–82.
31. Li Y, Feng HL, Cao YJ, Zheng GJ, Yang Y, Mullen S, *et al.* Confocal microscopic analysis of the spindle and chromosome configurations of human oocytes matured *in vitro. Fertil Steril* 2006;85:827–32.
32. Requena A, Bronet F, Guillén A, Agudo D, Bou C, García-Velasco JA. The impact of *in-vitro* maturation of oocytes on aneuploidy rate. *Reprod Biomed Online* 2009;18:777–83.
33. Khoueiry R, Ibala-Rhomdane S, Méry L, Blachère T, Guérin JF, Lornage J, *et al.* Dynamic CpG methylation of the *KCNQ1OT1* gene during maturation of human oocytes. *J Med Genet* 2008;45:583–8.
34. Wells D, Patrizio P. Gene expression profiling of human oocytes at different maturational stages and after *in vitro* maturation. *Am J Obstet Gynecol* 2008;198:455.e1–9.

17

Chapter 17

Acupuncture and/or herbal therapy as an alternative or complement for relief of polycystic ovary syndrome-related symptoms

Elisabet Stener-Victorin

Introduction

The theory of traditional Chinese medicine (TCM) and its clinical application has a long tradition and gynaecology is one of four major clinical sciences of TCM (the other three being internal medicine, surgery and paediatrics). Western medicine and TCM are opposites in many respects: Western medical science works from basic science and a clinical evidence-based perspective while TCM evolves from a holistic and macroscopic perspective.

Acupuncture (Latin *acus* meaning needle and *punctura* meaning puncture) is a method of treatment that dates back at least 3000 years. It is an integral part of TCM and over the past decade it has become established in Western medicine. Herbal medicine is another important part of TCM. However, owing to the mix of different herbs and the lack of studies of specific mechanism of action, it is difficult to interpret the results.

Attempts to merge Western and Chinese medical systems have not, in general, been successful and, owing to the lack of scientific documentation or poor research methodology, there is scepticism over the effects claimed for acupuncture and for various herbs and herbal formulations. One reason may be that the underlying mechanisms of acupuncture are most often described in the language of TCM and are rarely discussed in terms of biological events. However, in recent years the effect of particularly acupuncture on various conditions (pain and diseases) has been studied from a Western scientific perspective and the results show that acupuncture may have both a physiological and a psychological impact. Still, the many different styles of acupuncture practice and lack of agreement on the optimal acupuncture treatment for any particular condition may mean that some patients do not receive the best treatment. This uncertainty also makes the negative results of sham-controlled trials difficult to interpret. Unless we can be sure that both adequate acupuncture and an inactive sham were used in a particular trial, then that trial should not be interpreted as dismissing acupuncture for that condition.[1]

The use of acupuncture, herbs and herbal mixtures in the treatment of symptoms related to polycystic ovary syndrome (PCOS) has not been well investigated to date. A review of the literature reveals only a few studies, most of which are flawed by poor design and a lack of valid outcome measures and diagnostic criteria, which makes it difficult to interpret the results. This chapter's focus will be on describing possible mechanisms of action, experimental data and available clinical data of acupuncture treatment in women with PCOS. Examples of various herbs and herbal mixtures used for symptoms associated with PCOS are also briefly discussed.

Treatment of PCOS

Many women with PCOS require prolonged treatment and, owing to unclear aetiology, the treatment is most often symptom orientated. Treatment focuses on restoration of reproductive abnormalities with the aim of reducing clinical and biochemical hyperandrogenism, restoring menstrual cycles, inducing ovulation and improving reproductive outcomes. Treatment should also address metabolic disturbances, including hyperinsulinaemia, insulin resistance and obesity, which worsen many of the typical PCOS-related symptoms and affect long-term metabolic morbidity. In addition, women with PCOS appear to have poorer psychological health-related quality of life than women without PCOS[2] and symptoms of anxiety and depression are more prevalent in women with PCOS than in those without this disorder.[3–8] Eating disorders and suicidal behaviour are also overrepresented among women with PCOS.[8] Therefore, treatment focusing on improvement of psychological variables is important.

First-line therapy in PCOS is often oral contraceptives, which reduce hirsutism and acne but adversely affect glucose tolerance, coagulability and fertility.[9] Lifestyle intervention (diet or exercise alone or combined diet, behavioural and/or exercise modification) is proposed as the first-line therapy in overweight and obese women with PCOS for the treatment of metabolic disturbances.[10] There are indications that lifestyle modification may improve ovulatory function and pregnancy but further research is needed.[10]

Treatment strategies such as acupuncture, described from a Western medical perspective, may improve reproductive, metabolic and psychiatric abnormalities with no adverse effects in women with PCOS.

The physiological basis for acupuncture

Intramuscular needle insertion and stimulation cause a particular pattern of afferent activity in peripheral nerve (Aδ and C) fibres.[11] After insertion of acupuncture needles, they are stimulated by manual manipulation and/or electrical stimulation, so-called electro-acupuncture (EA), for 20–40 minutes. During EA, needles are attached to electrodes so they can pass an electrical current. It has been suggested that low-frequency EA (1–15 Hz) with repetitive muscle contraction results in activation of physiological processes similar to those resulting from physical exercise (Figure 17.1).[12]

Peripherally, stimulation of acupuncture points located in muscle tissue causes the release of a number of neuropeptides, such as substance P, calcitonin gene-related peptide (CGRP), vasoactive intestinal peptide (VIP) and nerve growth factor (NGF), from the peripheral nerve terminals into the surrounding area, resulting in increased microcirculation and glucose uptake, the latter most likely via a reflex response from muscle twitches during manual or electrical stimulation.[13]

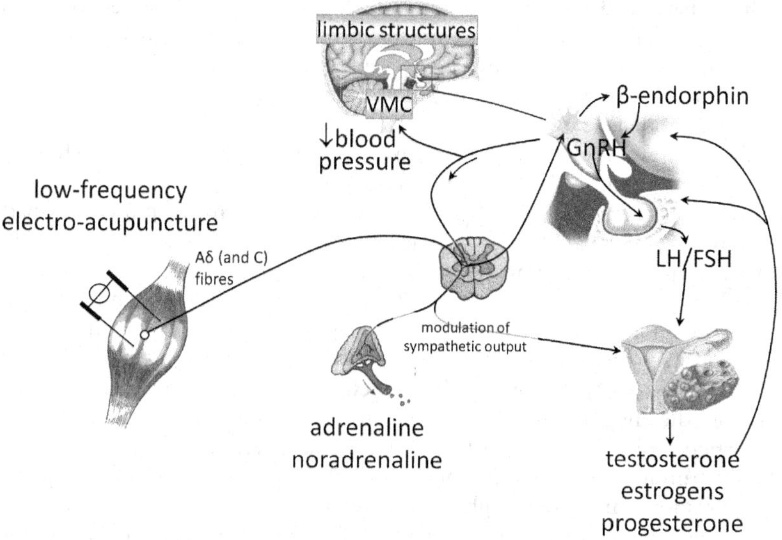

Figure 17.1 A hypothetical model of the effects of low-frequency electro-acupuncture (EA) in polycystic ovary syndrome (PCOS). Needle insertion in to the skin and muscle excite ergoreceptors and cause afferent activity in Aδ and C fibres. Needles placed and stimulated in the same somatic innervation area as the ovary decrease sympathetic nerve activity, which leads to decreased secretion and release of ovarian androgens. In parallel, the activity of higher control systems are modulated either directly or via the release of opioids, in particular β-endorphin, that induce functional changes in various organ systems. In women with PCOS, we suggest an increased sympathetic nerve activity and an increased β-endorphin production/release. Low-frequency EA decreases the central β-endorphins, providing a decreased sympathetic tone and a decreased luteinising hormone (LH) pulse frequency and amplitude that, in turn, will decrease ovarian androgen production. DHEA = dehydroepiandrosterone; DHEAS = dehydroepiandrosterone sulfate; FSH = follicle-stimulating hormone; GnRH = gonadotrophin-releasing hormone; VMC = vasomotor centre; adapted with permission from Stener-Victorin and Wu[110]

Depending on the number and location of the acupuncture needles and the intensity and type of stimulation of the needles, activation of muscle afferents also results in modulation of the transmission of signals in the spinal cord (segmental level) and in the central nervous system (CNS).[1] At segmental (spinal) level, acupuncture may modulate organs that are located in the same innervation area, for example the ovaries, as the stimulated acupuncture points via sympathetic reflexes.[14] Simultaneously, the nervous system transfer signals to the brain, which then yields the response that may affect the organ. Both segmental (spinal) and central mechanisms of acupuncture are most likely involved in the total effect of acupuncture treatment. In addition, the CNS regulates the release of hormones from the pituitary and thus acupuncture may also modulate the endocrine system.

Specifically, low-frequency EA causes the release of a large number of neuropeptides, serotonin, endogenous opioids and oxytocin in the CNS, which seem to be essential for inducing functional changes in various organ systems.[15,16] Of particular interest is β-endorphin, an endogenous opioid with high affinity for the μ-receptor.[17] The central hypothalamic β-endorphin system has a regulatory role in a variety of functions, including reproduction and autonomic function.[15,18] β-endorphin is produced and released from the hypothalamic arcuate nucleus and the nucleus of the solitary tract in the brain stem, which project to a number of sites within the brain, including to all parts of the hypothalamus.[19]

β-endorphin is a key mediator of changes in autonomic functions such as effects on the vasomotor centre (VMC) which results in a general decrease of sympathetic tone shown as regulation of blood pressure and also by decreased muscle sympathetic nerve activity (MSNA).[15,20] Hypothalamic β-endorphin also interacts with the hypothalamic–pituitary–ovarian (HPO) axis by exerting a tonic inhibitory effect on the gonadotrophin-releasing hormone (GnRH) pulse generator and on pituitary luteinising hormone (LH) release.[21,22] β-endorphin is also released into peripheral blood from the hypothalamus via the anterior pituitary,[23] a process regulated by corticotrophin-releasing factor (CRF), which is secreted from the paraventricular nucleus of the hypothalamus.[24] CRF promotes the release of β-endorphin, adrenocorticotrophic hormone (ACTH) and melanocyte-stimulating hormone into the bloodstream in equimolar amounts by stimulating the synthesis of their precursor pro-opiomelanocortin. β-endorphin in plasma is thought to be related to the hyperinsulinaemic response[25] and to stress.[26] Stress increases hypothalamic–pituitary–adrenal (HPA) axis activity and decreases reproductive functions. Thus, hormones of the HPA axis are closely related to those of the HPO axis. CRF, ACTH, β-endorphin and adrenal corticosteroids modulate the effects of stress on reproductive functions.[27]

Acupuncture may hypothetically affect the HPA axis by decreasing cortisol concentrations[28] and the HPO axis by modulating central β-endorphin production and secretion, thereby influencing the release of hypothalamic GnRH and pituitary secretion of gonadotrophin.[16,29] It may also decrease hyperinsulinaemia by decreasing high circulating β-endorphin concentrations.[30] The central and peripheral β-endorphin systems operate independently but both can be stimulated by afferent nerve activity, that is, by manual acupuncture and EA.[15]

How may acupuncture act in women with PCOS?

The primary aetiology of PCOS is not completely understood and remains a chicken-and-egg mystery, despite the high prevalence of the syndrome. While ovarian hyperandrogenaemia, which is the most consistent endocrine feature of PCOS, probably plays a key role in its aetiology,[31,32] hyperinsulinaemia and insulin resistance as well as abdominal obesity are also thought to be important aetiological factors in PCOS.[33,34] Also, neuroendocrine defects play an important role with persistently rapid LH pulsatility and increased amplitude, which further augment ovarian androgen production (Figure 17.2).[35] The role of β-endorphin as an inhibitory modulator of the GnRH pulse generator and on pituitary LH release suggests that PCOS may partly be a result of an insufficient central β-endorphin inhibition of GnRH. Evidence that β-endorphin does play a role in the pathogenesis of PCOS and in the dysregulation of GnRH/LH secretion comes from studies in which naltrexone or naloxone, μ-receptor antagonists, improved menstrual cyclicity and induced ovulation, and decreased insulin and LH levels, the LH to follicle-stimulating hormone (FSH) ratio and testosterone levels.[36–41] Because acupuncture effects may be mediated, at least partly, via modulation of β-endorphin production and secretion, which in turn affect GnRH/LH secretion, it is hypothesised that acupuncture may improve ovulatory dysfunction and thus decrease secretion of ovarian androgens in women with PCOS.

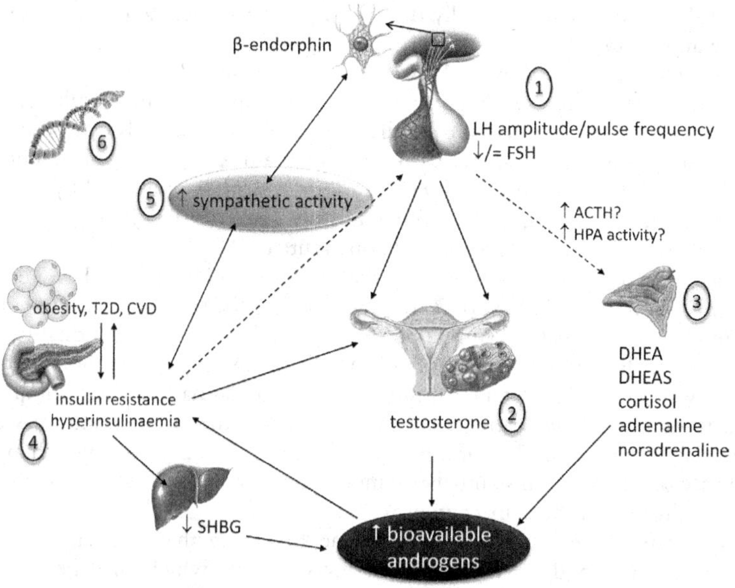

Figure 17.2 The pathogenesis of polycystic ovary syndrome (PCOS) is unclear and the heterogeneity of PCOS may well reflect multiple mechanisms. The most common theories that have been proposed to explain the pathogenesis of PCOS are as follows. (1) A neuroendocrine defect with altered β-endorphin secretion and release which together with altered feedback mechanisms lead to increased pulse frequency and amplitude of luteinising hormone (LH). (2) A defect in ovarian androgen synthesis, resulting in increased production of ovarian androgens. (3) Altered glucocorticoid metabolism, resulting in increased production of adrenal androgens. (4) Women with PCOS typically have a defect in insulin action and hyperinsulinaemia, and insulin acts synergistically with LH to enhance the androgen production of the theca cells. Insulin also acts on the liver to inhibit the production of sex hormone-binding globulin (SHBG). A reduction in SHBG leads to an increase in the biologically available free testosterone. (5) Women with PCOS have increased sympathetic nerve activity which may directly or indirectly contribute to increased androgen secretion. (6) There is a suggested genetic component in PCOS. ACTH = adrenocorticotrophic hormone; CVD = cardiovascular disease; DHEA = dehydroepiandrosterone; DHEAS = dehydroepiandrosterone sulfate; FSH = follicle-stimulating hormone; HPA = hypothalamic–pituitary–adrenal; T2D = type 2 diabetes; adapted with permission from Stener-Victorin *et al.*[111]

The finding of elevated circulating β-endorphin levels in women with PCOS[42] suggest that a dysregulated peripheral opioid system may play a role in the pathophysiology of insulin resistance and compensatory hyperinsulinaemia in PCOS. Opioids can stimulate the production of insulin by the pancreas[43] and inhibit the clearance of insulin by the liver,[39] thereby contributing to the hyperinsulinaemia often observed in PCOS. Several studies have shown that inhibition of the opioid tone with naltrexone or naloxone results in a reduction of hyperinsulinaemia in women with PCOS,[37–39] probably owing to an increased rate of insulin clearance or an increased sensitivity to insulin in target tissues.[38,39] Interestingly, low-frequency EA has been shown to decrease high circulating β-endorphin concentrations in women with PCOS and may hypothetically decrease hyperinsulinaemia and increase insulin clearance and/or insulin sensitivity.[30,44]

Many factors associated with PCOS, such as disturbed central and peripheral β-endorphin release, hyperandrogenaemia, hyperinsulinaemia and insulin resistance, as well as abdominal obesity and cardiovascular disease, are also associated with increased activity in the sympathetic nervous system.[45–49] The involvement of the sympathetic nervous system in PCOS pathology is further supported by the greater density of catecholaminergic nerve fibres in polycystic ovaries (PCO).[50,51] Increased ovarian sympathetic nerve activity might contribute to PCOS by stimulating androgen secretion.[52] It has been demonstrated that women with PCOS have enhanced ovarian NGF production.[53] NGF is a strong marker for sympathetic nerve activity. These results suggest that overproduction of ovarian NGF is a component of PCO morphology in humans. In a transgenic mouse model overexpressing NGF in the ovaries, it was found that that a persistent elevation in plasma LH levels is required for the morphological abnormalities to appear.[53] Taken together, these results may explain why ovarian wedge resection or laparoscopic laser cauterisation,[54] which probably temporarily disrupt ovarian sympathetic innervation, increase ovulatory function and decrease androgen synthesis in women with PCOS.

It has recently been demonstrated for the first time that women with PCOS have high activity in the sympathetic nervous system, which may be relevant to the pathophysiology of the syndrome.[55] Interestingly, testosterone was the strongest independent factor explaining high sympathetic nerve activity in women with PCOS. As the degree of androgen concentration can reflect the severity of PCOS, the relationship between MSNA and testosterone concentration indicates that the degree of sympatho-excitation is related to the degree of PCOS severity. The augmented sympathetic activity in PCOS may contribute to the vascular risk factors associated with the condition and therapies aimed at reducing sympathetic activity in this condition need to be studied.

Figure 17.1 illustrates the hypothesis of how acupuncture and specifically low-frequency EA may improve PCOS-related symptoms via modulation of endogenous regulatory systems, including the sympathetic nervous, the metabolic, the endocrine and the neuroendocrine systems.[15,16]

In the treatment of women with PCOS according to Western medical acupuncture, the needles are placed in the abdominal muscles and in the muscles below the knee in somatic segments according to the innervation of the ovaries (Th12-L2, S2-S4).[56] Additionally, points are selected bilaterally, extra-segmental to the ovaries, in muscles of the arm below the elbow to strengthen and lengthen the effect on the central nervous systems.[57,58] According to this hypothesis, classical acupuncture points are not the only places where the nervous system can be stimulated. However, acupuncture points are well described with respect to their anatomical location and innervations and they are thus often used in research. Classical acupuncture points are not specific, and needling of non-acupuncture points in the same segmental innervations most likely causes similar effects.

Evidence for the use of acupuncture in PCOS

Effects on ovulation

The effects of acupuncture on ovulatory dysfunction in women with PCOS have only been evaluated in case–control studies (Table 17.1).

Table 17.1 Acupuncture trials on ovulatory dysfunction in women with polycystic ovary syndrome (PCOS) and/or in women with undefined menstrual disturbances

Study	Design	Sample	Intervention	Main outcome measures	Results
Chen and Yu (1991)[44]	Case–control	11 women: 9 PCOS, 1 hypogonadotrophic amenorrhoea, 1 oligomenorrhoea	LF (4–5 Hz) EA, 30 minutes per treatment, 3 consecutive days over 13 cycles; approximately 39 treatments	Ovulation induction and plasma β-endorphin	Ovulation was induced in 6 of 13 cycles; plasma β-endorphin decreased after treatment
Gerhard and Postneek (1992)[59]	Two groups, no randomisation	45 women: 27 oligomenorrhoea, 18 luteal phase insufficiency; results were compared with those of 45 women receiving hormone treatment	Auricular acupuncture, 1 treatment per week over 3 months versus hormone treatment; approximately 12–14 treatments	Ovulation induction and pregnancy	Auricular acupuncture: 22 pregnancies – 11 after acupuncture, 4 spontaneous and 7 after additional hormone stimulation Hormone treatment: 20 pregnancies – 5 spontaneous and 15 in response to therapy
Mo *et al.* (1993)[60]	Uncontrolled	34 women with ovulatory dysfunction	Manual acupuncture, 20–30 minutes per treatment, 3 times per week over 3 months; approximately 30 treatments	Ovulation induction and endocrine measures	Ovulation was induced in 12 (35%). Modulation of endocrine measures
Stener-Victorin *et al.* (2000)[30]	Uncontrolled	24 women with PCOS	LF (2 Hz) EA, 30 minutes per treatment, 2 times per week for 2 weeks and thereafter once a week; 14 treatments	Ovulation induction and endocrine measures	Nine women (38%) experienced repeated ovulation or became pregnant; EA decreased the LH : FSH ratio, testosterone and β-endorphin concentrations 3 months after the last treatment
Stener-Victorin *et al.* (2009)[82]	RCT	84 women with PCOS	Group 1: LF (2 Hz) EA, 30 minutes per treatment, 2 times per week for 2 weeks and thereafter once a week; 14 treatments Group 2: physical exercise Group 3: untreated control group	MSNA	LF EA and physical exercise decreased MSNA compared with the untreated control group. LF EA reduced sagittal diameter, while physical exercise reduced body weight and BMI as compared with the untreated control group. Sagittal diameter was related to MSNA burst frequency in the EA group

BMI = body mass index; EA = electro-acupuncture; FSH = follicle-stimulating hormone; LF = low-frequency; LH = luteinising hormone; MSNA = muscle sympathetic nerve activity; RCT = randomised controlled trial

In one study, 11 anovulatory women (nine with PCOS) received low-frequency EA (3 days per cycle, over 13 cycles) to induce ovulation.[44] Ovulation was induced in six of the 13 menstrual cycles. EA had no effect in women with regular cycles. In the anovulatory women, high plasma β-endorphin levels and low hand skin temperature, indicating increased sympathetic nervous activity, were improved by EA, which probably reflected inhibition of the sympathetic nervous system.

Auricular acupuncture, once a week over 3 months, given to 45 infertile women with hormonal disturbances was compared with hormone treatment in 45 women in a non-randomised trial.[59] Auricular acupuncture yielded pregnancy rates equivalent to those induced by hormone treatment but with fewer adverse effects and miscarriages.

In another study, 12 of 34 women with undefined ovulatory dysfunction treated with manual acupuncture (average 30 treatments) had marked improvements in menstruation and biphasic basal body temperature for more than two cycles or became pregnant.[60] Regulatory effects on LH, FSH and estradiol (E_2) were shown, indicating an influence on the HPO axis.

In an uncontrolled trial, the effects of 14 low-frequency EA treatments on endocrinological and neuroendocrinological parameters and anovulation in 24 anovulatory women with PCOS were evaluated.[30] In nine women (38%), EA increased ovulation. The mean monthly rate of ovulation per woman increased from 0.15 before EA to 0.66 during and afterwards ($P=0.004$). Three months after the last treatment, the LH : FSH ratio and testosterone concentrations were significantly decreased.

To prevent the exacerbation of ovarian hyperstimulation syndrome (OHSS) caused by the combined use of human menopausal (hMG) and human chorionic gonadotrophin (hCG), acupuncture rather than hCG was given after hMG treatment. One single acupuncture treatment after hMG treatment induced ovulation in infertile women as effectively as the combination of hMG and hCG.[61] Importantly, acupuncture had the advantage of reducing the occurrence of OHSS.

Experimental studies support clinical findings of an effect of acupuncture on the HPO axis. Female rats continuously exposed to 5α-dihydrostestosterone (DHT) from puberty displayed reproductive and metabolic features of PCOS.[62] This DHT-induced PCOS disrupted oestrous cyclicity and caused PCO morphology and an increased number of hypothalamic cells expressing GnRH, most likely mediated by androgen receptor (AR) activation. Repeated low-frequency EA (3 days per week over 4–5 weeks) and physical exercise improved ovarian morphology, as reflected in a higher proportion of healthy antral follicles and a thinner theca interna cell layer than in untreated PCOS rats.[63]

Low-frequency EA in rats given 5 days per week over 4–5 weeks (a higher intensity than in previous studies) normalised oestrous cyclicity and restored GnRH and AR protein expression.[64]

These results may help explain the beneficial neuroendocrine effects of low-frequency EA in women with PCOS. It also indicates that more intensive treatment results in more pronounced effects.

Effects on metabolic abnormalities

There are no clinical trials in women with PCOS evaluating the effects of acupuncture on metabolic abnormalities. However, low-frequency EA with repetitive muscle contractions activate physiological processes similar to those resulting from physical exercise, thus hypothetically it may influence metabolic variables.

In female rats with DHT-induced PCOS,[62] both repeated low-frequency EA treatment and 4–5 weeks of voluntary exercise improve insulin sensitivity.[65] Furthermore, the DHT-induced PCOS resulted in increased production of leptin and interleukin 6 (IL-6) and decreased expression of uncoupling protein 2 (*UCP2*) in mesenteric adipose tissue compared with controls. Low-frequency EA restored the production of leptin and UCP2 while exercise normalised adipose tissue leptin and IL-6 production in PCOS rats. Thus, both EA and exercise ameliorate insulin resistance in rats with PCOS. This effect may involve regulation of adipose tissue metabolism and production since EA and exercise each partly restore divergent adipose tissue gene expression associated with insulin resistance, obesity and inflammation. In contrast to exercise, EA improves insulin sensitivity and modulates adipose tissue gene expression without influencing adipose tissue mass and cellularity.

Muscle contraction during low-frequency EA may hypothetically stimulate glucose uptake via an insulin-independent pathway and may, at least partly, be mediated via similar signalling pathways in skeletal muscle as after chronic exercise.[66,67] Low-frequency EA given 5 days per week over 4–5 weeks has been found to increase insulin sensitivity dramatically and to increase expression of glucose transporter 4 (*GLUT4*) in the soleus muscle of rats with DHT-induced PCOS compared with those without treatment.[68] These results indicate that low-frequency EA treatment induces both systemic and local effects involving intracellular insulin signalling pathways in muscle which may account for improved insulin sensitivity.

In other studies not related to PCOS, daily low-frequency EA treatment over 4 weeks reduced food intake and weight, possibly by increasing leptin levels, in both rats[69] and humans.[70–73] Low-frequency EA in rats also stimulated glucose transport in skeletal muscle independently of insulin and increased the insulin sensitivity of glucose transport.[74–76] Acute effects of low-frequency EA in rats with a prednisolone-induced insulin-resistant state demonstrated improved glucose tolerance and insulin sensitivity and decreased free fatty acids.[77] Skeletal muscle expression of insulin receptor substrate 1 and *GLUT4* was also increased.[77]

In 2009, it was demonstrated that the responsiveness to EA of plasma concentrations of insulin in streptozotocin-induced diabetic rats is mediated via mechanisms that involve somatic afferent nerves.[13] Peripheral β-endorphin secretion may also be involved in the regulation of glucose concentrations.[78–80]

A systematic review of 31 randomised controlled trials (RCTs) of acupuncture for obesity concluded that acupuncture may be an effective treatment for obesity[81] but there is a need for well-conducted RCT evaluating the efficacy of acupuncture in the treatment of obesity.

Effects on mental health

There are no clinical trials in women with PCOS evaluating the effects of acupuncture on symptoms of anxiety and depression or on health-related quality of life.

Acupuncture has been used as an alternative treatment for depressive disorders but its effectiveness and safety have not been well defined. In a systematic review with meta-analysis published in 2010, acupuncture as monotherapy was found to be comparable with antidepressants alone in reducing symptom severity of major depressive disorder but it did not differ from sham acupuncture.[82] There was insufficient evidence to demonstrate that acupuncture in combination with antidepressants results in better outcomes than antidepressants alone in the treatment of major depressive disorder. The incidence of adverse events in acupuncture intervention was significantly lower than with antidepressants. The review concluded that acupuncture is safe and effective in treating major depressive disorder and post-stroke depression, and could be considered an alternative option for the two disorders.

This is an important field to explore further with a focus on women with PCOS.

Effects on the sympathetic nervous system

In 2009, it was demonstrated for the first time that low-frequency EA and physical exercise lower high sympathetic nerve activity in women with PCOS.[83] Thus, treatment with low-frequency EA or physical exercise with the aim of reducing MSNA may be of importance for women with PCOS.

In an estradiol valerate (EV)-induced rat PCO model, transection of the superior ovarian nerve reduced the steroid response, increased β_2-adrenoceptor expression to more normal levels and restored oestrus cyclicity and ovulation.[84] Also, blockade of endogenous NGF action restored the EV-induced changes in ovarian morphology and expression of the sympathetic markers α_1- and β_2-adrenoceptors, p75 neurotrophin receptor $p75^{NTR}$, NGF-tyrosine kinase receptor (TrkA) and tyrosine hydroxylase. These data confirm that there is a close interaction between NGF and the sympathetic nervous system in the pathogenesis of steroid-induced PCO rats.[85]

In line with these observations, repeated low-frequency EA was found to reduce high ovarian concentrations of NGF,[86,87] CRF[88] and endothelin 1[86] in EV-induced PCO rats. It also modulated hypothalamic β-endorphin concentrations and immune function in the same rat PCO model.[89]

To investigate the hypothesis that repeated low-frequency EA treatments and physical exercise modulate sympathetic nerve activity in rats with EV-induced PCO, we studied the expression of mRNA and protein of α_{1a}-, α_{1b}-, α_{1d}- and β_2-adrenoceptors, the NGF receptor $p75^{NTR}$ and immunohistochemical expression of TH. Four weeks of physical exercise almost normalised ovarian morphology,[90] and both EA and exercise normalised the expression of NGF, NGF receptors, and α_1- and α_2-adrenoceptors.[85,90]

Low-frequency EA has been found to increase ovarian blood flow in rats. The needles were placed in the abdominal and hind limb muscles, which have the same somatic innervation as the ovaries and uterus.[91–93] The response was mediated via ovarian sympathetic nerves as a reflex response and the reflexes was controlled by supraspinal pathways, that is, the central nervous system.[91,93]

In mesenteric adipose tissue, expression of beta-3 adrenergic receptor (*ADRB3*), nerve growth factor (*NGF*) and neuropeptide Y (*NPY*) mRNA was higher in untreated DHT-induced PCOS rats than in controls. Low-frequency EA and exercise downregulated mRNA expression of *NGF* and *NPY*, and EA also downregulated expression of *ADRB3*, compared with untreated rats with DHT-induced PCOS. EA and exercise improved ovarian morphology, as reflected in a higher proportion of healthy antral follicles and a thinner theca interna cell layer than in untreated PCOS rats. These findings support the theory that increased sympathetic nerve activity contributes to the development and maintenance of PCOS and that the effects of EA and exercise may be mediated by modulation of sympathetic outflow to the adipose tissue and ovaries.

Continuing or completed RCTs on the effects of acupuncture in PCOS-related symptoms

There are currently four relevant RCTs in the trial registries:

- 'An RCT evaluating acupuncture versus non-penetrating sham acupuncture with primary outcome menstruation at the conclusion of the treatment period and secondary outcome changes in LH/FSH ratio and androgens'; www.anzctr.org.au: ACTRN12609000073202 (open for recruitment); target sample size 99
- 'Acupuncture for polycystic ovarian syndrome. An RCT evaluating acupuncture versus sham acupuncture with primary outcome ovulation and secondary outcome changes in LH and FSH'; clinicaltrials.gov: NCT00602940 (estimated study completion date: June 2010); target sample size 78
- 'Polycystic ovary syndrome (PCOS) – effect of physical exercise and electro-acupuncture'; clinicaltrials.gov: NCT00484705 (completed, $n=84$); an RCT evaluating low-frequency EA versus physical exercise versus an untreated control group; the primary outcomes were changes in androgen concentrations and menstrual pattern and secondary outcomes were changes in sympathetic nerve activity, insulin sensitivity, adipose tissue-related variables, coagulation factors, ovarian morphology and uterus peristalsis; published in 2009[83]
- 'Low-frequency acupuncture and gonadotrophin-releasing hormone pulse generator and stress axis in polycystic ovary syndrome'; clinicaltrials.gov: NCT00921492 (estimated study completion date: December 2010); an RCT evaluating acupuncture versus meeting a therapist to control for the increased amount of attention; target sample size 28.

Herbal therapy for the relief of PCOS-related symptoms

The list of herbs and herbal mixtures used for the relief of PCOS-related symptoms is extensive but few of these have been evaluated in women with PCOS. The herbs or herbal mixtures reviewed below are those commonly prescribed and recommended by TCM doctors and people working with complementary and alternative medicine.

Herbs for ovulation induction

Vitex agnus-castus

The extract of the whole fruit of the chaste tree plant (*Vitex agnus-castus*, also called chasteberry or monk's pepper) is considered to modulate endocrine and reproductive systems. In a trial in women with undefined irregular menstruation, *Vitex agnus-castus* restored menstrual cycles and increased pregnancy rates compared with the placebo-controlled group.[94] The effect of this plant has not been tested in women with PCOS.

White peony

Paeonia is derived from the dried roots of *Paeonia lactiflora* Pall. and there are indications that it decreases testosterone concentrations. Unkei-to, which contains paeonia, has been shown to stimulate estrogen and progesterone secretion in human granulosa cells, indicating that it might affect steroidogenesis and the ovulatory process.[95] In an uncontrolled trial, 34 women with PCOS were treated with a herbal mixture containing *Glycyrrhiza glabra* and *Paeonia lactiflora* called Shakuyaku-Kanzo-To (TJ-68) over 24 weeks.[96,97] TJ-68 decreased serum androgens by 35% in women who become pregnant without any adverse effects.

Sairei-to

Sairei-to is a Chinese herbal mixture containing twelve active ingredients (Saiko, Kanzou and Keihi, etc.) that has been shown to decrease androgens and induce ovulation in an uncontrolled trial in women with PCOS.[98]

Mentha spicata Labiatae

Mentha is a member of the Labiatae family and *Mentha spicata* Labiatae (spearmint) is one of two forms. Spearmint is common in eastern Asian and Indian diets. The effect of spearmint teas on hirsute women (12 with PCOS and nine with idiopathic hirsutism) has been evaluated in an uncontrolled trial, which found a significant decrease in free testosterone and LH concentrations.[99] Whether it reduced hirsutism or not was not evaluated.

Herbs for metabolic abnormalities

Berberine

Berberine is found in plants such as *Berberis*, goldenseal (*Hydrastis canadensis*) and *Coptis chinensis*. Clinical studies demonstrate that berberine has a hypoglycaemic effect in people with type 2 diabetes[100] and modulates lipid metabolism.[101] In an experimental model of dexamethasone-induced insulin resistance and increased thecal cell androgen synthesis, berberine decreased the degree of insulin resistance and androgen synthesis, thus indicating that it may improve PCOS-related symptoms.[102]

Cinnamon

Cinnamon is a spice derived from the bark of a small evergreen tree native to Sri Lanka. It has been used as a supplement in people with type 2 diabetes and studies have demonstrated a decrease in blood glucose.[103,104] In a small study, the effect of cinnamon was evaluated in women with PCOS and it was found to improve glucose response and insulin sensitivity.[103,104]

Labisia pumila

Labisia pumila is a Malaysian herb derived from a herbaceous plant with creeping stems. It has been used as a herbal medicine for various purposes, including treating menstrual irregularities. In experimental trial in rats, *Labisia pumila* reduced body weight, most likely via regulation of leptin secretion.[105] In another study in rats with DHT-induced PCOS, it improved insulin sensitivity and lipid profile.[106] The effect of this plant has not been tested in women with PCOS.

The list of herbs and herbal mixtures discussed in this chapter is not complete. They are examples of herbs used for the relief of symptoms in women with PCOS. However, many herbs are used on a speculative basis and little information and attention is given regarding safety and potential interactions with conventional pharmacological treatment.

Future perspectives

The effects of acupuncture depend on the stimulation and number of needles, the frequency, duration and number of treatments, and also environmental and psychological factors. With this in mind, standardisation and fixed study protocols, in which all patients receive the same treatment, will increase the validity of acupuncture studies. Fixed study protocols may bias the outcome but we believe that they are necessary.

More precise standards for reporting RCTs of acupuncture are needed to overcome difficulties in analysis and interpretation. The revised recommendations for improving the quality of reports of parallel-group randomised trials (CONSORT) statement addresses general difficulties.[107] However, certain aspects are insufficiently covered. The Standards for Reporting Interventions in Clinical Trials of Acupuncture (STRICTA) group have made recommendations to improve reporting of interventions in controlled trials of acupuncture. The STRICTA checklist should be used in conjunction with CONSORT to improve critical appraisal, analysis and replication of trials.[108]

There is a great need to evaluate further whether herbs and various herbal mixtures may be an alternative or complement in the treatment of PCOS-related symptoms. RCTs should include safety issues, and mechanistic studies are needed to search for the active compound in each source.

Conclusion

Despite the lack of a large body of evidence, we should not ignore the fact that many women with PCOS use acupuncture and various herbs and herbal mixtures. This alone is a compelling reason to investigate these methods. In the hands of competent registered health practitioners, acupuncture is safe.[109] Clinical and experimental evidence shows that acupuncture can be a suitable alternative or complement to pharmacological induction of ovulation in women with PCOS and may also relieve other symptoms, without adverse effects. Clearly, acupuncture and certain herbs modulate endogenous regulatory systems, including the sympathetic nervous system, the endocrine system and the neuroendocrine system. However, RCTs are needed to evaluate acupuncture and herbal mixtures in women with PCOS.

References

1. White A, Cummings M, Barlas P, Cardini F, Filshie J, Foster NE, *et al.* Defining an adequate dose of acupuncture using a neurophysiological approach – a narrative review of the literature. *Acupunct Med* 2008;26:111–20.
2. Coffey S, Bano G, Mason HD. Health-related quality of life in women with polycystic ovary syndrome: a comparison with the general population using the Polycystic Ovary Syndrome Questionnaire (PCOSQ) and the Short Form-36 (SF-36). *Gynecol Endocrinol* 2006;22:80–6.
3. Kerchner A, Lester W, Stuart SP, Dokras A. Risk of depression and other mental health disorders in women with polycystic ovary syndrome: a longitudinal study. *Fertil Steril* 2009;91:207–12.
4. Hollinrake E, Abreu A, Maifeld M, Van Voorhis BJ, Dokras A. Increased risk of depressive disorders in women with polycystic ovary syndrome. *Fertil Steril* 2007;87:1369–76.
5. Elsenbruch S, Benson S, Hahn S, Tan S, Mann K, Pleger K, *et al.* Determinants of emotional distress in women with polycystic ovary syndrome. *Hum Reprod* 2006;21:1092–9.
6. Himelein MJ, Thatcher SS. Depression and body image among women with polycystic ovary syndrome. *J Health Psychol* 2006;11:613–25.
7. Benson S, Arck PC, Tan S, Hahn S, Mann K, Rifaie N, *et al.* Disturbed stress responses in women with polycystic ovary syndrome. *Psychoneuroendocrinology* 2009;34:727–35.

8. Månsson M, Holte J, Landin-Wilhelmsen K, Dahlgren E, Johansson A, Landén M. Women with polycystic ovary syndrome are often depressed or anxious – a case control study. *Psychoneuroendocrinology* 2008;33:1132–8.
9. Lanham MS, Lebovic DI, Domino SE. Contemporary medical therapy for polycystic ovary syndrome. *Int J Gynaecol Obstet* 2006;95:236–41.
10. Moran LJ, Pasquali R, Teede HJ, Hoeger KM, Norman RJ. Treatment of obesity in polycystic ovary syndrome: a position statement of the Androgen Excess and Polycystic Ovary Syndrome Society. *Fertil Steril* 2009;92:1966–82.
11. Kagitani F, Uchida S, Hotta H, Aikawa Y. Manual acupuncture needle stimulation of the rat hindlimb activates groups I, II, III and IV single afferent nerve fibers in the dorsal spinal roots. *Jpn J Physiol* 2005;55:149–55.
12. Kaufman MP, Waldrop TG, Rybycki KJ, Ordway GA, Mitchell JH. Effects of static and rythmic twitch contractions on the discharge of group III and IV muscle afferents. *Cardiovasc Res* 1984;18:663–8.
13. Higashimura Y, Shimoju R, Maruyama H, Kurosawa M. Electro-acupuncture improves responsiveness to insulin via excitation of somatic afferent fibers in diabetic rats. *Auton Neurosci* 2009;150:100–3.
14. Sato A, Sato Y, Schmidt RF. *The Impact of Somatosensory Input on Autonomic Functions*. Heidelberg: Springer-Verlag; 1997.
15. Andersson S, Lundeberg T. Acupuncture – from empiricism to science: functional background to acupuncture effects in pain and disease. *Med Hypotheses* 1995;45:271–81.
16. Stener-Victorin E, Jedel E, Manneras L. Acupuncture in polycystic ovary syndrome: current experimental and clinical evidence. *J Neuroendocrinol* 2008;20:290–8.
17. Basbaum AI, Fields HL. Endogenous pain control systems: brain-stem spinal pathways and endorphin circuitry. *Annu Rev Neurosci* 1984;7:309–38.
18. Eyvazzadeh AD, Pennington KP, Pop-Busui R, Sowers M, Zubieta JK, Smith YR. The role of the endogenous opioid system in polycystic ovary syndrome. *Fertil Steril* 2009;92:1–12.
19. Ferin M, Van Vugt D, Wardlaw S. The hypothalamic control of the menstrual cycle and the role of endogenous opioid peptides. *Recent Prog Horm Res* 1984;40:441–85.
20. Yao T, Andersson S, Thoren P. Long-lasting cardiovascular depression induced by acupuncture-like stimulation of the sciatic nerve in unanaesthetized spontaneously hypertensive rats. *Brain Res* 1982;240:77–85.
21. Genazzani AR, Genazzani AD, Volpogni C, Pianazzi F, Li GA, Surico N, *et al.* Opioid control of gonadotrophin secretion in humans. *Hum Reprod* 1993;8 Suppl 2:151–3.
22. Jenkins PJ, Grossman A. The control of the gonadotrophin releasing hormone pulse generator in relation to opioid and nutritional cues. *Hum Reprod* 1993;8 Suppl 2:154–61.
23. Crine P, Gianoulakis C, Seidah NG. Biosynthesis of beta-endorphin from beta-lipotropin and a larger molecular weight precursor in rat pars intermedia. *Proc Natl Acad Sci U S A* 1978;75:4719–23.
24. Chan JS, Lu CL, Seidah NG, Chretien M. Corticotropin releasing factor (CRF): effects on the release of pro-opiomelanocortin (POMC)-related peptides by human anterior pituitary cells *in vitro*. *Endocrinology* 1982;111:1388–90.
25. Carmina E, Ditkoff EC, Malizia G, Vijod AG, Janni A, Lobo RA. Increased circulating levels of immunoreactive beta-endorphin in polycystic ovary syndrome is not caused by increased pituitary secretion. *Am J Obstet Gynecol* 1992;167:1819–24.
26. Lobo RA, Granger LR, Paul WL, Goebelsmann U, Mishell DR Jr. Psychological stress and increases in urinary norepinephrine metabolites, platelet serotonin, and adrenal androgens in women with polycystic ovary syndrome. *Am J Obstet Gynecol* 1983;145:496–503.
27. Rivier C, Rivest S. Effects of stress on the activity of hypothalamic–pituitary–gonadal axis: peripheral and central mechanisms. *Biol Reprod* 1991;45:523–32.
28. Harbach H, Moll B, Boedeker RH, Vigelius-Rauch U, Otto H, Muehling J, *et al.* Minimal immunoreactive plasma beta-endorphin and decrease of cortisol at standard analgesia or different acupuncture techniques. *Eur J Anaesthesiol* 2007;24:370–6.
29. Liang F, Koya D. Acupuncture: is it effective for treatment of insulin resistance? *Diabetes Obes Metab* 2010;12:555–69.

30. Stener-Victorin E, Waldenström U, Tägnfors U, Lundeberg T, Lindstedt G, Janson PO. Effects of electro-acupuncture on anovulation in women with polycystic ovary syndrome. *Acta Obstet Gynecol Scand* 2000;79:180–8.
31. Gilling-Smith C, Story H, Rogers V, Franks S. Evidence for a primary abnormality of thecal cell steroidogenesis in the polycystic ovary syndrome. *Clin Endocrinol (Oxf)* 1997;47:93–9.
32. Abbott DH, Dumesic DA, Franks S. Developmental origin of polycystic ovary syndrome – a hypothesis. *J Endocrinol* 2002;174:1–5.
33. Dunaif A, Thomas A. Current concepts in the polycystic ovary syndrome. *Annu Rev Med* 2001;52:401–19.
34. Barber TM, McCarthy MI, Wass JA, Franks S. Obesity and polycystic ovary syndrome. *Clin Endocrinol (Oxf)* 2006;65:137–45.
35. Blank SK, McCartney CR, Helm KD, Marshall JC. Neuroendocrine effects of androgens in adult polycystic ovary syndrome and female puberty. *Semin Reprod Med* 2007;25:352–9.
36. Ahmed MI, Duleba AJ, El Shahat O, Ibrahim ME, Salem A. Naltrexone treatment in clomiphene resistant women with polycystic ovary syndrome. *Hum Reprod* 2008;23:2564–9.
37. Fruzzetti F, Bersi C, Parrini D, Ricci C, Genazzani AR. Effect of long-term naltrexone treatment on endocrine profile, clinical features, and insulin sensitivity in obese women with polycystic ovary syndrome. *Fertil Steril* 2002;77:936–44.
38. Hadziomerovic D, Rabenbauer B, Wildt L. Normalization of hyperinsulinemia by chronic opioid receptor blockade in hyperandrogenemic women. *Fertil Steril* 2006;86:651–7.
39. Fulghesu AM, Ciampelli M, Guido M, Murgia F, Caruso A, Mancuso S, *et al.* Role of opioid tone in the pathophysiology of hyperinsulinemia and insulin resistance in polycystic ovarian disease. *Metabolism* 1998;47:158–62.
40. Lanzone A, Fulghesu AM, Cucinelli F, Ciampelli M, Caruso A, Mancuso S. Evidence of a distinct derangement of opioid tone in hyperinsulinemic patients with polycystic ovarian syndrome: relationship with insulin and luteinizing hormone secretion. *J Clin Endocrinol Metab* 1995;80:3501–6.
41. Ciampelli M, Fulghesu AM, Guido M, Murgia F, Muzj G, Belosi C, *et al.* Opioid blockade effect on insulin beta-cells secretory patterns in polycystic ovary syndrome. Oral glucose load versus intravenous glucagon bolus. *Horm Res* 1998;49:263–8.
42. Wortsman J, Wehrenberg WB, Gavin JR 3rd, Allen JP. Elevated levels of plasma beta-endorphin and gamma 3-melanocyte stimulating hormone in the polycystic ovary syndrome. *Obstet Gynecol* 1984;63:630–4.
43. Bruni JF, Watkins WB, Yen SS. beta-Endorphin in the human pancreas. *J Clin Endocrinol Metab* 1979;49:649–51.
44. Chen BY, Yu J. Relationship between blood radioimmunoreactive beta-endorphin and hand skin temperature during the electro-acupuncture induction of ovulation. *Acupunct Electrother Res* 1991;16:1–5.
45. Fagius J. Sympathetic nerve activity in metabolic control – some basic concepts. *Acta Physiol Scand* 2003;177:337–43.
46. Ojeda S, Lara H. *Role of the Sympathetic Nervous System in the Regulation of Ovarian Function.* Berlin: Springer-Verlag; 1989.
47. Sir-Petermann T, Maliqueo M, Angel B, Lara HE, Pérez-Bravo F, Recabarren SE. Maternal serum androgens in pregnant women with polycystic ovarian syndrome: possible implications in prenatal androgenization. *Hum Reprod* 2002;17:2573–9.
48. Reaven GM, Lithell H, Landsberg L. Hypertension and associated metabolic abnormalities – the role of insulin resistance and the sympathoadrenal system. *N Engl J Med* 1996;334:374–81.
49. Dissen GA, Garcia-Rudaz C, Ojeda SR. Role of neurotrophic factors in early ovarian development. *Semin Reprod Med* 2009;27:24–31.
50. Semenova II. Adrenergic innervation of the ovaries in Stein-Leventhal syndrome. *Vestn Akad Med Nauk SSSR* 1969;24:58–62.
51. Heider U, Pedal I, Spanel-Borowski K. Increase in nerve fibers and loss of mast cells in polycystic and postmenopausal ovaries. *Fertil Steril* 2001;75:1141–7.
52. Greiner M, Paredes A, Araya V, Lara HE. Role of stress and sympathetic innervation in the development of polycystic ovary syndrome. *Endocrine* 2005;28:319–24.

53. Dissen GA, Garcia-Rudaz C, Paredes A, Mayer C, Mayerhofer A, Ojeda SR. Excessive ovarian production of nerve growth factor facilitates development of cystic ovarian morphology in mice and is a feature of polycystic ovarian syndrome in humans. *Endocrinology* 2009;150:2906–14.
54. Balen A. Surgical treatment of polycystic ovary syndrome. *Best Pract Res Clin Endocrinol Metab* 2006;20:271–80.
55. Sverrisdottir YB, Mogren T, Kataoka J, Janson PO, Stener-Victorin E. Is polycystic ovary syndrome associated with high sympathetic nerve activity and size at birth? *Am J Physiol Endocrinol Metab* 2008;294:E576–81.
56. Bonica J. *The Management of Pain*. Philadelphia, London: Lea & Febiger; 1990.
57. Thomas M, Lundberg T. Importance of modes of acupuncture in the treatment of chronic nociceptive low back pain. *Acta Anaesthesiol Scand* 1994;38:63–9.
58. Thomas M, Lundeberg T. Does acupuncture work? *Pain Clinical Updates* 1996;4:1–4.
59. Gerhard I, Postneek F. Auricular acupuncture in the treatment of female infertility. *Gynecol Endocrinol* 1992;6:171–81.
60. Mo X, Li D, Pu Y, Xi G, Le X, *et al.* Clinical studies on the mechanism for acupuncture stimulation of ovulation. *J Tradit Chin Med* 1993;13:115–19.
61. Cai X. Substitution of acupuncture for HCG in ovulation induction. *J Tradit Chin Med* 1997;17:119–21.
62. Mannerås L, Cajander S, Holmäng A, Seleskovic Z, Lystig T, Lönn M, *et al.* A new rat model exhibiting both ovarian and metabolic characteristics of polycystic ovary syndrome. *Endocrinology* 2007;148:3781–91.
63. Mannerås L, Cajander S, Lönn M, Stener-Victorin E. Acupuncture and exercise restore adipose tissue expression of sympathetic markers and improve ovarian morphology in rats with dihydrotestosterone-induced PCOS. *Am J Physiol Regul Integr Comp Physiol* 2009;296:R1124–31.
64. Feng Y, Johansson J, Shao R, Mannerås L, Fernandez-Rodriguez J, Billig H, *et al.* Hypothalamic neuroendocrine functions in rats with dihydrotestosterone-induced polycystic ovary syndrome: effects of low-frequency electro-acupuncture. *PLoS One* 2009;4:e6638.
65. Mannerås L, Jonsdottir IH, Holmäng A, Lönn M, Stener-Victorin E. Low-frequency electro-acupuncture and physical exercise improve metabolic disturbances and modulate gene expression in adipose tissue in rats with dihydrotestosterone-induced polycystic ovary syndrome. *Endocrinology* 2008;149:3559–68.
66. Goodyear LJ, Kahn BB. Exercise, glucose transport, and insulin sensitivity. *Annu Rev Med* 1998;49:235–61.
67. Deshmukh AS, Hawley JA, Zierath JR. Exercise-induced phospho-proteins in skeletal muscle. *Int J Obes (Lond)* 2008;32 Suppl 4:S18–23.
68. Johansson J, Yi F, Shao R, Lönn M, Billig H, Stener-Victorin E. Intense acupuncture normalizes insulin sensitivity, increases muscle GLUT4 content, and improves lipid profile in a rat model of polycystic ovary syndrome. *Am J Physiol Endocrinol Metab* 2010 Jul 27. [Epub ahead of print]
69. Kim SK, Lee G, Shin M, Han JB, Moon HJ, Park JH, *et al.* The association of serum leptin with the reduction of food intake and body weight during electroacupuncture in rats. *Pharmacol Biochem Behav* 2006;83:145–9.
70. Lee M, Kim J, Lim HJ, Shin BS. Effects of abdominal electroacupuncture on parameters related to obesity in obese women: a pilot study. *Compl Ther Clin Pract* 2006;12:97–100.
71. Cabioglu MT, Ergene N. Electroacupuncture therapy for weight loss reduces serum total cholesterol, triglycerides, and LDL cholesterol levels in obese women. *Am J Chin Med* 2005;33:525–33.
72. Cabioglu MT, Ergene N. Changes in levels of serum insulin, C-peptide and glucose after electroacupuncture and diet therapy in obese women. *Am J Chin Med* 2006;34:367–76.
73. Cabioglu MT, Ergene N. Changes in serum leptin and beta endorphin levels with weight loss by electroacupuncture and diet restriction in obesity treatment. *Am J Chin Med* 2006;34:1–11.
74. Holmang A, Mimura K, Lonnroth P. Involuntary leg movements affect interstitial nutrient gradients and blood flow in rat skeletal muscle. *J Appl Physiol* 2002;92:982–8.
75. Chang SL, Tsai CC, Lin JG, Hsieh CL, Lin RT, Cheng JT. Involvement of serotonin in the hypoglycemic response to 2 Hz electroacupuncture of zusanli acupoint (ST36) in rats. *Neurosci Lett* 2005;379:69–73.

76. Chang SL, Lin KJ, Lin RT, Hung PH, Lin JG, Cheng JT. Enhanced insulin sensitivity using electroacupuncture on bilateral Zusanli acupoints (ST 36) in rats. *Life Sci* 2006;79:967–71.
77. Lin RT, Tzeng CY, Lee YC, Ho WJ, Cheng JT, Lin JG, *et al.* Acute effect of electroacupuncture at the Zusanli acupoints on decreasing insulin resistance as shown by lowering plasma free fatty acid levels in steroid-background male rats. *BMC Complement Altern Med* 2009;9:26.
78. Chang SL, Lin JG, Chi TC, Liu IM, Cheng JT. An insulin-dependent hypoglycaemia induced by electroacupuncture at the Zhongwan (CV12) acupoint in diabetic rats. *Diabetologia* 1999;42:250–5.
79. Lin JG, Chang SL, Cheng JT. Release of beta-endorphin from adrenal gland to lower plasma glucose by the electroacupuncture at Zhongwan acupoint in rats. *Neurosci Lett* 2002;326:17–20.
80. Lin JG, Chen WC, Hsieh CL, Tsai CC, Cheng YW, Cheng JT, *et al.* Multiple sources of endogenous opioid peptide involved in the hypoglycemic response to 15 Hz electroacupuncture at the Zhongwan acupoint in rats. *Neurosci Lett* 2004;366:39–42.
81. Cho SH, Lee JS, Thabane L, Lee J. Acupuncture for obesity: a systematic review and meta-analysis. *Int J Obes (Lond)* 2009;33:183–96.
82. Zhang ZJ, Chen HY, Yip KC, Ng R, Wong VT. The effectiveness and safety of acupuncture therapy in depressive disorders: systematic review and meta-analysis. *J Affect Disord* 2010;124:9–21.
83. Stener-Victorin E, Jedel E, Janson PO, Sverrisdottir YB. Low-frequency electroacupuncture and physical exercise decrease high muscle sympathetic nerve activity in polycystic ovary syndrome. *Am J Physiol Regul Integr Comp Physiol* 2009;297:R387–95.
84. Barria A, Leyton V, Ojeda SR, Lara HE. Ovarian steroidal response to gonadotropins and beta-adrenergic stimulation is enhanced in polycystic ovary syndrome: role of sympathetic innervation. *Endocrinology* 1993;133:2696–703.
85. Manni L, Lundeberg T, Holmang A, Aloe L, Stener-Victorin E. Effect of electro-acupuncture on ovarian expression of alpha (1)- and beta (2)-adrenoceptors, and p75 neurotrophin receptors in rats with steroid-induced polycystic ovaries. *Reprod Biol Endocrinol* 2005;3:21.
86. Stener-Victorin E, Lundeberg T, Cajander S, Aloe L, Manni L, Waldenström U, *et al.* Steroid-induced polycystic ovaries in rats: effect of electro-acupuncture on concentrations of endothelin-1 and nerve growth factor (NGF), and expression of NGF mRNA in the ovaries, the adrenal glands, and the central nervous system. *Reprod Biol Endocrinol* 2003;1:33.
87. Stener-Victorin E, Lundeberg T, Waldenström U, Manni L, Aloe L, Gunnarsson S, *et al.* Effects of electro-acupuncture on nerve growth factor and ovarian morphology in rats with experimentally induced polycystic ovaries. *Biol Reprod* 2000;63:1497–503.
88. Stener-Victorin E, Lundeberg T, Waldenstrom U, Bileviciute-Ljungar I, Janson PO. Effects of electro-acupuncture on corticotropin-releasing factor in rats with experimentally-induced polycystic ovaries. *Neuropeptides* 2001;35:227–31.
89. Stener-Victorin E, Lindholm C. Immunity and beta-endorphin concentrations in hypothalamus and plasma in rats with steroid-induced polycystic ovaries: effect of low-frequency electroacupuncture. *Biol Reprod* 2004;70:329–33.
90. Manni L, Cajander S, Lundeberg T, Naylor AS, Aloe L, Holmäng A, *et al.* Effect of exercise on ovarian morphology and expression of nerve growth factor and alpha(1)- and beta(2)-adrenergic receptors in rats with steroid-induced polycystic ovaries. *J Neuroendocrinol* 2005;17:846–58.
91. Stener-Victorin E, Kobayashi R, Kurosawa M. Ovarian blood flow responses to electro-acupuncture stimulation at different frequencies and intensities in anaesthetized rats. *Auton Neurosci* 2003;108:50–6.
92. Stener-Victorin E, Kobayashi R, Watanabe O, Lundeberg T, Kurosawa M. Effect of electro-acupuncture stimulation of different frequencies and intensities on ovarian blood flow in anaesthetised rats with steroid-induced polycystic ovaries. *Reprod Biol Endocrinol* 2004;2:16.
93. Stener-Victorin E, Fujisawa S, Kurosawa M. Ovarian blood flow responses to electroacupuncture stimulation depend on estrous cycle and on site and frequency of stimulation in anesthetized rats. *J Appl Physiol* 2006;101:84–91.
94. Westphal LM, Polan ML, Trant AS. Double-blind, placebo-controlled study of Fertilityblend: a nutritional supplement for improving fertility in women. *Clin Exp Obstet Gynecol* 2006;33:205–8.
95. Sun WS, Imai A, Tagami K, Sugiyama M, Furui T, Tamaya T. *In vitro* stimulation of granulosa cells by a combination of different active ingredients of unkei-to. *Am J Chin Med* 2004;32:569–78.

96. Takahashi K, Kitao M. Effect of TJ-68 (shakuyaku-kanzo-to) on polycystic ovarian disease. *Int J Fertil Menopausal Stud* 1994;39:69–76.
97. Takahashi K, Yoshino K, Shirai T, Nishigaki A, Araki Y, Kitao M. Effect of a traditional herbal medicine (shakuyaku-kanzo-to) on testosterone secretion in patients with polycystic ovary syndrome detected by ultrasound. *Nippon Sanka Fujinka Gakkai Zasshi* 1988;40:789–92.
98. Sakai A, Kondo Z, Kamei K, Izumi S, Sumi K. Induction of ovulation by Sairei-to for polycystic ovary syndrome patients. *Endocr J* 1999;46:217–20.
99. Akdogan M, Tamer MN, Cüre E, Cüre MC, Köroglu BK, Delibas N. Effect of spearmint (*Mentha spicata* Labiatae) teas on androgen levels in women with hirsutism. *Phytother Res* 2007;21:444–7.
100. Stumvoll M, Goldstein BJ, van Haeften TW. Type 2 diabetes: principles of pathogenesis and therapy. *Lancet* 2005;365:1333–46.
101. Wang YX, Wang YP, Zhang H, Kong WJ, Li YH, Liu F, *et al.* Synthesis and biological evaluation of berberine analogues as novel up-regulators for both low-density-lipoprotein receptor and insulin receptor. *Bioorg Med Chem Lett* 2009;19:6004–8.
102. Gao L, Li W, Kuang HY. [Of berberine and puerarin on dexamethesone-induced insulin resistance in porcine ovarian thecal cells]. *Zhongguo Zhong Xi Yi Jie He Za Zhi* 2009;29:623–7.
103. Pham AQ, Kourlas H, Pham DQ. Cinnamon supplementation in patients with type 2 diabetes mellitus. *Pharmacotherapy* 2007;27:595–9.
104. Wang JG, Anderson RA, Graham GM 3rd, Chu MC, Sauer MV, Guarnaccia MM, *et al.* The effect of cinnamon extract on insulin resistance parameters in polycystic ovary syndrome: a pilot study. *Fertil Steril* 2007;88:240–3.
105. Fazliana M, Wan Nazaimoon WM, Gu HF, Ostenson CG. *Labisia pumila* extract regulates body weight and adipokines in ovariectomized rats. *Maturitas* 2009;62:91–97.
106. Mannerås L, Fazliana M, Wan Nazaimoon WM, Lönn M, Gu HF, Ostenson CG, *et al.* Beneficial metabolic effects of the Malaysian herb *Labisia pumila* var. alata in a rat model of polycystic ovary syndrome. *J Ethnopharmacol* 2010;127:346–51.
107. Moher D, Schulz KF, Altman D; CONSORT Group. The CONSORT Statement: revised recommendations for improving the quality of reports of parallel-group randomized trials 2001. *Explore (NY)* 2005;1:40–5.
108. Prady SL, Richmond SJ, Morton VM, Macpherson H. A systematic evaluation of the impact of STRICTA and CONSORT recommendations on quality of reporting for acupuncture trials. *PLoS One* 2008;3:e1577.
109. Vincent C. The safety of acupuncture. *BMJ* 2001;323:467–8.
110. Stener-Victorin E, Wu X. Effects and mechanisms of acupuncture in the reproductive system. *Auton Neurosci* 2010 Mar 27. [Epub ahead of print]
111. Stener-Victorin E, Jedel E, Mannerås L. Acupuncture in polycystic ovary syndrome: current experimental and clinical evidence. *J Neuroendocrinol* 2008;20:290–8.

Chapter 18

Consensus views arising from the 59th Study Group: Current Management of Polycystic Ovary Syndrome

Diagnosis/pathophysiology

1. The Rotterdam European Society of Human Reproduction and Embryology (ESHRE)/American Society for Reproductive Medicine (ASRM) consensus definition for polycystic ovary syndrome is the most pragmatic and appropriate one.
2. There are significant ethnic differences in the expression of hyperandrogenism and metabolic disease.
3. A definitive diagnosis of polycystic ovary syndrome can be difficult to achieve in adolescence and an early diagnosis should be re-evaluated in adulthood.
4. Psychological wellbeing is adversely affected by polycystic ovary syndrome. Health-related quality of life (HRQoL) assessment should be considered as part of the woman's routine clinical care.

Management

Lifestyle and metabolic aspects

5. The management of polycystic ovary syndrome (including its long-term health risks) is best delivered by a multidisciplinary approach, including dietary and educational counselling, exercise training, stress management and psychosocial support.
6. All women with polycystic ovary syndrome should be assessed for the risk of developing impaired glucose tolerance and type 2 diabetes.
7. Preconception counselling in women with polycystic ovary syndrome seeking fertility should include potential obstetric risks.
8. Weight loss should be emphasised in the treatment of women with polycystic ovary syndrome who are overweight and for the prevention of type 2 diabetes. There is no evidence of superiority of a particular type of diet for women with

polycystic ovary syndrome. If the woman's body mass index is greater than 35 kg/m^2, bariatric surgery should be considered. Fertility treatment should be deferred until after the initial period of rapid weight loss.

Treatments

9. The management of severe or persistent acne is best performed by a dermatologist. Seborrhoea is a common finding in polycystic ovary syndrome, the severity of which is predictive of poor clinical response to conventional topical and antimicrobial acne therapies. Strategies for management include topical therapies, oral antiandrogens and, for severe cases, isotretinoin.
10. The management of hirsutism may require a combination of cosmetic and topical treatments and oral antiandrogens (for example, combined oral contraceptive pills containing cyproterone acetate or drospirenone, or the antiandrogens spironolactone and finasteride). Women should be counselled on the risk of venous thromboembolism with the third-generation combined oral contraceptive pills.
11. Female-pattern hair loss can be halted and may respond to 2% topical minoxidil and systemic antiandrogens.
12. Clomifene citrate is the first-line therapy for anovulatory polycystic ovary syndrome. Further choices, including low-dose gonadotrophin therapy or laparoscopic ovarian diathermy, can be selected taking into consideration age and other predictors of outcome. It is essential to minimise the risks of multiple pregnancy and ovarian hyperstimulation syndrome.
13. Metformin is overused in the treatment of polycystic ovary syndrome and is ineffective as a solo agent or in combination to treat infertility and to achieve live births. The use of metformin to prevent miscarriage or to prevent pregnancy complications is unproven.
14. Although metformin delays the development of diabetes in women with impaired glucose tolerance, its long-term effects in women with polycystic ovary syndrome are not yet clear.
15. *In vitro* maturation of oocytes collected from unstimulated ovaries is a promising treatment option for women with polycystic ovaries requiring assisted reproductive technology. It is simpler and safer for women but less successful than *in vitro* fertilisation.
16. Women with menstrual cycle disturbance not wishing fertility should have endometrial assessment and receive protection against developing endometrial hyperplasia and adenocarcinoma.

Research

17. Large cross-sectional studies are required of different ethnic communities to assess the prevalence of polycystic ovary syndrome and longitudinal studies are required of its evolution over time, from puberty and throughout life.
18. More studies are required to assess HRQoL using validated tools such as the PCOS Questionnaire. Clinical trials should incorporate a quality of life questionnaire during assessment of the impact of treatment.

19. Better understanding of the pathogenesis of polycystic ovary syndrome will help to identify credible candidate pathways for future genetic studies.
20. Investigations of candidate genes are appropriate but studies of plausible candidates need to be adequately powered and replicated in independent series. International genome-wide association studies should be encouraged and supported.
21. Research on predictive factors in early childhood for later development of polycystic ovary syndrome is recommended.
22. The use of anti-Müllerian hormone in assessing polycystic ovary syndrome needs to be evaluated further.
23. The determination of reference ranges for testosterone and other hormones should be established for each analytical method using criteria established by the International Federation of Clinical Chemistry and Laboratory Medicine.
24. Current definitions of polycystic ovary syndrome use the terms clinical and laboratory evidence of hyperandrogenism. There is a need for more robust and transparent definitions of clinical scoring systems for acne and hirsutism as well as normal ranges for serum androgen measurement.
25. Studies are required to evaluate the benefits of psychological therapies, such as cognitive behavioural therapy, for improving the emotional wellbeing of women with polycystic ovary syndrome.
26. There are insufficient randomised controlled trials on the management of polycystic ovary syndrome, particularly of treatments used in adolescence.
27. The long-term benefits of lifestyle modification and pharmacotherapy for management of women with polycystic ovary syndrome who are overweight should be evaluated.
28. Bariatric surgery provides a research opportunity to investigate changes in polycystic ovary syndrome independent of weight loss.
29. Individualised approaches to the management of anovulatory infertility are likely to render ovulation induction more effective and safer. Prospective cohort follow-up studies are required in well-defined patient categories and of adequate sample size looking at singleton live birth rates over a given period of time.
30. More research is required into the use of aromatase inhibitors such as letrozole for ovulation induction.
31. Continued work is needed to optimise scientific and clinical aspects of *in vitro* maturation to improve efficacy and safety. Long-term follow-up studies with appropriate controls are required for children born after *in vitro* maturation.
32. Complementary therapies such as acupuncture need further evaluation in the management of endocrine, reproductive and metabolic disorders.

Index

Notes

ASRM = American Society for Reproductive Medicine
ESHRE = European Society of Human Reproduction and Embryology
FSH = follicle-stimulating hormone
hCG = human chorionic gonadotrophin
HDL = high-density lipoprotein
hMG = human menopausal gonadotrophin
HRQoL = health-related quality of life
IDF = International Diabetes Federation
IVF = *in vitro* fertilisation
IVM = *in vitro* maturation of oocytes
NICE = National Institute for Health and Clinical Excellence
OHSS = ovarian hyperstimulation syndrome
PCOS = polycystic ovary syndrome
RCT = randomised controlled trial
SHBG = sex hormone-binding globulin
WHO = World Health Organization

Printed in the United States
By Bookmasters